Feeling Smarter and Smarter

Harold N. Levinson, MD

Feeling Smarter and Smarter

Discovering the Inner-Ear Origins and Treatment for Dyslexia/LD, ADD/ADHD, and Phobias/Anxiety

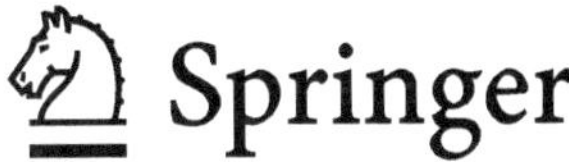

Harold N. Levinson, MD
Levinson Medical Center for Learning Disabilities
Great Neck, NY
USA

ISBN 978-3-030-16207-8 ISBN 978-3-030-16208-5 (eBook)
https://doi.org/10.1007/978-3-030-16208-5

This Copernicus imprint is published by the registered company Springer Nature Switzerland AG
The registered company address is: Gewerbestrasse 11, 6330 Cham, Switzerland

To my wife Diggy; she has literally been the loving wind beneath my—and our family's—wings.

To my wonderful daughters, Laura and Joy, and their great spouses, Rob and Roger.

To my six very special grandkids, Hannah, Josh, Emily, Sophia, Natalie, and, of course, Arianna.

To my very dear philanthropic dyslexic friend, Peter Alfond, whose recent untimely death motivated me to rapidly complete this life-helping book in record time.

And to all my many patients. They have taught me how best to understand and help them.

Why I Became an MD and Medical Researcher

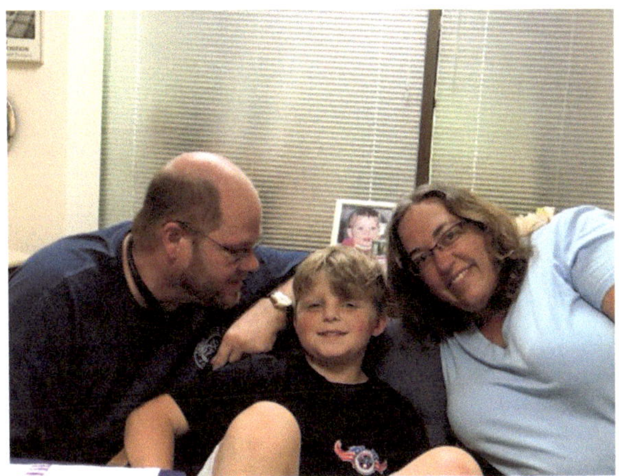

One half-hour after giving 10-year-old Michael Shultz a small dose of an inner-ear-enhancing medication and testing him for tiredness, he began crying hysterically for the first time ever. He ran over to me and tightly hugged me—refusing to let go, still sobbing: "I'm better. So much! You really helped me. I can think. I can concentrate. The noise and clicking in my ears are gone. I don't feel so stupid anymore." He then grabbed my book, *The Upside-Down Kids: Helping Dyslexic Children Understand Themselves and Their Disorder*, from his mother, and started reading the adult introduction. His parents were stunned—as were we all. He had never read so spontaneously or so rapidly before—especially words he never before appeared to know. It was truly an amazing moment! Tears rapidly spread throughout the office.

A second "night-and-day improvement" was reported following continued treatment, as you'll see later in the book.

Maria

Having studied thousands of dyslexics for over 50 years, I'm still amazed how my understanding of their symptoms and their complex "four-dimensional" disorder deepens with every new patient I listen to, examine, and successfully treat. So just after completing this book's Closure, a gifted dyslexic adult, named Maria, *spontaneously* provided me—and now you—with one of the best descriptions of the dyslexia syndrome that I've ever encountered:

> *Whereas many dyslexics may get disoriented and lost when leaving their house—explaining their agoraphobia (and mine)—I get lost inside my own home. And the reason is that my directional coordinates keep changing within my mind's inner-ear—so that even the rooms within my house keep switching, as if moved around by an unseen drunken architect playing disorientation games on a broken computer.*
>
> *The same jumbling happens to me when I read, write, talk, and move, rendering me both mentally and physically klutzy. And so I spend all of my efforts trying to outsmart the untiring error-machine within me. At least I did so before receiving your life-changing treatment.*
>
> *I felt as if someone were spinning me around faster and faster. But I didn't feel the dizziness, just the effects. And once I was mentally disoriented and physically destabilized in this way, I was rendered unable to properly input most of what I experienced. Nor could I concentrate, think, talk, remember, and navigate without fears of messing everything up. Rather than being spun around externally, however, it was my demon—my faulty inner-ear—creating my symptoms.*
>
> *Can you imagine how dumb and inept I felt, especially when I'd been previously told my dyslexia was due to a thinking-brain impairment. All I heard was "brain damage." Then I was certain I would forever remain this crazy way. Had I not stumbled onto your research and treatment, I shudder to think that I might never have recovered.*
>
> *Your simple explanations and inner-ear-improving meds awakened me from my confused dyslexic dream—nightmare, really. And fixed almost everything. Just really understanding that I had only one simple and treatable fine-tuning inner-ear dysfunction that was creating my total jumble made me feel significantly better. But then when the meds kicked in, the words I read and used suddenly stopped scrambling and moving on the page. My thinking, actions, and orientation became clearer—I actually know where I am, both inside and outside of my house. Much less anxiety! Best of all, I no longer feel dumb, misunderstood, lost in space. And I no longer feel controlled by a drunken demon. I'm amazed I made it this far, considering…*

Thank God, you helped guide me safely to Earth. No one can really understand the enormous relief—and gratitude—I now feel, except for all the others you've similarly helped.

When I look back, I don't know whether to laugh or cry. Laugh because I now really know what's wrong with me, and am all but cured. Cry because I'm saddened that so many others like me still believe this brain damage nonsense to be true—and so will never get better as I did… unless your treatment becomes more commonplace.

Having a nephew with ASD, I was both interested and shocked to learn that you can now also help some autistics with the same meds I took. But after some reflection, it made perfect sense—that is, if autistics have two demons, the same one as mine, plus another one causing their autism. So if you get rid of my demon, then they might feel much better. Wow!

Thanks for providing me with both your understanding and treatment. Both were really, really "lifesaving." And thanks for now enabling me to help others as I was helped. Perhaps even my nephew.

—Maria S.

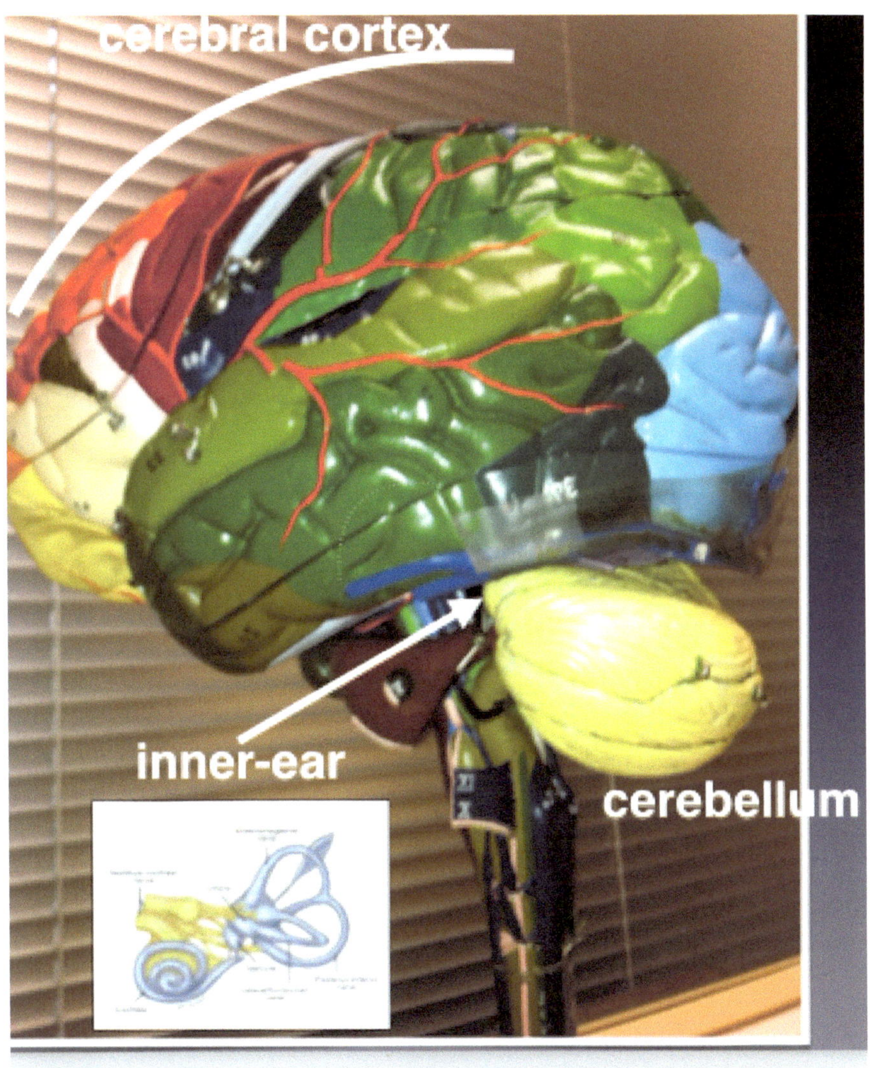

Consider this illustration as only a general "treasure map" needed to initially visualize and understand the anatomical terms used during my—and your—solution to the dyslexia riddles throughout this book. Refer to Appendix 1 *only afterwards* for a more detailed neuroanatomical explanation—unless you happen to be a professional.

Preface: An Essential Overview

Sit down before fact as a little child, be prepared to give up every preconceived notion, follow humbly wherever and to whatever abyss nature leads, or you shall learn nothing.

—Thomas Huxley

Initially understanding dyslexia after examining only a few cases—or even a roomful—is akin to meeting several strangers—or even a very large group—and comprehending humanity.

Unmasking dyslexia was like peeling an onion, but one in which each layer was found to be another onion.

—Harold N. Levinson, MD

Feeling Smarter and Smarter is a book about dyslexic children as well as those diagnosed with disorders akin to the ones found on this book's cover: children who suffer from varied combinations and severities of a wide range of heretofore unexplained and perplexing inner-ear-determined symptoms affecting their reading, writing, spelling, math, memory, speech, sense of direction and time, and also their grammar, concentration and activity levels, balance, and coordination; children who have disturbing headaches, dizziness, ringing ears, and motion sickness; children who invariably become frustrated and begin to feel dumb, ugly, klutzy, anxious/phobic, and depressed; children who are impulsive, cut class, become truant, and drop out of school and therefore may often drift to drugs, violence, and crime; children who bully and are bullied; and children who often grow up to become emotionally traumatized and scarred dysfunctional adults.

And so *Feeling Smarter and Smarter* is also *about* and *for* the millions of frustrated and failing adults who are often overwhelmed by unknown dyslexia-related "demons" dating back to their birth or later acquired.

Perhaps the most devastating of the many and varied symptoms characterizing dyslexics is impaired self-esteem. As a rule of thumb, the smarter dyslexics are, the more frustrated they become by their struggles—and so the dumber and uglier they feel. Unfortunately, compliments do not significantly help dyslexics, since they cannot inwardly believe them to be true. Quite often, they view themselves as impostors—even those who attain fame and success. They feel dumb on the inside while acting smart enough, they believe, to fool others outwardly.

From my 50-plus years of clinical experience, I've determined that there are only two sure ways to help dyslexics and those with other related neurophysiological impairments overcome their many frustrating symptoms—especially impaired self-esteem:

1. They *need* to know, and *truly feel*, that their symptoms and failures are not their own fault—that they are not lazy, stupid, rebellious, dumb, or just *bad*, terms often used to label or denigrate them. They *need* a simple, logical, scientific explanation for their many symptoms and the resulting frustrations. And this explanation *must* be of sufficient force, scope, and depth to replace their own devastating inner convictions—drawn from either repeated failures—and/or an inner sense of functioning below their own expected par. They also require loving parents and/or partners and caring professionals to help them fully benefit from the scientific breakthroughs presented in this book.
2. Most importantly, they *need* a medical treatment that can rapidly improve their functioning—as well as helpful nonmedical add-on therapies. As you will soon learn from many of my thousands of successfully treated dyslexics and those with other related inner-ear disorders, *improved overall functioning rapidly triggers enhanced self-esteem while minimizing anxiety and depression, often regardless of age.*

Thus, it became essential to also provide this groundbreaking understanding to as wide an audience of concerned healers as possible—and so to potentially enable all who have the dyslexia syndrome to obtain the best possible holistic help ASAP before existing symptoms intensify and secondary emotional scarring and irreparable harm occur.

This book is the one that many have asked me to write—a book providing a general overview of the vital discoveries that were absolutely needed to meaningfully understand, diagnose, and successfully treat those with this previously mystifying impairment. However, knowing what to say and how to write it successfully were two separate problems. Fortunately, my writing dilemma was easily resolved. Having spent most of my medical career—more than 50 years—diagnosing and successfully treating bright, frustrated, and often devastated dyslexics of all ages, I decided that the best way for you to learn about their disorder was the same way I did: by simply listening to real dyslexics, as well as those with related disorders, describe all their reading and non-reading symptoms—the "demons" characterizing their *total* disorder, not just their reading impairment.

By far, my greatest understanding of dyslexia and its complex syndrome came from studying the favorable—often dramatic—responses of over 35,000 dyslexic children and adults to a "life-saving" medical treatment.

The process of observing and recording these improvements was truly amazing—and highly rewarding. When the root cause of the dyslexia syndrome was discovered and medically treated, patients began reporting the rapid disappearance of a wide range of *reading and non-reading* symptoms—scores of them—that no one had ever realized were part and parcel of their disorder. And the analysis of these favorable treatment responses, all of which are presented in this book, allowed me to gain a uniquely accurate and far-ranging panorama of this previously oversimplified and completely misunderstood four-dimensional dyslexia hologram.

Because we often see and truly believe what we are initially taught to expect, new and challenging breakthrough solutions, such as those characterizing this book, are frequently resisted—and therefore, scientific discovery and acceptance are slowed. But fortunately, my patients will rapidly and convincingly provide you with the same overwhelming, indisputable facts and vital insights that I initially needed to override both my own prior mistaken—biased—dyslexia-related convictions and my corresponding resistance to changing them. Only then was I eventually freed to solve the many century-old riddles about dyslexia and its syndrome of symptoms that had eluded all others.

Accordingly, this is a book replete with discoveries and *solutions*—many of which you will likely find both surprising and fascinating:

- A *solution* clearly demonstrating that dyslexia is not just a reading disorder but a large cluster of reading *and* non-reading symptoms caused by one simple and treatable signal-scrambling impairment within the inner-ear and its supercomputing cerebellum—man's lower brain—often leading to emotional/behavioral fallout
- A *solution* suggesting that all the primary symptoms characterizing the dyslexia syndrome—such as those highlighted in the first few paragraphs of this preface—arise when initially normal brain structures fail to adequately process the scrambled signals received from a dysfunctional inner-ear/cerebellar fine-tuner
- A *solution* leading to a highly effective inner-ear-enhancing medical treatment capable of rapidly and often dramatically improving scores of symptoms and many differently named disorders
- A *solution* unmasking a previously hidden link that connects such differently appearing and defined disorders as d*yslexia (or SLD)*, *ADD/ADHD*, and *phobias/anxiety* to a common inner-ear/cerebellar origin—thereby explaining why these and so many other impairments frequently co-occur with one another, along with some mood disorders
- A *solution* capable of fully explaining *all* dyslexic symptoms and their causative mechanisms with sufficient depth and clarity so as to enable dumb-feeling and self-blaming dyslexics to feel smarter
- A *solution* that completely debunks the century-old mistaken conviction that dyslexia is a pure reading comprehension disorder akin to alexia, resulting from a proven acquired thinking-brain impairment in adults—an alluring and "addic-

tive" theoretically based fantasy failing to explain 100 percent of dyslexia's true panoramic reality[1]

However, to really solve the many riddles characterizing dyslexia—all resulting from a false conviction that stuck like crazy glue ever since bright reversal-prone dyslexics were first described in English by Morgan in 1896[2]—many other important resolutions were required, including the following:

- A *solution* resolving the seeming paradox, whereby the American Psychiatric Association's official Diagnostic and Statistical Manual of Mental Disorders (DSM-V) now justifiably indicates that dyslexia does not exist as traditionally conceptualized and defined, despite the indisputable fact that dyslexics abound
- A *solution* that can lead to partial improvements in a wide range of *major brain processing impairments* such as autistic spectrum disorder (ASD), mental retardation, Down syndrome, cerebral palsy, brain injury, epilepsy, schizophrenia, and other disturbances where the cerebellum is a coexisting determinant

---

[1]Alexia with and without agraphia was first described by Dejerine in 1891 and 1892, respectively, depending on the location of the acquired brain injury. Previously normal reading adults then suddenly lost their ability to recognize viewed letters and words. This is the concept used throughout this book for reasons to follow—despite later modifying insights.

Many variations of alexia have since been described. They have been properly referenced in this book and are best summarized in an Internet review by Mendez Manuel (https://clinicalsciences.wordpress.com/article/alexia-1bbsle13m97c0-111/).

Despite all these later modifications, there is a night-and-day qualitative, severity-related, and prognostic distinction between the reading and related neurological symptoms of alexia and dyslexia. This is why they were initially so differently termed. My dyslexia theory suggests that their similarities are due to the fact that alexia is a proven primary cerebral impairment, whereas dyslexia—the syndrome—results when these very same, but initially normal (alexia-related), cerebral processors secondarily fail to compensate for the distorted or dizzy signals received from a fine-tuning impairment within the CVS system. Thus, the terms acquired alexia and developmental dyslexia highlight their distinct causative and so also their differing qualitative/quantitative origins.

With this clarification in mind, and to avoid the century-old confusion that dyslexia = alexia and so also that alexia = acquired dyslexia, I chose to oversimplify the current alexia concepts presented so that nontechnical and nonprofessional readers lacking neurological expertise might best understand dyslexia and its major differences with alexia—not with "acquired dyslexia." (The latter mistakenly suggests that the only difference between alexia and dyslexia is that the former is acquired.) As you will learn, dyslexia can also be acquired by any disorder impairing the CVS system—further refuting the above equation and misconcepts.

Quite clearly, it has taken this somewhat lengthy book to eventually describe only dyslexia. And even its neuroanatomy was displaced to the very end (in Appendix 1) to avoid overloading and confusing readers too early. What if I had to also fully explain (acquired) alexia and its neuroanatomy/neurophysiology as well as variations before even getting to dyslexia? I'm sure that even unforgiving purists would agree that some sort of writer's/teaching compromise was needed. As a clinician, not a writer, I hope my compromise works—especially since my clarifications which distinguish dyslexia and alexia remain the same, despite my intended oversimplification. One more insight: although the neurological concepts of alexia became more complex over time, the equation dyslexia = alexia as used through this book didn't change.

[2]This disorder was initially identified and overlooked in a German publication by Berkhan in 1881 and termed "dyslexia" by Berlin in 1887. However, I chose to use the date it first appeared in English.

- An *explanatory solution* as to why independent scientific validation for many of the above findings occurred *very belatedly*—more than two decades after they were initially proposed—and why the initial support for these cerebellar-related solutions by Nobel Laureate and cerebellar neuroscientist Sir John Eccles, and outstanding others, went unheeded
- Also a related *explanatory solution* as to why and how subconscious bias mechanisms played havoc with most dyslexia researchers, regardless of their brilliance, determination, and altruism—and so created and maintained century-old riddles rather than solved them
- And finally, a likely biological *explanation* of psychological bias (refer to Chap. 11) and how its derailing effects were recognized, analyzed, and overcome—solved

Based on my therapeutic success and perspective, I believe that the combined discoveries and resulting solutions, as well as the fascinating insights presented within this book, will vastly improve the lives of countless individuals suffering from the dyslexia syndrome and a score of related previously misunderstood disorders—all of which result from a simple and treatable signal impairment within the inner-ear/cerebellum. Incredibly, the total of all those obviously afflicted with these varied but related disorders likely exceeds 25 percent of the population—not counting all those falling below the radar.

And as the many patients presented in this book will clearly reveal—as already exemplified by Michael and Maria—this breakthrough medical treatment really, really works for both young and old. So when improvements suddenly occur, *smart but dumb-feeling dyslexics* rapidly begin *feeling smarter and smarter*—hence the title of this book.

I truly hope my endeavor has been successful. I certainly gave it my very best shot.

Great Neck, NY, USA Harold N. Levinson, MD

Contents

Chapter 1
Dyslexia by Any Other Name

It's a bird! It's a plane! No, it's Superman.

If only dyslexia were so simple. It's a learning disorder! It's a language disorder! It's brain damage! Is it alexia? Congenital word blindness? Minimal brain damage? Minimal cerebral dysfunction? No, it's strephosymbolia (twisted symbols), specific learning disorder, specific learning disability… No one has it! Everyone has it!

It's a gift! It's a tragedy! It's normal! It's abnormal! It exists! It doesn't exist!

You're probably wondering what in the world Superman has to do with dyslexia. Nothing really, except to highlight an intriguing contrast. We all know who Superman is and what he looks like, even though he exists only as a fantasy. We know about his fatal kryptonite flaw, and his image is instantly recognized by all. His name and character are clearly defined. No synonyms are needed.

By comparison, dyslexia describes a very real impairment that tragically affects countless millions. And despite over a century of dedicated research efforts, this disorder has defied all prior attempts at a meaningful description and in-depth understanding. Its accepted causation has turned out to be as pure a fantasy as Superman. And medical treatment has remained a hopeless dream— until now.

As a result of its elusive nature and form, dyslexia became whatever experts, and even non-experts, fantasized it was. It thus accrued many superficial identities—and many, many names, causes, and definitions. So it remained devoid of any comprehensive, dependable, and holistic portrait. In many ways it almost seems as if this disorder and many of its experts have unwittingly conspired to resist its clarification and solution. Thus, it has raised infinitely more questions than answers.

Sadly, all of the answers and theories you may be acquainted with are most likely incorrect, either totally or substantially so. And to add further confusion, the official American Psychiatric Association's (APA) diagnostic manual now *justifiably* claims dyslexia doesn't exist as a diagnostic entity, despite the presence of countless dyslexics. Has not some kind of anti-scientific force disabled the collective superpowers geared toward dyslexia's unmasking?

Fortunately, this book intends to clarify all the existing confusions while solving the dyslexia riddles. Quite a challenging undertaking! Although a Superman-like

H. N. Levinson, *Feeling Smarter and Smarter*,
https://doi.org/10.1007/978-3-030-16208-5_1

task, I can assure you that my patients and I will provide you with more discoveries, solutions, and insights than you ever thought possible. My dyslexic cases have now finally neutralized the "kryptonite flaw" that has been befuddling us all for decades. And so they will even fully explain why the APA was *correct*, but very incomplete, in its attempted diagnostic "clarification."

An Astonishing Variety and Combination of Symptoms

If you're thumbing through these pages, odds are that you, your child, or someone else you love or care about may have problems with reading, writing, spelling, math, memory, speech, and other related symptoms that suggest the presence of some kind of *named* learning, linguistic, or concentration difficulty. Possibly you or your loved one is experiencing phobias or panic attacks. Even mood disorders. And you may have come across the terms "dyslexia," learning disability/disorder (LD), attention deficit disorder (ADD), attention deficit hyperactivity disorder (ADHD), and even developmental coordination disorder (DCD).

Unfortunately—as with many disorders that science wishes it could better explain—these diagnostic terms primarily *describe symptoms*; they don't clarify causes, at least not accurately or comprehensibly. And because these diversely named disorders, based on varied clusters of symptoms, are given different names and "diagnoses," their common origins and interconnections, as well as an overall integrated portrait, have remained significantly hidden.

Thus, chances are high that a bright and relatively healthy loved one with multiple and seemingly unrelated symptoms is being mistakenly labeled with a mishmash of confusing diagnostic terms such as those mentioned above, instead of being treated for a single, all-encompassing, and substantially "curable" syndrome. Can you imagine the frustration and despair felt by those told that they suffer from four to ten different diagnoses, with at least one of them linked to brain damage or dysfunction? And that there's nothing that can be done medically to help!

Chances are even better that you haven't found satisfactory answers to the following questions: What is the exact cause and explanation of the typically present reading, writing, spelling, and math problems, especially those characterized by reversals? Why does someone who is so bright have such a poor memory for sequential tasks and have difficulty recalling words, names, and/or important dates? Why might a dyslexic also be experiencing difficulties with sense of direction and time? Why might he, or she, have issues with grammar, concentration, and even activity levels, ranging from underactive to hyperactive? How are brain fog and superfocusing compatible with one another? How can dyslexia be called a language impairment when so many dyslexics are linguistically gifted (e.g., Winston Churchill)? Is there an important diagnostic distinction between speech and severe language disorders caused by strokes or injury? Why do differing dyslexics manifest such diverse symptomatic combinations and severities?

Why are poor balance and coordination as well as rhythm issues and accident-proneness, however minimal, *invariably* present in those with the above diversely named disorders—even in individuals who are good at sports? Did you know, for example, that Magic Johnson, Muhammad Ali, Caitlyn (formerly Bruce) Jenner, and other superbly gifted dyslexic athletes invariably have poor eye coordination when reading and poor hand coordination when writing, even though they excel on the field and court?

Might expressive speech and auditory processing problems, as well as the so-called Freudian slips of the tongue, be part of the same dyslexic symptomatic complex? Stuttering and stammering too? What do headaches, stomachaches, dizziness, motion sickness, and excessive sensitivity to light, noise, taste, and touch have to do with learning and attention as well as with anxiety and mood disorders? Why do bright, handsome boys and pretty, gifted girls often feel dumb and ugly? And why do so many dyslexics—even those who are world-famous and highly accomplished—inwardly feel inept and like "klutzy" imposters?

Most important, if the above problems and/or many, many others—such as spatial/directional symptoms; delays in learning simple motor tasks like speech clarity and tying shoes; catching, batting, and throwing a ball; riding a bike, even blowing one's nose; and later on driving a car—are present, what do they indicate and what can be done to help? Can these symptoms be medically treated? And if they're overcome, is their cause still present?

Must their symptoms be treated separately? And if most or all of them stem from a common core, is it possible to find a "cure all" similar to antibiotics for a generalized bacterial infection? If not a cure, then perhaps at least a major overall improvement such as using insulin to treat the diverse symptoms of diabetes? And in addition to medical treatment, are there nonmedical add-on or even stand-alone therapies that can be helpful—and how do they work?

Rest assured that all of these questions and many, many others will be fully answered by the time you're finished reading this book. And an amazing array of other important insights will pop up as the paragraphs fly by and the pages turn. Guaranteed: You will be provided with the clearest and best "super-face" of dyslexia and its many synonyms to date. And most importantly, you'll know how to best understand and treat *all* these symptoms, not just "tutor" one or two or "suck it up" and "learn to live and suffer with them."

Names Lead Us Astray: Just Another Wild Goose Chase

Let's get back to the names and synonyms. Do you think the list I provided at the beginning of the chapter was confusing? Did you know there were fully *36* synonyms for dyslexia when I last counted them in 1969 while reading *The Dyslexic Child*, written by world-renowned neurologist and dyslexia researcher, MacDonald Critchley? Yet none of his brilliant neurological descriptions of dyslexic reading and non-reading symptoms provided any of the real answers and solutions I had been looking for—or that you require now. That's because Critchley, and countless others before and after him, many of them also truly gifted, were simply looking for the "dyslexia needle" in the wrong theoretical haystack. And since I was clinically inexperienced at the time,

I, too, initially joined his tantalizingly simple, but vastly mistaken, "theoretical bubble." That is, until my many patients pointed me in the right scientific direction—down a road never before scientifically traveled. And I went there.

The *Dyslexia = Alexia* Misconception

A fundamental and irresistible misconception, you see, was leading us all astray. That is, we all believed that the reading problem experienced by dyslexics was identical to the severe and irreversible reading comprehension impairment characterizing those *rare* adults who have developed *alexia* following a brain injury.

For those of you who may be unfamiliar with this term, alexia is a rare, complete inability of adults to comprehend the meaning of letters and words they clearly see. It is caused by an acquired impairment within the left or dominant thinking brain's reading processor, and there is no reasonable chance of improvement. Thus, the reasoning for over a century was that dyslexia must also have its roots in the very same area of the thinking brain. And that dyslexics must also have severe alexia-like reading comprehension problems.

An addictive concept Perhaps it would be beneficial at this point to explain more clearly why we were all so addicted to the alexia theory of dyslexia. It was as simple as believing that what goes up comes down. Since we knew, via autopsy studies, the exact processor responsible for adults losing their reading comprehension for words seen, it was natural to assume that this very same impaired thinking-brain processor was responsible for otherwise normal children failing to naturally acquire reading functioning. It was just too easy and perfect an explanation to resist—or scientifically question. Sadly, this assumption became a conviction without checking it out with dyslexics. And I'm sure you all know what the acronym for ASSUME stands for.

Five deadly flaws However, by carefully listening to, observing, and examining, dyslexic children, I slowly came to recognize that the assumptions maintaining this theory had at least *five deadly flaws*. And to maintain this "theoretical addiction" to the *dyslexia = alexia* concept, major refuting data had to be unwittingly sidestepped by its followers. And sidestepped they were—unchallenged—until now.

What were these five deadly flaws? In short, after examining thousands of dyslexics, it became obvious that, unlike alexics: (1) dyslexics had absolutely no evidence of a primary cerebral or thinking-brain dysfunction, minimal or otherwise. (2) They did not have a reading comprehension impairment. (3) Their reading capability and scores often improved, either spontaneously or with medical and nonmedical interventions. (4) Dyslexics were recognized by nearly all experts to have so-called "soft" balance, coordination, and rhythmic neurological signs, which I and a few others identified to be of a definitive inner-ear and cerebellar origin. And

(5) dyslexia was recognized to be a developmental syndrome—one you're born with—having many reading and non-reading symptoms, whereas alexia is a "pure," severe, and rare reading comprehension impairment invariably acquired by adults following a brain injury.

Slightly modifying vs. discarding a mistaken theory However, with dyslexia, even "five strikes and your favorite theory is out" didn't apply. Thus, even the world-renowned dyslexia expert, McDonald Critchley, did not find the neurological evidence within the thinking brain to support his believed cerebral or alexia-like cause of dyslexia. He did, however, insightfully acknowledge that the reading disorder in dyslexia (vs. in alexia) might improve over time and could be "cured." And he noted the "soft" neurological signs that came along with dyslexia—but were absent in alexia. Despite all this, he completely failed to recognize that dyslexia and alexia were completely separate disorders having different origins, manifestations, and outcomes.

Guess how he reconciled his apparent dilemma—enabling him to stick to his addictive *dyslexia* = *alexia* theory? He added yet another intriguing synonym—"developmental dyslexia"— to the list, bringing his grand total to 37. He proposed that a developmental lag within their cerebral reading processor, rather than a defect, explained the fact that dyslexics had no cerebral neurological signs and that their reading eventually got better—even to the point of a "cure."

But Critchley failed—as did most others before and after him—to recognize that dyslexia was not just a pure reading disorder, as was alexia, but rather part of a much larger syndrome comprising scores of symptoms, many of which he himself described in his outstanding book! He also overlooked the important significance of the many inner-ear/cerebellar signs found among his dyslexic patients.

Critchley also ignored or denied the fact that dyslexics did not have an alexia-like reading *comprehension* impairment. Thus, for example, he claimed that the clumsy to-and-fro eye movements typical of dyslexics when they read were merely random searching movements similar to those seen in the blind. *But he failed to test his conviction.* Had he simply asked his dyslexic patients, they would have told him that they habitually skip over letters, words, and sentences and thus require a compensatory finger or marker to help their fixation and sequential tracking problem when reading. And had he used his finger and/or larger print and observed their immediate reading improvement, Critchley would have been forced to recognize that dyslexia had a primary inner-ear-determined ocular-motor causation rather than an alexia-like, cerebral incomprehension one. But he never went there.

Clearly, if reading comprehension was truly impaired in dyslexia as in alexia, using a finger or marker or larger print would be completely powerless to bring improvement. In the end, Critchley's new synonym was a very good try. But as you will learn in more detail, he fell far afield from the solution he desperately sought. And so received no prize.

You are probably wondering at this point: Considering the data available to Critchley, how could this esteemed neurological clinician—and most others to date—have accepted the clinically nonsensical equation that *dyslexia = alexia*? And even worse that *dyslexia = severe reading comprehension impairment? Then unscientifically called both the disorder and only severe degrees of its reading symptom—of the many other reading intensities and non-reading symptoms you've read about so far—by the same name, thus indicating that: dyslexia = "dyslexia"*? Nonsensical? I believe so.

That's like *illogically equating* both the complex diabetic disorder with only severe degrees of a single one of its many symptoms—"very high blood sugar levels." And then similarly naming them both diabetes—thus creating the false equation: *diabetes = severely high or comatose blood sugar levels = "diabetes."*

No doubt you are also wondering: Why were Critchley and most all of the traditionalist dyslexia experts so blinded to their own extensive clinical realities? Were group-think and denial possibly in play? Might these bias-related phenomena also explain why tiny segments of the dyslexia disorder are differently labeled rather than holistically understood? And also why the easy, dyslexia-synonym road-to-nowhere is so often taken, adding confusion vs. insight?

Neurological rationalizations Perhaps you are also considering how and why the word *minimal*—as in "minimal brain damage" and "minimal cerebral dysfunction"—came to be used in connection with dyslexia? Stated another way: How can a defect in our highest brain structure be considered minimal—especially if it causes so many dyslexic symptoms? As Maria noted in the opening pages, most patients when told they have minimal brain damage or dysfunction are so traumatized that they don't even hear the word *minimal*.

Because of my psychoanalytic training, answers explaining the distorted dyslexic-like reasoning I was seeing in the dyslexia field eventually became as obvious to me as they were critical to understanding this syndrome. Thus, I also realized that the word *minimal* was employed because no one could ever find "hard" or *definitive* neurological signs indicative of the thinking-brain damage or dysfunction similar to that found in alexia. Not Critchley nor any of his brilliant colleagues!

Rather, dyslexics invariably exhibit an abundance of mistakenly labeled "soft" balance, coordination and rhythmic as well as directional neurological signs—the latter simply explaining the typical reversals never found in alexics. In fact, these signs, when objectively viewed, are hard and fast indicators that clearly point to a dysfunction within the inner-ear and its "supercomputer," the cerebellum—man's lower or "little brain."

However, instead of looking at where the symptoms and neurological signs were pointing to, and thus where the dyslexic disorder was likely stemming from, dyslexia professionals used these inner-ear signs, in a pseudoscientific manner, to infer the presence of hard evidence of a thinking-brain impairment—even though no such hard evidence could be found. Confused by this circular or reversed dyslexic-like logic? I certainly was initially!

A Scientific Neurosis: How So Many Experts Went Astray

Maybe now you're starting to understand why it took a psychiatrist with both psychoanalytic and neurological training to unravel the riddles characterizing dyslexia. In many ways, I believe a "scientific neurosis"—even a "psychosis" at times—was at work here. In order to maintain the mistaken belief that *dyslexia = alexia = severe reading incomprehension or "dyslexia"* in the complete absence of any confirming evidence, and in the presence of overwhelming refuting data, "thinking-brain believers" were forced—unwittingly and with the best of intentions—to deny a vast array of scientific and clinical realities. And they simultaneously and rigorously resisted any and all genuine solutions before their very eyes. Instead, they all seemed compulsively fixated on a tantalizing old theory from which they just couldn't shake loose and backtrack.

Sadly, they even resisted—and continue to resist—the new and all-encompassing CVS/dyslexia theory and approach that this book describes, one that has been clearly shown to provide successful medical methods of screening and diagnosis. And as you will read in the pages ahead, the traditionalists have also actively resisted reviewing and fact-checking the discovery of a "lifesaving" and often dramatically effective medical treatment (and even prevention)—despite the fact that their own concepts have essentially led nowhere scientifically since reversal prone dyslexics were first described in an English-language publication in 1896. Some of them even failed to show up at my clinic after requesting in writing to observe my therapeutic methods and successes firsthand. None spoke to my patients—nor perhaps even to their own.

Might they have feared that checking would prove they were wrong—or seemingly worse, that I was right? And so they unwittingly pulled an "ostrich"—stuck their heads in the sand? Was kryptonite to blame after all, or its psychological equivalent: bias and its enforcer—denial.

Toward Solving the Dyslexia Riddle: The DDD Synonym and Concept

Believe it or not, I actually ended up adding another tongue-twisting synonym to the dyslexia lexicon in what has been called a "highly original... challenging...decades ahead of its time" 1973 research publication entitled, *Dysmetric Dyslexia and Dyspraxia (DDD)—Hypothesis and Study*. To date, DDD is the only synonym that is completely capable of explaining and encompassing *all* dyslexic reading and non-reading symptoms as well as all their many determining mechanisms and inner-ear/cerebellar neurological signs.[1]

---

[1] *Dysmetric* indicates a CVS-spatial/temporal dysfunction. *Dyslexia* initially represented the *visual reading impairment that I mistakenly equated with this total disorder, but later updated.* And *dyspraxia* highlights the CVS-determined scrambled eye movements I initially considered secondarily scrambling the visual reading input—thus causing "dyslexia"— as well as accounting for all the other balance/coordination signs and symptoms found characterizing dyslexics.

"How could such a super-claim be possible?" skeptics are no doubt wondering. Well, as I said up front, I plan to let my patients answer this question for you as this book unfolds. But first, let me briefly satisfy your curiosity and summarize what I discovered.

Independent validation In the 1973 publication I previously noted, many well-known and outstanding clinicians independently, and without any potentially biasing knowledge of the study's design, verified my neurological findings that *only* an inner-ear/cerebellar problem appeared present among dyslexics. There was absolutely no evidence of the thinking-brain cerebral neurological signs that are invariably present in alexia—and mistakenly believed present in dyslexia.

Finding an explanatory theory Now all I needed was a logical theory to explain how an inner-ear/cerebellar-determined motor coordination output impairment might cause a sensory input cognitive problem—dyslexia. Finding this explanation might sound like a simple task, especially in retrospect. But I can assure you it wasn't initially simple at all, since most other researchers were either opposed to or shocked by my "challenging" ideas and findings at the time.

So here's the short version of the *updated DDD* theory that *eventually* emerged after my first try: Due to a hypothesized fine-tuning impairment within the inner-ear and its supercomputing cerebellum, scrambled or "dizzy" signals were being sent up to various parts of the thinking brain. A *secondary inability* of these and other diverse, initially normal, brain areas to adequately process the *scrambled multisensory and motor signals* they were receiving and then sending readily explained the multitude of differing resulting symptoms that characterize dyslexics.

Additionally, I reasoned that the severity of the individual symptom depended upon (1) the degree of signal-scrambling and (2) the ability of the processors within the thinking brain and other central nervous system (CNS) structures to descramble the "dizzy signals" received via compensatory processes, one of which is likely neuroplasticity. Since IQ is not significantly determined by the inner-ear or cerebellum, this simple theory easily explained why there are so many bright and gifted dyslexics—despite many and severe symptoms. Indeed, this theory, when finally updated, explained just about 100 percent of what we now know about dyslexia—the syndrome.

Differences Between DDD and *Dyslexia = Alexia* Concepts

No doubt, a simple illustration of CVS signal-scrambling and how the normal reading and non-reading processors within the dyslexic brain attempt to descramble them will be helpful here in clarifying my DDD concept as well as the dyslexia syndrome it encompasses. A failure to descramble results in symptoms, whereas compensation, if successful, may minimize or completely mask symptom formation. (Refer to Chap. 9 for a more complete explanation.)

Thus, for example, according to my DDD theory, dyslexics compensate and so learn to decode and understand the following scrambled reading and non-reading signals, just as you are now doing, because their processors are normal: **7H15 M3554G3 53RV35 7O PR0V3 H0W 0UR M1ND5 C4N D0 4M4Z1NG 7H1NG5!**

By sharp contrast, the traditionalist *dyslexia* = *alexia* = *"dyslexia"* theories mistakenly postulated the presence of an alexia-like cerebral *reading processing and comprehension problem* ("*dyslexia*") they mistakenly believed was the essence of the dyslexia disorder, while explaining *absolutely none of the other numerous symptoms* and characteristics most dyslexics manifest.

Thus, according to the *mistaken* traditionalist theories, both alexics and dyslexics clearly see the following sentence, but its symbols or signals have no meaning for them whatsoever since their reading processors are thought to be similarly impaired. In reality, only alexics have lost the meaning of the following clearly seen signal: **THIS MESSAGE SERVES TO PROVE HOW OUR MIND CAN DO AMAZING THINGS!**

The cause of dyslexia vs. its compensation As previously mentioned, observing and testing dyslexics reveals that the CVS causes the dyslexia syndrome but that the decoding ability of the cerebral cortex or thinking brain is largely responsible for compensatory improvements. By contrast, alexia is caused by a proven lesion within the left thinking brain's dominant reading processor—as demonstrated by testing and, sadly, by autopsy. And so any possible improvement would be mainly due to improvements within this very same impaired processor, exceptions aside. This simple insight explains alexia's poor prognosis—there is no compensatory super-cerebral cortex to help out.

Multiple dyslexic reading symptoms and mechanisms As also previously noted, dyslexics do not have a primary alexic reading comprehension disorder at all. Rather, they have *multiple dysfunctioning reading symptoms and mechanisms*, including those involving spatial-temporal functions (reversals), fixation-tracking (losing their place), word movement and double vision, tunnel vision (seeing only one letter at a time in a multi-lettered word), light and glare sensitivity, memory, phonological capability, concentration, delayed processing, etc.

These and a number of other impaired reading mechanisms, determined to be of *primary* inner-ear/cerebellar origin, *secondarily* lead to dyslexics experiencing difficulty grasping what is read, despite normal reading processors. So even the true dyslexic reading disorder was never explained by the *dyslexia* = *alexia* theories. Unfortunate—since dyslexics would happily have told the theorists all of this had they been asked (refer to Chap. 16).

One CVS dysfunction vs. multiple brain impairments Additionally, traditionalist theory would be forced to suggest that each one of the overlapping—or comorbid—symptoms that most dyslexics experience, and that clinicians such as Critchley have observed and reported over the years, was due to a correspondingly impaired but different brain processor, one brain impairment per one or more symptoms. The problem was that most dyslexics also have many, many issues with reading, writing, spelling, math, and speech, as well as concentration, balance, coordination, rhythm, etc. As a result, if ten or more separate brain processors were impaired in dyslexics, their IQs would approach zero. Improvements would then be impossible—certainly not improvements like Michael's. And the idea of a normal-IQ dyslexic, or especially a bright, gifted one like Maria and many others that follow in this book and are elsewhere reported, would be an oxymoron.

By contrast, DDD postulates only one CVS signal-scrambling impairment that may radiate to multiple normal brain processors, including some within the CVS itself, and thus result in multiple symptoms when the latter fail to properly decode the distorted signals received and transmitted. As a result, this DDD concept is consistent with, and readily explains, why dyslexics have a favorable prognosis and why this disorder, despite multiple symptoms, is independent of IQ—while also clarifying and encompassing 100 percent of all dyslexic symptoms and manifestations.

Therefore, traditionalist theorists were wrong unless, of course, they presented persuasive counter-explanations!

Satisfied for now? Or still skeptical?

"*Still skeptical!*" I hear you whispering. "*How was it that you alone, Dr. Levinson, and a consulting psychoanalytic colleague, were able to discover what all others failed to do?*"

The answer is as simple as the question: because I used a simple and readily available clinical tool ignored by all others. I'll share a bit of that story shortly. But first it's time to meet some of the real experts, my most illuminating and insightful teachers. Dyslexics themselves! They often confused me and forced me to find new and intriguing solutions. But—unlike the scientific literature and traditionalist theorists—they never, ever misled me.

Chapter 2
The Bottom Line

Of all the questions parents and patients ask, two of them form their real bottom line: What is dyslexia all about? And what help can be realistically expected from medical treatment?

Dyslexia is what dyslexics experience Before we go any further with theories and clinical proofs, I want you to meet some "real live" dyslexics, for they will answer these questions better than I can. As you will soon learn from the three case presentations in this chapter and the many others that follow, *dyslexia is what dyslexics experience and reveal*—not what experts have previously believed or published about this baffling disorder and not what reading and other tests have measured.

Only dyslexics have real experiential knowledge of this syndrome's four-dimensional cauldron of symptoms. In short, you will soon learn that you can't define this highly complex, multifaceted mental/physiological syndrome by relying only on reading scores, writing scores, and other scores—especially as they often vary in extremes among dyslexics. In doing so, you are missing the entire forest for a few scraggly twigs.

Med benefits By listening to Paula West and her description of her dyslexic son Ron's favorable responses, you will be well on your way toward gaining an in-depth feel for the many symptoms underlying this multidimensional disorder. And by reading about Meg Fex's rapid and dramatic improvements as well as observing her handwriting before and shortly after starting on medication, you will quickly grasp what medical treatment has to offer dyslexics. These and many other favorable responses to treatment are what have provided the greatest and deepest *bottom line* understanding and benefits to those suffering from the dyslexia syndrome. Sadly, most of these vital insights have been largely overlooked by researchers and therapists to date.

Synergy Importantly, a vital therapeutic force—a synergy, if you will—is catalyzed for dyslexics when a true and meaningful understanding of their disorder

H. N. Levinson, *Feeling Smarter and Smarter*,
https://doi.org/10.1007/978-3-030-16208-5_2

replaces prior confusion and helplessness, and when previously frustrating and debilitating symptoms suddenly disappear with CVS enhancers.

Creating this synergy is *my* bottom line! Pay careful attention to the words of the patients and/or their loved ones that follow, especially the descriptions related to rapid favorable responses to a groundbreaking medical treatment. For I'm certain that these truly amazing observations will enlighten and inspire you as they have me. And so they will more than fulfill your bottom line.

Listening to a Few Favorably Responding Dyslexics

Mrs. Paula West's letter, below, shows how her efforts to help her son enjoy a family vacation at Disneyland substantiated, in an unsuspecting and thus objective way, the inner-ear/cerebellar origin and treatment of dyslexia. And the description of her own struggles point to a fact the experts have consistently overlooked—that one can read well and still be "dyslexic." Or, more accurately, one can read well and still suffer from the inner-ear/cerebellar syndrome from which dyslexia stems.[1]

Ron West

Ron's mother wrote these words to me before I even met her son[2]:

As a mother who has watched her eleven-year-old son struggle for years with reading and speech difficulties, I cannot adequately express the relief and excitement that I felt after reading your book, A Scientific Watergate—Dyslexia. *Every testimony that I read revealed more to me about my son. With every word the pieces of Ron's life came together for the very first time. It was a remarkable awakening to the reality of his condition. It seemed so simple. It was as if I should have known the answer all along.*

Sadly, I did not know what was wrong with him before, and neither did the other experts that I took Ron to visit year after frustrating year. Their answers were always the same: "There is no treatment for dyslexia. With special help and tutoring he may improve..." Certainly I received no encouragement or constructive advice.

Lately we began to realize that no matter what we did, it simply would not be enough to keep Ron afloat within the public school structure. Our hope of sending him to college was fading in our hearts. Ron could not even explore his intense interest in science and math—because he could not read.

---

[1] The crucial point that I hope you understand and remember is this: Regardless of whether you use the term dyslexia or any of its many synonyms, dyslexia represents a *syndrome* of many and diverse symptoms rather than just a reading disorder. Reading difficulties are just one of the syndrome's many symptoms, as fever may be just one symptom of the flu. And some with the flu may not evidence fever.

[2] Direct quotes in the book may have been minimally edited for grammar, punctuation, spelling, formatting, clarity, and conciseness. Also, in order to convey the continuity of my research, only Meg Fex was taken from an earlier presentation.

Our desire to see Ron achieve his best led us to your office door. A few weeks ago, I convinced myself that there must be a treatment for Ron and I became determined to find it. I started with the public library. There I found many, many books about dyslexia. Their message was all the same: "Learn to live with your brain malfunction." I didn't bother to read more than the jacket covers of these books—I knew that they didn't have the answer for me. I wanted treatment, not lifestyle adjustments.

Then I saw A Scientific Watergate—Dyslexia. *Clearly written across the front cover was the tagline, "How and why countless millions are deprived of breakthrough medical treatment." I almost wept with joy just holding your book. I rushed home and began to read it until I had completed all 417 pages. At times your book was very technical. But I didn't stop reading because I could fully understand the gist of your work and your patients' testimonials.*

After all these years, it seems as if we are finally going to receive some real help for Ron. Our hearts are filled with expectations about our upcoming appointment. You might think that we are placing too much hope in our visit to your office but we have already seen the results that motion-sickness medications have had on Ron's mood and anxiety levels.[3]

Last fall, while visiting Disney World, I gave Ron non-drowsy Dramamine every day so he would not become nauseated on the rides. Normally, Ron is afraid of amusement park motion activities. But I had hoped, with the medication, that he would enjoy at least a few of them. To my great delight, by the fourth day of our vacation Ron was like a different little boy. He no longer seemed afraid of anything. He rode on all the rides and even laughed while rocketing around on a wild roller coaster. He kept asking to ride again and again.

After we returned home, I kept telling people how different Ron had seemed on our vacation. I showed everybody the happy pictures that I had taken of him on a roller coaster—smiling from ear-to-ear.

As you can guess, this positive change in Ron did not continue. I naturally blamed his returning fears and anxieties on the everyday frustrations that he felt at school. I certainly would never have credited a daily dose of Dramamine II for his fast improvement. At least not until I read your book.

Although our experience with Ron's taking this medication was completely unexpected, the results were significant enough that I could immediately recognize the importance of your therapeutic findings for others with similar symptoms, myself included.

Paula West

Paula West herself, it turned out, was no stranger to the CVS (cerebellar-vestibular system) syndrome. She describes herself and her symptoms as follows:

After reading your books, I have come to realize that I too have many symptoms of a CVS or inner-ear disorder.[4] *While I have always excelled in reading and writing, I cannot*

[3] The unexpected favorable responses of dyslexics to anti-motion sickness medication, noticed in hindsight, clearly, independently, and "blindly" confirm its efficacy. I noted many such cases, and some were included in *A Scientific Watergate: Dyslexia. To date, the exact role and frequency of favorable placebo responses is unknown. But they assuredly are involved to some relatively minor extent and contribute to the overall 75–85 percent improvement rate.*

[4] The shorthand term "inner-ear" is used throughout this work to represent not only the inner-ear itself but also its neuronal super-computer called the cerebellar-vestibular system (CVS). The CVS is the highest brain structure of many animals and is thus capable of modulating many complex or "higher" functions in man.

spell. I can still remember high school algebra down to the smallest detail, but I cannot add without a calculator. I understand north and south, but I always confuse left and right without careful thought. I cannot even look at a merry-go-round without becoming nauseated.

I was not able to go to college because I would not take the SAT test. I could not spell without a dictionary or complete the math portion without a calculator. My superior IQ was useless without the tools on which I had learned to rely. Even this letter would not have been possible were it not for a computer.

When younger, I learned computer programming in a technical school. At that time a college degree was not required. Although I was remarkably proficient in this profession, I still had to carefully hide my inability to spell lest it be mistaken for lack of intelligence.

I feel very fortunate to have succeeded in the business world without a college degree and with my spelling/math difficulties. I worked in the banking industry for many years and it would be a great surprise to my former employers if they knew that I could not even add without a calculator!

Sincerely,
Mrs. Paula West

Meg Fex

All too often, professionals tend to mistakenly view dyslexia as if it were only a reading disorder of educational rather than medical or neurophysiological origin. As a result, they believe that tutoring, although very helpful, holds the primary key to treatment. Without the clinical experience obtained from listening to scores of dyslexics, it is difficult for many to understand that simple and safe medications can often trigger greater degrees of reading, writing, spelling, etc. improvements than hours and hours of frustrating tutoring. More important, even when tutoring does improve reading, writing, spelling, etc., it remains completely unable to "cure" the mechanisms that underlie symptom formation. Nor can tutoring alone, however helpful and necessary, come close to also rapidly improving many of the other devastating nonacademic perceptual, balance, coordination, psychosomatic, etc. symptoms that characterize dyslexics and their underlying CVS syndrome.

Only by reading how Meg Fex no longer sees words jumping around on the page and by observing how substantially and rapidly her writing has improved following treatment can you truly grasp the neurophysiological vs. educational origins of dyslexic or SLD symptoms—and the significant *compensatory* benefits often derived by tutoring dyslexics *after* medical treatment is initiated.

I anticipate that Mrs. Katy Fex's following description of her daughter's improvements will help convince you that this book provides all dyslexics in need of help with genuine medical understanding and therapeutic solutions as opposed to empty, fragmented diagnostic terms and "Band-Aids" for coping strategies.

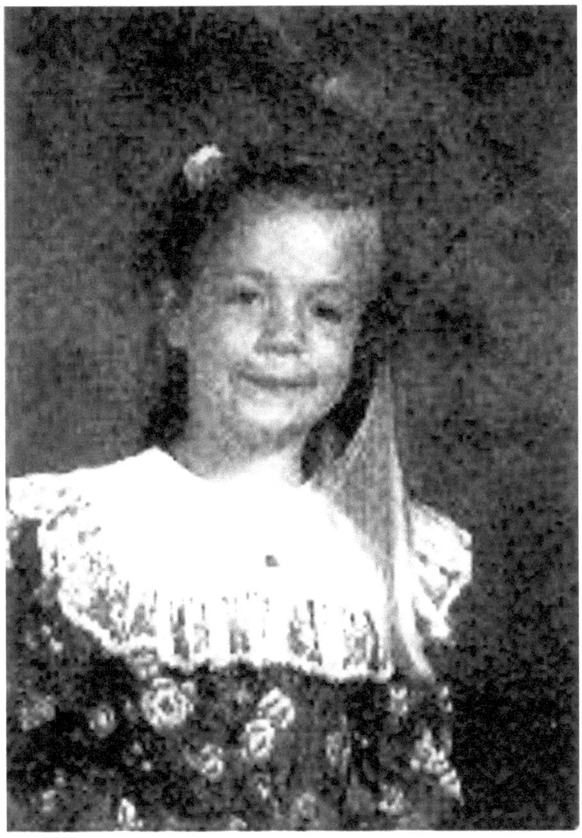

Mrs. Katy Fex related her 6-year-old daughter's improvements to me as follows:

As I write this letter to you, I am sitting in the children's section of the public library. Few people would appreciate the significance of this. Megan has been taking meclizine[5] *for only six days now. And her response to the medication has been nothing short of miraculous. So much has happened in this short time that I have had difficulty getting everything into my journal. I now face the task of condensing this into a letter to you without writing a novel... Here goes:*

Meg had to postpone beginning medication because she had another severe ear infection (detected by your staff). She took her first one-quarter of an antihistamine pill Saturday morning and went to ballet in the afternoon. I was very concerned that, with all the physical activity, Meg might have some kind of reaction.

[5] Meclizine is one of several anti-vertigo inner-ear medications found helpful in treating the many and varied symptoms of dyslexia. As you will soon read, some dyslexics, like Meg, became compulsive readers. So their doses had to be reduced. In these and many other cases, the role of placebos is considered to be clinically minimal.

Meg does not know why she is taking the medication—she believes it is for her ear. As a result, I told her, "Meg, you took your ear medicine today so if you feel bad you have to let Mommy know."

Meg replied, "I don't feel bad Mommy, I feel great… You know Mommy, I can't explain it, but I'm not so mixed up today.'

"David (Meg's father) and I tried to be cautiously optimistic, trying to pass it off as a good day—David being the greater skeptic. But this was the beginning of the most incredible week. Meg has done nothing but write and read all week. We find her with books or pencil and paper in the morning. And we have to take them out of her bed at night after she has fallen asleep.

When I asked Meg if her reading had gotten any easier, she said, "Yes." I asked her how. She explained it this way: "It's like the letters are glued down. The letters are glued on the paper. Now they don't jump around."

Sitting in your office a few weeks ago, you asked me what I wanted from all this. And I said that I wanted to eliminate her frustration. This treatment has made that possible, and so much more.

I have come to realize that her problem was much more complex than we ever imagined, affecting all parts of her life. Her ability to compensate was incredible… masking most of her symptoms from us.

Throughout this, I continue to read all the literature I can on the subject. I have read the criticism of your work— attributing its success to a placebo effect. But no placebo could accomplish this. Not all the positive thinking in the world could do this. This is real. This all makes sense.

Meg's Graphomotor Response to Medication

To further illustrate Meg's improvement, I thought it would be helpful to provide samples of her writing prior to inner-ear-enhancing medications and *after only two days* on medication.

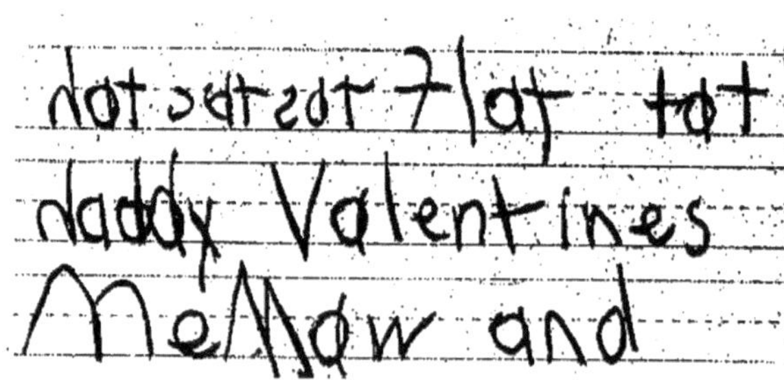

Prior to treatment Meg's letter (above) took over one and a half hours to complete. And it was just too much for her to add Elizabeth's name.

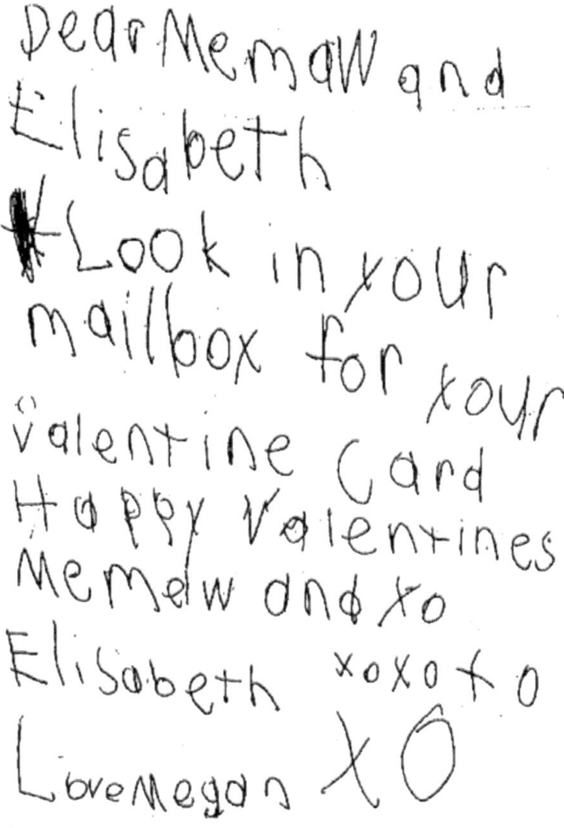

Dear Memaw and
Elisabeth
Look in your
mailbox for your
valentine Card
Happy Valentines
Memaw and to
Elisabeth xoxoxo
Love Megan XO

Two days after treatment After only two days on medication (meclizine), Meg completed the above letter in about 15 to 20 minutes. Meg wrote it independently and asked only how to spell words.

Concluding Thoughts

Although rapid changes in writing are *visual evidence* that can readily be demonstrated and grasped, readers should know that similar improvements in all the diverse symptoms characterizing dyslexics are possible—and do occur when medical therapy is successful. And these improvements may take place over a wide range of reading and non-reading functions. Perhaps now you will better understand how unexpected improvements in successfully treated patients serve to illuminate the many hidden but related symptoms defining the dyslexic syndrome.

Successfully treated patients, in fact, served as the greatest trove of information for me when I was trying to unmask this disorder. Why? Well, when the root cause of the "dyslexia syndrome" was correctly addressed with medication, patients began reporting the rapid disappearance, or improvement, of a wide range of symptoms that no one initially realized were part of the syndrome. Often those who suffer from the CVS disorder are not consciously aware of many of their own impairments. Their symptoms often seem "normal" to them; they've always had them and never had anything to compare them to—and so didn't always know what normal was. Or, these patients may have compensated for their deficits so well, and for so long, that those around them are not even aware they have so many issues.

Patients' rapid posttreatment responses A great many similarly rapid and amazing improvements arose during my treatment of dyslexics. And they allowed me to gain an infinitely more accurate and far-ranging picture of this previously hidden, multi-dimensional, and multi-symptomatic disorder than I would have gained by listening to, and/or observing, their pretreatment symptoms or by testing them via any and all other means combined.

Most importantly, by medically illuminating all the varied but previously hidden dysfunctioning elements characterizing the dyslexia syndrome, I was able to utilize this vital "therapeutic dissecting tool" for more definitive diagnosis and analysis. By reading on, you will see for yourself just how this "therapeutic tool" illuminates the four-dimensional (4-D) dyslexia hologram with a clarity and certainty never before thought possible.

At this point, though, you are probably a bit curious as to how I discovered the CVS cause of this complex disorder when all of my training and study were telling me to look to the psyche and then the thinking brain for explanations.

So let's take a brief trip back to my early days in the dyslexia field.

An Important Zag: Explaining Additional Insights

But wait a second. Before we go back there, I'd like to zag and thereby highlight a fascinating observation or two. Do you recall, in the very first page, how Michael Shultz impulsively grabbed a book from his mother and began reading adult content, unable to stop, after taking a test dose of a med? And, similarly, how Meg just started reading spontaneously, almost compulsively, and was found asleep with a book in hand?

Well, I've had a few other patients who just couldn't stop reading at bedtime following treatment. So I decreased their med doses—and thus eliminated their compulsive-like reading side effect. Amazed? I certainly was, as with every new unexpected insight that came my way.

And another related insight occurred to me: Have you wondered how Michael Shultz began reading words he didn't previously know? Thanks to my having come across similar therapeutic responses,[6] I had already formed a few assumptions. Is it possible that some dyslexics absorb much more information than they are consciously aware of? And that the meds enable dyslexics to recover these blocked memories—free them from over-inhibition? And/or that treated dyslexics are now suddenly able to read and understand new content normally—spontaneously, as do gifted readers? Certainly no one can realistically dispute the insightful value of these observations and anecdotal responses. Indeed, these clinical insights, when properly pursued and tested, have led me to dyslexia solutions that could not have been obtained in any other way.

So now I'm finally ready to go back in time and tell you how my career in dyslexia got started—and how my zigzagging research effort evolved.

[6] For, example, I recall a 13-year-old severely dyslexic girl who chewed a test dose of a CVS enhancing med. A half-hour later, she rapidly and accurately read the highway signs and airport directions for her parents who were late for their plane trip home.

Chapter 3
A Bit of History and Discovery

A Chance Event

In the tradition of most scientific discoveries, my research in dyslexia started by chance rather than design, in 1964. Following my psychiatric residency at Kings County Hospital, Brooklyn, NY, I needed a job. I was newlywed and had not the proverbial penny to my name. Poring through the *Times* classifieds, I learned that the Bureau of Special Reading Services (SRS) within the New York City Board of Education needed a psychiatrist to help the young reading-disabled kids within their purview.

At that time, reading disability was thought by all SRS experts to be psychologically determined. So I was hired. My credentials and training were excellent. I was young, ambitious, psychologically minded, and brimming with energy and dedication.

There was only one minor problem. I knew nothing about reading or learning disabilities and had never heard of dyslexia. No big deal. I devoured the entire scientific literature of the era before showing up for work on day one. At that time there were two major theories attempting to explain the severe reading and learning difficulties experienced by the children within the Bureau, one psychological and one neurological.

The SRS accepted otherwise normal children from other schools for extra tutoring and counseling who were two or more years behind in reading. But, believe it or not, they did not accept disruptive kids at the time. And I was tasked to treat only those reading impaired who failed to benefit from remediation and social work intervention.[1]

[1] The basic criteria for acceptance into the SRS program and the diagnostic definition of dyslexia were identical: two or more years behind one's peers in reading scores. Frankly, this "magic" dividing line seemed arbitrary to me, at best, and silly at worst. Yet everyone else seemed content to march to its diagnostic tune. So I went along with it until I belatedly confirmed my initial instinct. However, the fact that the SRS criteria and the accepted definition of dyslexia were identical certainly made my research easier, perhaps even possible.

Also, I did not yet know that most of these psychological or psychosomatic symptoms were either CVS-determined or secondary reactions to this CVS impairment and its encompassing dyslexia and ADD/ADHD segments.

H. N. Levinson, *Feeling Smarter and Smarter*,
https://doi.org/10.1007/978-3-030-16208-5_3

Psychological vs. Neurological Theories

Because I had zero independent clinical experience at the time, I had absolutely no quarrel with the SRS view that the reading impaired were behind because of psychological causes—especially since I was psychiatrically and psychoanalytically trained and therefore biased toward that type of belief.

I was gung ho, though, just rearing to help these kids and their parents who were desperate for the very benefits I was trained to provide them. I had no idea at that point in my career that everything I had belatedly read about those with severe reading impairments, or dyslexia, was drastically in error.

And so, I began psychiatrically examining hundreds of anxious and frustrated reading-disabled kids who were feeling dumb, ugly, and hopeless. Some were phobic, school phobic especially. Others were too anxious to concentrate and sit still—at least so I thought. Still others were in complete denial, refusing to admit they had any reading and learning problems at all. Many had typical psychosomatic-related symptoms, such as headaches, lightheadedness, dizziness, nausea, or stomachaches. Some were nail-biters, a few had tics, while others stuttered and stammered. Many had sleep disturbances of various types, including insomnia, night terrors, and sleepwalking. Frustration outbursts and minimal impulsivity were not uncommon, nor were moodiness, boredom, opposition, and defiance—but only mild versions of these, or else these kids would have been disqualified from admission to the SRS program. And then there were those with a past history of bed-wetting and soiling. And among the youngest, a very few still thumb-sucked at night, although most had stopped.

As a group, these children evidenced a challenging enough array of mental and behavioral symptoms to keep a young, eager, and conscientious psychiatrist's schedule filled to the max. So I busily went about attempting to psychologically help these kids as well as their concerned, and sometimes "overconcerned," parents.

Incorrect psychological theories But I soon stumbled upon a scientific dilemma, one that was difficult for me to initially solve. Although many well-recognized psychoanalysts of that era were explaining reading, writing, spelling, and even math problems on the basis of underlying primary psychological mechanisms having to do with issues such as aggression, sibling rivalry, childhood sexual conflicts, and voyeurism, I could not clinically verify the psychological cause-and-effect relationship of these Freudian-related mechanisms within the patients I was examining. Nor did my psychotherapeutic treatment result in any significant change in their reading and related academic performance—despite my committed attempts to minimize or resolve the allegedly causative psychological mechanisms or triggers proposed by psychoanalytic experts.

I did, however, provide the children with some emotional benefit and stability, but their basic academic problems remained unchanged. Naturally, I felt inadequate because of my failure to elicit and resolve the emotional conflicts deemed by experts to be critical determining factors.

I coped with my frustration by trying harder and harder. I examined and treated more and more patients until my experience became exponentially wider and deeper than that of the psychoanalysts writing the books about these disorders. With increasing clinical experience, my confidence in my own findings steadily grew.

One thing became crystal clear: the authors of the scientific papers and books I read did not understand the reading-disabled or dyslexic kids that I was examining. For the first time, I began to seriously question both the experience and expertise of many "experts."

Over time, I began to gather and analyze a large set of my own clinically based observations on the kids I attempted to help. Some of these observations defied psychological explanation. For example, why were so many severely impaired readers coming to the SRS for tutoring from the "best" homes and the top schools? And by contrast, why were so many less impaired readers coming from the most troubled and disadvantaged families and the worst schools?

Thus, I was forced to wonder: Was it possible that reading disability or dyslexia was not of a primary psychological origin? Was it possible that psychological experts, by analogy, were blindly throwing theoretical darts at their preconceived fantasized image of the reading-disabled and their assumed symptom-determining mechanisms? In other words, were they mistakenly creating and then connecting psychological dots to fit their expectations? Was it possible that the mental and behavioral symptoms of these kids reflected the *result* rather than the *cause* of their reading and learning issues? Was it possible that child-rearing, teaching, and environment played only important *secondary* roles in reading disability or dyslexia—roles that could be positive or negative?

Was it also possible that these kids' poor self-esteem resulted from their academic failures? Is that why the smartest kids often felt the dumbest? Because their instinctive expectations were higher, and so their failure and frustration were much more difficult to palate? More devastating? Was that why they flunked my psychotherapy so badly? Or was it I who had flunked by misapplying my efforts to their psyches rather than to their probable core neurological problems? Was it also likely that the primary origins of reading and learning disorders were neurological rather than psychological?

At that time, these ideas and questions about neurological causes were blasphemous to my SRS colleagues.

Resolving a Clinical Paradox or Two

After examining and psychologically treating hundreds and hundreds more kids—alleged to be neurologically normal by others, meaning cerebral signs were absent, I began to wonder more and more: Was it scientifically sound to assume these children suffered from a primary psychological problem just because there was an absence of obvious and/or reported cerebral neurological findings? Probably not.

Logically, I was also forced to reason that in order for reading disability or dyslexia to be psychologically caused, there had to be positive observable evidence of specific psychological determining mechanisms that were sufficient to explain *all* of the typical reading and related symptoms that characterized the kids I examined—as well as the *specific quality* of these symptoms, e.g., reversals, losing one's reading place, word movement, slanted writing, difficulty recalling the multiplication tables, and more. Yet I could find none—despite having gained considerable clinical experience since my initial doubts. This disturbing absence eventually led me to further believe that there had to be a neurological origin escaping our detection and thus that psychoanalysts had fantasized mechanisms not there.

Looking for a neurological origin I was finally forced to conclude that the absence of reported neurological findings in dyslexics meant only that we had to try harder to find the missing diagnostic signs that were somehow eluding our capability to detect them. And that once found, these neurological signs would lead us to discover dyslexia's elusive neurological origin.

So I began rereading the neurological literature on dyslexia. At first glance, the reading processor/thinking-brain theory of dyslexia (discussed in Chap. 1) seemed perfectly logical and sound. Indeed, it seemed irresistible; alluringly simple. And I was determined and headstrong enough to believe that I could find what others could not—the hidden cerebral neurological signs.

As a result, I proceeded to examine 1000 consecutive dyslexic kids within the SRS way back in the late 1960s in the hope that I could find the thinking-brain neurological signs that had been missed by all prior neurologists studying this disorder, Critchley and gifted others included.

What did I find? Nothing! Nada! Zip!

An Unexpected Discovery

In retrospect, I may have been one of the most gung ho proponents of the thinking-brain theory of dyslexia—at least at first—so determined and committed was I to finding the cerebral signs that all others had somehow overlooked. I knew the neurological signs were there, just waiting for me to find them. So I examined and reexamined these kids repeatedly—fully expecting that I would somehow succeed by sheer dint of my dauntless determination and efforts. No such luck. I was eventually forced to a point of humility, best stated by Goethe: "With all my sweated lore, I stand no wiser than before."

Hiding in plain sight However, upon carefully reviewing all the combined clinical data characterizing these one thousand kids, I accidentally stumbled on a surprising realization: Over 75 percent of the dyslexic kids had some difficulty with balance/coordination/rhythm, either by past and/or current history and/or upon neurological examination.

For example:

- Some were late crawlers, late sitters, late walkers, and late talkers.
- Some had difficulties with fine motor coordination: tying shoelaces; buttoning; zippering; and holding and using pencils, crayons, scissors, and eating utensils.
- Many had eye-hand coordination issues with activities such as catching, throwing, and batting a ball.
- Some had gross motor coordination problems with running, skipping, hopping, climbing, or difficulties with sports—group as well as individual.
- Accident proneness was not unusual: tripping, falling, bumping, and dropping.
- Many had balance-related problems with walking a beam or curb, or riding a bike; some often bumped into others walking alongside them when distracted by conversation.
- Speech coordination symptoms, such as difficulties with articulation and even stuttering and stammering, were not infrequent.
- Freudian slips of the tongue frequently occurred. Indeed, I later recognized that many of these kids frequently manifested "slips" or errors of various kinds, leading me to recognize them to be caused by dyslexic mechanisms, usually intensified when the kids were fatigued, distracted, and/or anxious.
- Many appeared to have "clumsy" eyes, repeatedly losing their place when reading.
- Some held their pencils awkwardly and experienced difficulties writing in a smooth, straight, and coordinated manner.

And many of the specific neurologic signs I was unexpectedly finding were those often exhibited by dizzy and off-balance individuals, as well as by drunken drivers:

- Difficulty following/tracking a moving target accurately and smoothly
- Difficulty reading letters, words, and sentences in a smooth, rhythmic manner
- Difficulty standing on one foot, especially with eyes closed
- Difficulty touching finger to nose with eyes closed and arms initially fully extended
- Difficulty rotating outstretched arms in opposite directions rhythmically and rapidly
- Difficulty with tandem or heel-to-toe walking while maintaining balance
- Difficulty moving the thumb to each of the other four fingers in sequence repetitively, without skipping or losing direction

So in the final analysis, my gut instinct was right. I did find the missing signs. They just weren't the ones I was looking for. But at least I'd found definitive neurological signs. And they'd been hiding in full view all along.

Circular Logic

Now here's another shocking discovery I stumbled across: upon re-reviewing the neurological literature, I realized that other traditionalist dyslexia experts had also found similar balance/coordination/rhythmic neurological signs—just as I had.

However, they had simply ignored or minimized the diagnostic significance of these signs—often even leaving them out of their reports and/or not even examining dyslexics for them. And the reasoning used by experts in doing so was as simple as it was mistaken.

Since these "motor" signs were not the hard and fast evidence of a thinking-brain dysfunction that we were all searching for, my colleagues and predecessors were led to deny their true neurologic importance, using unwitting bias mechanisms to do so. Thus, these definite inner-ear/cerebellar motor signs were called "soft" rather than "hard." And amazingly, gifted clinicians were found reasoning in circles so as to maintain their thinking-brain theory of dyslexia. Although previously discussed, we'll go into more detail about this circular and distorted reasoning in a later chapter. Why? Because recognizing and overcoming my own scientific bias and denial as well as that of all my colleagues was absolutely crucial to my solving the dyslexia riddles.

For now, the important questions that should be jumping out at you are the following: Shouldn't the neurological traditionalists have reasoned that their thinking-brain/reading processor dyslexia convictions may have been wrong since no supporting evidence was found? And shouldn't they have explored the significance of the balance/coordination/rhythmic—motor—signs that *were* found rather than denying their importance by calling them "soft" and "minimal" or even "atypical"? And finally, might there be a hidden or subconscious resistance force capable of often misleading the best, the smartest, and the most dedicated? It certainly appeared so.

Chapter 4
The Turning Point: Solving the Dyslexia Riddle

Somehow a super-laser of insight, launched presumably from my subconscious, finally penetrated and burst my traditionalist bubble. I was suddenly able to look at the clinical reality of dyslexics with fresh eyes and a new perspective. And I was finally capable of thinking nontraditionally—relatively resistance-free. Accordingly, I reasoned in a seeming atypical or nontraditionalist fashion:

1. If there exists no neurological evidence of a thinking-brain dysfunction in dyslexia, as confirmed present in alexia, then perhaps dyslexia is not of a thinking-brain origin.
2. If only balance/coordination/rhythmic neurological signs exist in dyslexia, then perhaps dyslexia is caused by the same impairment responsible for the balance/coordination/rhythmic signs.
3. If balance/coordination/rhythmic signs are known to be of inner-ear/cerebellar origin, then dyslexia is probably of a similar inner-ear/cerebellar origin.
4. If the reading impairment in dyslexics is often characterized by reversals, ocular fixation, and sequential tracking problems, as well as memory uncertainty, yet has a favorable outcome with tutoring over time, *and* if alexics show only a complete inability to comprehend clearly seen letters and words as well as a hopeless prognosis, are not their respective reading impairments completely different?

Therefore, I reasoned that these two disorders and their respective reading impairments must likely stem from completely separate neurological origins! And I thought: Have the traditionalists perhaps been confusing zebras with tigers—simply because both have stripes?

H. N. Levinson, *Feeling Smarter and Smarter*,
https://doi.org/10.1007/978-3-030-16208-5_4

Testing the Inner-Ear/Cerebellar Hypothesis

Neurological (CVS) validation Thus, I began to wonder: Since I had found balance/coordination/rhythmic inner-ear/cerebellar signs in over 75 percent of dyslexics *without even searching for them,* what percent of dyslexics would evidence such signs if I specifically went looking for them neurologically? And if the very same dyslexics were sent to gifted child neurologists and neurotologists (inner-ear specialists)—without these experts being told ahead of time the purpose of the referral so as to minimize bias— what percentage of these children would be found to have inner-ear/cerebellar dysfunctioning?

Since I had briefly mentioned this study in Chap. 1, you sort of know a little about what happened. Upon my own detailed neurological examinations, I found 96 percent of dyslexics to have definite evidence of inner-ear/cerebellar dysfunction. None had *any evidence of a thinking-brain impairment.* And famed Columbia-Presbyterian Hospital child neurologists also reported "cerebellar deficits" in *96 percent* of these very same children, without even looking for such findings. Again, *none* of the children were found to have any evidence of a thinking brain impairment despite the neurologists' stated belief that a cerebral deficit and "minimal cerebral dysfunction" had to be present in dyslexics.

Electronystagmography (ENG) validation And finally, without knowing anything at all about my research and its intent or the patients' symptoms, all of the leading neurotologists from the best medical centers in New York City reported that 90 *percent* of referred dyslexics had inner-ear dysfunctioning, based on electronystagmographic (ENG) inner-ear testing developed by Nobel Laureate Robert Barany.

My Initial Oversimplistic CVS Hypothesis

Okay, so having independently confirmed and scientifically published the evidence of only an inner-ear/cerebellar dysfunction in dyslexia (1973), which I termed DDD, I was left to explain how a *motor output* dysfunction can result in a *reading input* disorder.

To do so, I oversimplistically reasoned as follows within the same publication *before any updates*: If CVS dysfunctioning was causing poorly coordinated eye movements, then the visual reading input taken in by those uncoordinated "dyslexic eyes" might then become secondarily scrambled. And thus, the normal reading center within the thinking brain would have difficulty processing these scrambled visual signals—causing the reading impairment that I, and all others, mistakenly equated with the total dyslexia disorder or syndrome.

Although this initial hypothesis was logically consistent with many of the known neurological findings at the time, as well as with my clinical recognition that most dyslexics manifested visual letter and word reversals as well as difficulty fixating and tracking letters and words in sequence, I was still left with the task of proving it was true.[1]

Validating the CVS Hypothesis

The 3-D Optical Scanner To confirm my hypothesis, I needed to definitively demonstrate the existence of clumsy or discoordinated eye movements in dyslexics vs. non-dyslexics. That was the rub! I knew of no existing instrument that could do the job. So I designed the 3-D Optical Scanner. This instrument projects a series of moving letters and words onto a screen at measurably accelerating speeds until visual blurring eventually occurs (refer to Chap. 19, Appendices 6 and 7 for more). In order to see the projected symbols clearly, the eyes are reflexively forced to track these moving targets at increasing speeds until reaching their maximum tracking capacity. At this point, when the eyes cannot run any faster, the accelerating target escapes from view—resulting in a signal-scrambling or blurring-speed endpoint or marker that was reliably reproducible.

I reasoned that "clumsy" dyslexic eyes would not be able to efficiently—reflexly—race after or sequentially track the moving sequence. Thus, they would more rapidly scramble the accelerating moving targets and so reach "blur-out" at target speeds significantly lower than those of non-dyslexics. And this is exactly what happened, thus experimentally verifying my initially proposed—but oversimplistic and thus incomplete—inner-ear/cerebellar-determined visual fixation and tracking/processing hypothesis of dyslexia.

For the ease of testing young children, I eventually used pictures of elephant sequences instead of sentences, with similar results. I then added electrodes to monitor the tracking eye movements. Guess what I discovered? The eyes suddenly—reflexly—stopped moving after blurring was reported. This made perfect sense: Why would the eyes keep moving after blurring occurred if there was nothing to see and reflexly follow? So now I could more objectively *observe and demonstrate this blurring-speed endpoint or maximum reflex tracking capacity* on paper

[1] I still had not fully recognized that dyslexia was a complex syndrome, not just a reading disorder. That's because I had not yet fully escaped from the traditionalist bubble. And didn't realize it. Complete escape from misassumptions isn't easy. As they say, you can take the kid out of Brooklyn, but you can't take the Brooklyn out of the kid—Brooklyn being, in this case, your mental baggage: biased thinking.

Almost three decades later, Finnish neurotologist Tapani Rahko independently validated the presence of benign paroxysmal positional vertigo (BPPV) and abnormal involuntary eye movements in dyslexia—impairing reading. However, his reported frequency was far higher than that reported by independent neurotologists involved in my study and the incidence I later obtained in my own follow-up studies. Importantly, all the specific neurological and ENG signs were reported within the Appendices of *A Solution to the Riddle—Dyslexia*. And a chapter was devoted to discussing these findings.

rather than just taking the patient's word for it or relying on my observations of their eye movements during testing. So far, so good![2]

The 3-D Auditory Scanner With additional clinical experience, I soon recognized that there often coexisted —but not invariably—an auditory or phonetic component to the reading disorder. And so I developed a 3-D Auditory Scanner and demonstrated that dyslexics also—though not always—scrambled and then blurred-out *listened-to spoken words* much faster than did non-dyslexics, *using the limited measuring tools at my disposal.* This explained why so many dyslexics reported auditory delays in processing and/or difficulty in accurately perceiving and remembering things others told them. In other words, the normal thinking brain of dyslexics required extra time and concentration to *compensate* for the processing of the scrambled visual and auditory word signals sent to it.

Updating My Initial CVS Hypothesis

Based entirely on patient observations, Q&A methods, and simple logic "momentarily" freed of bias, I was forced to recognize that the reading disorder in dyslexia was far more complex than just ocular-motor visual scrambling. And that a valid theory of dyslexia had to also include compensation so as to account for cognitive and maturational improvements—eventually reasoning that the latter were mostly derived from the thinking brain and perhaps the higher cerebellum, both of which are connected via feedback circuits.[3]

Thus, I was led to re-conceptualize my initially oversimplistic visual fixation and tracking reading concept of dyslexia, albeit a major theoretical breakthrough at the time. Instead, I now viewed dyslexia as a primary multisensory and motor signal-scrambling CVS dysfunction *in dynamic equilibrium* with compensatory, and even destabilizing, mechanisms.

Restating my updated theory Accordingly, I was forced to reason: the initially normal thinking brain in dyslexics appears to be *secondarily* attempting to compensate for the *primary ocular-motor and multisensory input and motor output* signal-scrambling dysfunction triggered by an impaired fine-tuner within the inner-ear and cerebellum.

[2]There did appear to be many bewildering exceptions to this neat and tidy blurring-speed rule. For example, I encountered what I called "phantom tracking"—where the eyes of a few "atypical" dyslexics kept moving but saw only a blur. Analyzing all the exceptions and their mechanisms opened entirely new and unexpected research vistas, resulting in fresh insights into both dysfunctioning and compensatory tracking as well as an improved testing methodology. Amazing what happens when you *pay attention* to the exceptions rather than ignore them.

[3]This insight, among many others, also validated my gut feeling that the two-or-more-years-behind criteria for defining dyslexia was nonsensical—leading me to use the paradoxical term, "Dyslexics without dyslexia," challenging the mistaken belief of traditionalists that dyslexia is just a reading disorder. However, the "experts" reluctantly accepted my insight several decades later—so there's hope. But evolution moves very slowly—perhaps for good reasons.

Similar to many dyslexics, the experts just got the origins of dyslexia backward: they mistakenly blamed the thinking brain for being the primary *cause* of dyslexia rather than an important secondary compensating and processing force. And for a century, this fantasy was accepted reality—until my dyslexic patients forced me to challenge this mistaken illusion.

The Bias Factor

Why the experts got it wrong So I began to wonder, bringing my psychoanalytic training into play: *Might some experts have been hampered by tunnel-thinking, conceptual reversals, and other dyslexic mechanisms, as was I initially?* Might we all be influenced by psychologically motivated denial and other Freudian slips of logical reasoning, using dyslexic-like mechanisms? Might these same mechanisms within me have slowed down the speed at which I recognized my own unwitting and/or mistaken assumptions and those of others? Is kryptonite real?[4]

Eventually, I *completely* revised my initial oversimplistic dyslexia theory and its first update so that it proved capable of explaining 100 *percent* of dyslexia-related data, not just the visual, auditory, and other CVS neurological aspects. But it took thousands of patients to help me.

A Medical Solution

The abovementioned and related testing instruments proved reliable in significantly validating my inner-ear/cerebellar hypothesis of dyslexia and more. They also served as a medical means of screening, diagnosing, and even somewhat predicting those with inner-ear/cerebellar dysfunctioning who might then be predisposed toward developing the typical dyslexic academic symptoms later on when attending school.

Clinically validating the CVS med effects After recognizing the primary role of the inner-ear/cerebellar system in dyslexia, I went on to test and then clinically validate the efficacy of anti-motion sickness or inner-ear-enhancing medications in treating this disorder. The favorable responses of dyslexics led to the first and only medical treatment for this impairment. And when properly combining diverse

[4]Might we be in continuous denial, exceptional lapses aside? And might it be in the lapses that insights and discoveries consciously occur—explaining their infrequency? Might we be sleepwalking more than we know and so unwittingly confusing our (theoretical) dreams or fantasies with reality? Does Superman represent the force within us that overcomes kryptonite?

I was also *forced* to modify my initial CVS theory because of other considerations, such as why non-CVS individuals with nystagmus or abnormal eye movements didn't have dyslexia, etc.

groups of inner-ear-enhancing and related medications, as well as nutrients, I was *eventually* able to more effectively, rapidly, and often dramatically help 75–85 *percent* of treated subjects.

Prevention By successfully treating very young 3-to-4-year-olds who showed early signs of speech and other balance/coordination difficulties, I was even able to *prevent* their typical dyslexic reading and writing symptoms from ever surfacing later on.

How do I know this? Because the pre-treated kids developed typical reversal-prone "dyslexic" symptoms only when their meds were stopped in the second or third grades. And these academic symptoms rapidly disappeared once the meds were restarted. I also found that I could induce dyslexic symptoms in normal individuals by simply spinning the kids around till very dizzy—thus rendering their signals "dizzy." And by pre-treating them with inner-ear-enhancing meds before spinning, I could *prevent* or minimize their "temporary dyslexia" from occurring.

Compensation Moreover, I found that my diagnostic instruments, via function-enhancing repetitive and conditioning techniques, were minimally capable of improving the very mechanisms they were revealing to be impaired. These vital insights had more than just a therapeutic significance. They demonstrated a likely neuroplastic role of the brain in compensating for its own failures, and so explained, at least in part, how and why the symptoms of dyslexics often improved over time via mechanisms sometimes referred to simply as "maturation after delayed development" or "late blooming." Indeed, I've seen very, very late bloomers who suddenly started reading more "normally" in graduate school. Once again, such phenomena were *named* by observers but never properly explored and understood.

Related CVS disorders Following my successful treatment of thousands and thousands of dyslexics, I was later able to demonstrate that ADD/ADHD and phobias, as well as DCD or developmental coordination disorder, were also inner-ear/cerebellar-triggered phenomena. And that these variously named disorders, and many others, all substantially overlapped with one another in most referred dyslexics and so were reflections of a common CVS denominator. We'll get into the fascinating phobia, ADD/ADHD, and other connections to the CVS later on in the book.

Closing the "History Book"

As you might have guessed by now, the number of insights sparked by my research has already filled a number of scientific papers, books, and articles. The above presentation is merely a highly condensed and updated summary of many decades of research that culminated in the first and only comprehensive medical understanding, diagnosis, treatment, and even prevention of dyslexia and its related learning, ADD/ADHD, and phobic disorders.

I would love to go on and on with further details, but I think that's enough for now. You'll learn more about my work as this book unfolds. And if you become hooked and want to read more about these topics, you can refer to the many independently validating sources I've listed at the end of the book and on my website—*dyslexiaonline.com.*

Finally, I'd like to reemphasize a crucial insight in case you're unfamiliar with clinical research: atypical, paradoxical, or unexpected findings often appeared at my every scientific twist and turn. Although this data often appeared statistically insignificant—which meant that many researchers would have discarded them in favor of the majority rule—my psychoanalytic training had taught me to do the very opposite. My exploring the frustrating and perplexing *exceptions* to the apparent rule invariably led me to invaluable insights and a better and deeper comprehension of the total dyslexia/CVS gestalt. In fact, as you previously read, the CVS signs in dyslexics were mistakenly assumed by traditionalists to be "soft" and atypical exceptions until I demonstrated them to be the true rule. (See the ASSUME principle.)

How My Background Helped Guide Me to a Scientific Solution

No doubt you are still curious how one Brooklyn-born psychiatrist with Freudian psychoanalytic and neurological training was able to solve all the century-old dyslexia riddles that had long eluded all others. So allow me a small digression. Perhaps my sharing a few personal things about myself may more completely help answer this question.

Good with bias I was born to a hardworking, aspirational, Jewish immigrant family over 80 years ago. And so I became good at standing firm against biased opinions and tough odds, and better at dealing with atypical data and concepts than might more gifted "Mayflower Americans," no counter-bias intended.

Determined Having survived starvation and repeated Cossack killing sprees in Czarist Russia, my family imbued me with significant determination skills—no matter how great the obstacles appeared.

Liked challenges Combined with my stubborn determination were some other personal traits that I think turned out to be helpful as well. I enjoyed mental challenges—especially those leading me to relentlessly tackle, simplify, and solve complex math and related scientific issues. I later wondered if this trait led me, subconsciously of course, to a profession where I felt tirelessly driven to solve and treat complex mental and neurological problems, such as those within this book.

Street smart I think I was also a bit more conceptually agile and analytic than others. Maybe it was just "street smarts?" But I seemed, for whatever reason, better able to shift gears, zigzag, and self-correct, especially later on when my assumptions and those of others repeatedly led me and my research astray. And I can assure you, unwittingly made misassumptions are a dime a dozen. More often than not, it feels as if you're working in a universe where straight lines curve and parallel lines intersect.

Intuitive and challenging My intuition and somewhat oppositional nature often led me to question the convictions of others. For example, despite being schooled as a Freudian, I instinctively felt that all the psychoanalytic theories proposed in the 1960s to explain reading disorders or dyslexia were either significantly lacking or dead wrong. Some of them felt truly absurd, even when I was first learning about the topic. Although I trusted Freud's genius, I began to have serious doubts about the dyslexia-related concepts of many of his second- and third-generation followers, who often seemed to be trying to out-Freud Freud. As previously noted, that's when I first learned to doubt experts, despite their superb reputations and qualifications.

Two scientific supermen Just to be perfectly clear: Among the many scientific giants in history that shaped my research interests and truly inspired me, I believe there were two Supermen—Freud and Einstein. Whereas Freud miraculously explained our incredibly complex inner-subconscious world, his twin scientific genius, Einstein, amazingly captured our infinitely complex external universe. And I came to believe these two "separate" worlds may be far larger and more interconnected than most would think. Thus, these beliefs led me and my research to recognize that the CVS system, the subconscious, as well as gravity, the full moon, and other electromagnetic orienting mechanisms and signals interact (refer to Kathy in Chap. 11).

Freudian influences and reflections Why was Freud so important to me? Because I believe that my own Freudian psychoanalysis played a major role in eventually leading me and my research efforts to a soft and successful landing. Thus, for example, I learned how to better understand my motives, reasoning, and related errors as easily as those of my patients—and so also those of my scientific colleagues. And eventually I became significantly more adept at minimizing or sidestepping the unwitting Freudian and dyslexic slips leading us all astray—both of which, I discovered, used similar subconscious mechanisms (refer to Chap. 8).

Interestingly, my own analysis had also shown me how often we are *favorably* directed on a subconscious level. For example, have you wondered where in the world my analogy to Superman and his neutralizing kryptonite came from? Or why I used it?

Finding Superman and kryptonite I was looking for a simple, colorful way to portray the negative force of bias that I've encountered within myself and within many *super-bright* professionals throughout my research career. I trusted my subconscious to provide me with a desired analogy. And it did, just as it had solved many of my math problems while asleep. It wasn't a cognitively and consciously thought-out process of mine at all. Rather, solutions or clues just popped into my head—including many novel dyslexia insights—drawn from my unconscious, akin to a readily understandable dream.

"So what do these Superman and fatal kryptonite symbols mean?" I hear you asking. My guess: *That nature created both brilliant super-scientists to propel mankind forward as well as bias or kryptonite to slow down their advances.*

"Why," you may also be wondering, "the need for nature to neutralize our progress?" My assumption: *To prevent the inevitable chaos resulting from unchecked escalating advances before adaptations arise.*

A need for scientific simplicity I also believe that another personality trait of mine has significantly aided me in my scientific "quest." I like to keep my ideas as simple as possible. Thus, I always keep in mind the acronym: KISS (Keep It Simple, Stupid).

Most importantly, my need for simplicity somehow led me to the vital tool that was absolutely essential in solving the dyslexia puzzle—*listening to patients*. In fact, there would never have been a solution without its use. Thus, I will discuss this simple tool in the very next chapter.

My MD role model Before we move on, though, I'd like to share my most important career- and life-inspiring influence of all. I was, and still am, inspired by my old family MD, Dr. Rose. I still remember him traveling by subway from the Lower East Side of Manhattan to care for me as a child, even after my family moved to Brooklyn. I also recall that he often "forgot" or refused to charge us, despite our protestations. No doubt, my later "forgetting" to charge indigent patients while making house calls in Bed Stuy's housing projects during my residency in Brooklyn was also a Freudian slip—and certainly Dr. Rose-related.

Believe it or not, I still view Dr. Rose as my personal Hippocrates. And I have vowed to emulate his warmth, altruism, and dedication to healing the sick and suffering as best as I can until I'm gone—a goal that may not be attainable, but one I'm still pursuing. Why else would I now be writing this book? It's still pay-it-forward time. Thanks, Dr. Rose.

Chapter 5
Listening to Dyslexics: My Simple Clinical Path Proved Key to Discovery

When initially starting my research from ground zero, I instinctively determined that the best way—and perhaps the only way—to fully understand dyslexics, and so their disorder, is to *listen* patiently and carefully to their many and varied symptoms, including what has been reported by their parents, teachers, and testers. Then keenly observe their difficulties in performing reading, writing, etc. psychological and neurological tasks. And analyze everything you've obtained for important clues—and correlations—so as to find all of this disorder's key characteristics as well as their underlying determining origins.

Importantly, follow the facts wherever they lead. And try to recognize and so minimize the negative impact of any misassumptions made.[1]

Three Clinical Hurdles

Although the above may now seem obvious and simple, there were at least three major *initial* hurdles to overcome if you wished to use this psychoanalytic-like Q&A listening method, including having access to many hundreds—really thousands—of patients available for testing and evaluation.

First, to successfully perform this kind of in-depth "detective work," enormous time, patience, and determination—dedication—are required. How else would it be possible to initially collect, analyze, and reanalyze a huge amount of continually accruing descriptive/examination data from hundreds, and then thousands, of examined patients in order to find common manifestations and previously hidden

[1] I mistakenly assumed initially that dyslexia was just a reading disorder, first of psychological and then of cerebral origin. However, following the facts wherever they led saved my research efforts from dead ends. As you read on, you will see that just about all our initial conscious and unwitting assumptions about dyslexia were incorrect. And for good reason. Nature is just too complex and our thinking too "simplistic" to initially assume or guess correctly.

H. N. Levinson, *Feeling Smarter and Smarter*,
https://doi.org/10.1007/978-3-030-16208-5_5

denominators. And to initially do all of this before computers and smart programs were available to analyze and apply big data obtained from large samples and even from individual patients; also where the dyslexia in each and every dyslexic appeared clinically different?

Second, children are reluctant to open up to strangers, even those sincerely interested in helping them.

Third, the vast majority of dyslexic children, and also adults, did not consciously know what was specifically wrong with them. Thus, they didn't really know what to reveal, even when completely cooperative. Even worse, no professional initially knew what key questions to correctly ask them. And as you've read, most investigators, myself included, unwittingly denied rather than objectively followed the facts. Therefore, hundreds and hundreds of dyslexic patients were required to eventually obtain the needed insights which very slowly and disconnectedly, but repeatedly and convincingly, emerged in dribs and drabs, despite initial misassumptions and other resistance/bias factors.

Analyzing Observed Performance Errors Proved Helpful

Fortunately, I found a better way to obtain the vital information to which only dyslexics were privy. I personally observed the *errors and difficulties as well as compensatory strategies* of dyslexic children and adults when performing reading and related tasks and then used Q&As to obtain further information for analysis. This step turned out to be far easier and significantly more productive as you will readily see, especially in Chap. 16. That's where I illustrated just how all the many dyslexic reading symptoms, as well as their CVS dysfunctioning and compensatory determining mechanisms, were discovered, using all the steps.

Accordingly, I became more optimistic after gathering the data this observation step provided. Thus, for example, I recognized that dysfunctioning eye tracking, orientation (or reversals), as well as phonetic, concentration, and memory mechanisms, often triggered typical dyslexic reading problems and that the following compensatory, cerebrally determined methods helped improve reading performance: deliberately slowing down reading speed, using larger typeset and/or a marker, as well as repetition in one-to-one enhanced focusing situations to improve memory retention while minimizing distractibility.

However, I knew this overall process was still going to be long and tedious unless I found a better way to unmask this elusive disorder. But I really didn't much care at that point since each new insight served to catapult me forward. As I excitedly advanced, I remained in a highly focused, driven state in which time and effort seemed irrelevant. And challenging obstacles were seen as mere bumps in a road, adding even more excitement and new insights after overcoming and better understanding them as resistance barriers and solution blockers. The only scientific thing that mattered to me was progressing, advancing, succeeding.

Putting My Conviction to the Test: The Final Simple Step Needed for a Solution

The favorable response illuminator Fortunately, I found the best and *simplest* possible method to unmask the symptoms comprising the dyslexia syndrome—one overlooked by all others. As noted in prior chapters, I had developed the conviction that dyslexia was determined by inner-ear/CVS dysfunctioning based on initially analyzing the neurological and related mega-data I had collected from examining over a thousand dyslexic patients, and an independently validated follow-up study I initially published in 1973.

Then I quickly took the next game-changing clinical step that seemed logical to me. I offered my CVS-dysfunctioning dyslexic patients a trial treatment with safe CVS-improving medications. But I did so with my eyes wide, wide open—not blind or double-blind as many of my colleagues would have advised.

This crucial clinical step was the one that ultimately made a solution to the many dyslexia riddles more rapidly possible—even "elementary," as super-detective Sherlock Holmes might say. The collective reading and non-reading improvements—scores of them—derived from listening to thousands of dyslexics responding favorably to inner-ear-enhancing medication triggered the understanding that even the *reading segment* of the total dyslexic disorder was a multi-determined and symptomatically complex system within a far larger holistic world—the CVS syndrome.

As you will better realize in the following chapters, the dyslexia in each and every dyslexic is significantly different, despite having a common CVS origin—especially since the CVS is quite complex. Thus, illuminating, understanding, and reconciling all of these individual dyslexia-related variations as well as their commonalities were crucial to solving the dyslexia riddles. And so my initial qualitative listening method proved infinitely more productive and revealing than merely performing typical double-blind controlled studies examining single variables. That's because the latter studies were limited in scope and the "normal" control groups used were often found to be in error.

Finding the Multidimensional Face of Dyslexia: An Introductory Illuminating Sketch

During medical treatment, patients began experiencing and reporting dramatic improvements in a wide range of initially unexpected dyslexia-related reading and non-reading functions, as you have already been shown by Michael, Maria, Ron, and, of course, Meg. So I clinically reasoned that for every reported improvement, there must have been an impairment that preexisted it. And after neuroanalyzing (akin to psychoanalyzing) those improvements, I finally began to see a fascinating, but preliminary, 4-D sketch of the previously hidden dyslexia portrait as well as its CVS-determining neurophysiological mechanisms. Thus, the following syndrome of reading and non-reading dyslexic symptoms initially and surprisingly emerged at a "fast and furious" pace via improvements when using this rather simple and commonsense clinical research method I termed a *symptom-illuminating tool:*

> *A huge percentage of my patients reported improvements in overall reading capability as well as in such previously unrecognized reading symptoms as: impaired visual fixation and tracking, blurring, double vision, word movement, light sensitivity, overloading or flooding, and tunnel vision. There were even improvements in the delayed processing of reading content that is often mistaken for incomprehension. And phonetics spontaneously became easier.*
>
> *Favorably responding dyslexic children also noted that they were suddenly able to catch or throw a ball. Tripping, falling, and accident-proneness disappeared. Balance improved so patients were no longer fearful of riding a bike. Their writing no longer drifted all over the page like a drunk stumbling down the street, and became better coordinated. Articulation and/or pronunciation became clearer for some, and stuttering improved or disappeared for others. Adult dyslexics reported an enhanced feel for time and timing—and suddenly were able to dance or carry a tune. Some noted greater ease in driving a car while others were surprised that their golf and other sports skills dramatically improved.*
>
> *Concentration improved and distractibility substantially decreased. Brain fog and overactivity disappeared. Memory got better. Patients could suddenly hear more clearly, while understanding conversations at a faster speed. Many were becoming more social and were no longer fearful of speaking up.*
>
> *Fears of heights, elevators, escalators, and planes suddenly disappeared. Nightmares stopped. Moodiness often lightened, and depression not infrequently vanished. Spatial relations and directional sense improved; they no longer feared getting lost or becoming disoriented. Their headaches, dizziness, and motion sickness suddenly and unexpectedly disappeared.*
>
> *And importantly, the vast majority began feeling smarter and smarter.*

To reemphasize Since only inner-ear or CVS-enhancing medications were used to obtain the above improvement-based sketch in CVS dysfunctioning dyslexics, it was reasonable to assume that most of the symptomatic changes were CVS-related and/or essential components of the dyslexia syndrome. Fortunately, this "elementary" clinical assumption proved valid upon analysis, and this simple dissecting/clarifying research tool proved highly illuminating and successful.

And to completely explain and encompass 100 percent of the many and varied symptoms characterizing dyslexics, their underlying triggering and compensatory mechanisms, as well as all other related data that were eventually revealed, I was forced to repeatedly broaden the scope and depth of my initially conceived CVS-determined visual reading theory of dyslexia that I first postulated in 1973. But you'll have to wait until Chap. 9 to see my latest all-encompassing and fully explanatory CVS concept that was last modified just before this book's publication.

But one thing is now certain. Because just about all the past ideas about dyslexia were proven incorrect, had I pursued a double-blind comparative quantitative approach, most of my ensuing insights would have led me to the very same dead-ends traversed by my many distinguished traditionalist colleagues. And I would have certainly lost the complex 4-D "dyslexic forest."

The Qualitative Neuroanalytic Method Proved Capable of Unmasking Dyslexia

Eventually, my simple, commonsense Q&A, neuroanalytical (listening, observation, examination, dissection, analysis, deduction, and treatment) method paid off. And so I:

- Came to recognize the amazing complexity of the dyslexic reading disorder as well as its many co-determining dysfunctioning vs. compensatory mechanisms
- Discovered 17 other major non-reading areas of CVS or dyslexic impairments
- Identified scores of specific symptoms within each one of the eighteen major dysfunctional categories—the majority of these symptoms never before recognized or understood to be part of this dyslexia or CVS syndrome
- *Developed a specific list of questions I could reliably use for diagnostic and neuroanalytic purposes—a list previously missing, of course, when I first began questioning dyslexics*
- Discovered the many primary CVS mechanisms responsible for all the reading and non-reading symptoms characterizing the dyslexia syndrome
- Distilled the super-ten basic inner-ear/cerebellar functions at the root of *all* the many symptoms and determining mechanisms reported by dyslexics
- Finally saw and described the hidden face characterizing the dyslexia/CVS syndrome
- Developed a medical treatment capable of simply, safely, and rapidly helping 75–85 percent of treated dyslexic children and adults while also explaining the efficacy of most nonmedical therapies and their likely relationship to the CVS

Retrospective Insights

The Brooklyn method When I look back in time, it's even easier to see and explain why my *simple elementary* "Brooklyn method," especially the favorable response illuminator, worked in my equally simple "mom-and-pop-like," albeit sophisticated, Medical Dyslexia Treatment Center. I merely listened to, and recorded, the collective insights spontaneously provided by thousands of suffering patients with the dyslexia syndrome. Then I analyzed their determining mechanisms and reoccurring frequencies as well as their relationship to one another and their common origin. And, of course, I neurophysiologically tested patients for CVS impairments using many of the sophisticated diagnostic techniques described within Chap. 19.

Quite clearly, these evolving insights were far too many and diverse for any, and even all, involved professionals to have theoretically anticipated or conceived beforehand. Nor could they be found by investigating only single variables or by reading those studies unwittingly misdirected by mistakenly believed *dyslexia = alexia = severe reading incomprehension* misassumptions and definitions.

Finding and connecting the "dots" vs. publishing My desire to help patients enabled me to connect and integrate, rather than individually publish, the thousands of diverse initially puzzling and isolated clinical "dots" or insights dyslexics offered me. This important choice and effort eventually resulted in a multidimensional scattergram I called the 4-D Dyslexia/CVS portrait rather than an enhanced and impressive curriculum vitae.

The "triple-blind" methods By comparison, my psychoanalyst teachers likely saw only a few dyslexic patients and dots, misapplied Freud's psychoanalytic method, and listened to only themselves—as did the traditionalist neurologists and neurophysiologists. Since the latter believed *dyslexia = alexia = severe reading incomprehension,* they viewed research as merely a means to prove their century-plus-old ingrained cerebral convictions, as defined by the prior equation.

However, the post-Critchley neurophysiological investigators often used more sophisticated and statistically based research designs. And they collectively tested hundreds, likely thousands, of different dyslexic samples for single dots or variables in seemingly well-controlled double-blind studies to ensure "objectivity"—frequently overlooking and/or criticizing the positives offered by "simple" clinical eyes-wide-open studies and anecdotal methods such as mine.[2]

Thus, most other dyslexia investigators, as well as non-experts having no dots, were searching for and/or attempting to prove their respective preconceived images of dyslexia's portrait instead of following the facts wherever they led. And so they inevitably found their previously believed concept by looking through what Freud might call a *Projection telescope—having an unknown mirror attached to the other*

[2] No other neurological researcher chose to *follow this Q&A "neuroanalytic" (similar to psychoanalytic) investigative method.* And the reasons were simple. This was a psychoanalytic-like method—negatively/defensively referred to by some as merely clinical or anecdotal evidence, and neurologists were not geared to use it. And because neurological experts were initially certain that *dyslexia = alexia,* they saw no reason to further pursue and analyze a problem they believed was long ago solved in 1896. They just sought objective proof—finding the elusive cerebral neurological signs—to cement their irrefutable *dyslexia = alexia* conviction!

Glued to their alexia universe as well as their sophisticated double-blind investigative path, dyslexia researchers remained unable to see beyond themselves, nor willing to try. So they also defensively resisted listening to a challenging convert like me from planet "Brooklyn" who found and used a simple anecdotal method and investigatory route that significantly differed from theirs. *Never mind that my qualitative listening/neuroanalytic method worked—and so ultimately proved successful in unmasking and treating the previously hidden 4-D dyslexia syndrome and all its currently known causal mechanisms.* Kryptonite appeared to have them all spellbound. Thus, they continued to listen only to themselves and like-minded colleagues—not to my dyslexic patients, nor even their own!

end. In other words, because all of their double-blind so-called "objective" studies were mistakenly and unwittingly based on the erroneous equation and definition *dyslexia = alexia*, I referred to their flawed research as "triple-blind."

The Hidden Fallacies Underlying "Objectively" Controlled Dyslexia Studies

Because all traditionalist dyslexia researchers mistakenly believed that *dyslexia = alexia = severe reading incomprehension,* they attempted to contrast and so clarify the reading impaired or dyslexics from normal reading samples—the latter erroneously believed non-dyslexic, often in blind and double-blind studies to maximize objectivity. But this logical investigative method was fatally flawed from the very start.

Why, you might still wonder? Elementary! How can you accurately choose normal and/or non-dyslexic and even dyslexic samples if you don't really know what dyslexia is all about? You can't—not accurately so! But all traditionalists absolutely believed the misassumptions inherent in the above equation and so never questioned or looked at them with their eyes wide-open. Thus, for example, if all apples are mistakenly believed red, then objectively designed investigative studies using non-red look-alikes as control groups will unwittingly provide misleading results—even if performed double-blind.

The reading/dyslexia myth Clearly, even Critchley found "reading cured" dyslexics. Wasn't Mrs. Paula West, described in Chap. 2, obviously "dyslexic"—or suffering from the dyslexia syndrome, even though she read well? And you will soon recognize that Kathy, to be presented in the very next chapter, belatedly learned to read well enough to complete graduate school via compensation while still exhibiting severely impaired dyslexic mechanisms typical of most dyslexics. And when you get to super-reader Jenny in Chap. 20, you'll better understand that you can be "dyslexic without 'dyslexia'" ("dyslexia" meaning a [severe] alexic-like reading score/comprehension impairment). Thus, control groups using "normal" readers in dyslexia studies may, like red vs. non-red apples, result in triple-blind errors.

Although I was the first to refute the *dyslexia = alexia = dyslexia* equation based on these and many other clinical observations, as well as the fact that the reading scores and performance of dyslexics often rapidly normalized on meds, as did Meg's (in Chap. 2) and many others, this mistaken severe reading score-dependent definition of dyslexia persisted. And it still persists in influencing most of the objective double-blind controlled studies currently conducted, including those adding on a phonological requirement.

The phonological/dyslexia error As you will learn, even the *current definition* that dyslexics must have a phonological impairment is partially mistaken—and certainly inadequate. Thus, the previously mentioned dyslexic "super-readers" had this phonological impairment. And there exist reading impaired dyslexics with significant dysfunctioning visual mechanisms that are phonologically normal and even superior.

Dyslexia doesn't even exist, according to DSM-V And there's more. As you've just noted, dyslexia isn't even a reading disorder but a syndrome of many possible reading and non-reading symptoms existing within a larger CVS syndrome. No wonder why the DSM-V refuted the existence of dyslexia based on its traditionalist held mis-concepts and erroneous belief in the above mistaken equation. Because these triple-blind errors and the above erroneous equation were crucial in derailing a solution to the dyslexia riddles, they will be further highlighted and discussed in Chap. 8—Kathy and The Mistaken Theories of Dyslexia.

By comparison to the double-blind investigative designs, my simple Brooklyn listening Q&A method eventually exposed and clarified the abovementioned misassumptions because I first studied what dyslexia really was with open eyes before publishing eyes-closed studies utilizing flawed concepts and control groups.

Insights into Research Methods

So, what may we now conclude? Simply, that all investigative methods are helpful. However, some are better than others at specific stages/times for certain disorders and/or specific characteristics, often dependent on whether overall or macro qualitative/anecdotal descriptions are best initially—as for dyslexia, before double-blindly proceeding with proving and quantitatively measuring individual or micro "dots" in clinical darkness.

Thus, for example, the initial study of single variable double-blind dots in dyslexia, following a mistaken conviction that *dyslexia* = *alexia,* then additionally led to a further inevitable chain of oversights and mistaken assumptions and convictions—misleading us all for over a century. That's because they were mistakenly investigating alexia, which had nothing to do with dyslexia except having completely different reading disorders; hence, my *zebra* = *tiger* analogy—since they both also had dissimilar stripes in common.

By contrast, after first qualitatively sketching the multidimensional dyslexia portrait by listening to countless dyslexics describe their many and diverse symptoms—while also observing and examining their impairments and later med-triggered improvements, it then became possible to pointedly find and validate its vital dots.

I had always believed that the resulting synergy created by combining my more open-ended macro studies with ensuing highly focused, triple-blind-free validating microinvestigations, especially those using neuroimaging techniques, would more deeply and completely solve the dyslexia/CVS riddles and more rapidly lead to real cures. As you will read below, this process has already begun.

A Clarification: I Did Publish—But I Did It Two Ways

Publishing is important Don't get me wrong. Of course, it was important to have investigated and publish data in controlled studies, which usually examined one or two variables at a time. However, I did it the way I thought best, given my highly unique priorities, circumstances, and time/energy restraints—in both clinically based peer-reviewed and summary research papers as well as in books! In truth, these publications served to better clarify my own concepts rather than to satisfy others. And as you've just read, my clinical method enabled me to self-correct and so avoid the many unwitting errors that those critical of this path are still replicating. As I soon learned, some critics are often insatiable, mistakenly obsessed with their method vs. substance—and likely motivated by group-think bias. And thank God for those helpful critics who enabled me to see and correct my own unwitting errors—and there were many.

Working Alone

The negatives By contrast to highly trained and gifted research teams within the auspices of well-funded and endowed university research centers where scientific productivity is often justifiably measured by publications, I worked alone—with only my patients. That's the way psychiatrists and psychoanalysts were initially trained to clinically function many years ago. No grants or funding, no special research training or full-time research positions, no essential multidisciplinary teams or assistants, no statisticians, no advanced instruments, no independent consultations—except those personally paid for, no need to publish, no writers and editors to help, no tenure, no consensus—but also no/less group-think.

Not the best way to conduct research. But my 100 percent over-focused desire to neuroanalyze and successfully treat patients, as well as my time-saving clinical loner habit reinforced by preference and need, led me to continue in this rather unsophisticated manner.

My overload "So why did you feel so pressured for time?" I hear readers thinking. And the simple answer: Because I was overloaded, and refused to admit it. Yes, denial!

Thus, I needed to initially avoid any and all additional overloading "distractions," including those crucial positive ones just mentioned that most researchers depend upon. I felt that these "diversions," however invaluable, would derail or slow me and my accelerating and exciting research momentum down. This was especially so since I was clinically investigating multiple, rapidly appearing interrelated research leads and hundreds of novel insights popping up at the very same time among hundreds of dyslexics—most triggered by my highly productive symptom-illuminating therapeutic tool. And I needed time and energy to also design and use varied diagnostic and therapeutic instruments to measure, explain, and validate my insights as I progressed.[3]

I also maintained a voluntary academic position at NYU Medical Center, and large full-time psychiatric and dyslexia practices—the latter needed to fulfill my MD needs as well as to provide new clinical insights.

And I almost forgot to mention: my research and writing/publications were akin to hobbies. So I squeezed them in before, in-between, and after 12-plus hour therapeutic workdays, and weekends. Yes, I also worked many evenings and Saturdays to accommodate patients, as did my Hippocrates, Dr. Rose. Thus, I was belatedly, but reluctantly, forced to terminate my cherished psychiatric hospital and office practices to avoid burning out. There didn't seem to be a moment to spare.

Too many insights By contrast to all other dyslexia researchers fortunate enough to have one or two novel insights to pursue and formally publish in a timely and peer-acceptable manner with the help of funding, teams, etc., I had thousands of dots—but no time, funding, research associates, etc.

So How Did I Really Do It All?

A helpful partner Although I seemingly worked alone without colleagues, I had invaluable, albeit unseen, helpful partners. My wife Diggy made all my accomplishments possible. She was the whole football team and organization, allowing me to be the workaholic "healing physician and research quarterback." But Diggy is another miracle and book—the unseen force and "wind beneath my wings!" My super-enabler and emotional anchor! Clearly, I could never have succeeded alone or even come close without her. Indeed, this was a total family effort where all willingly and lovingly sacrificed to fulfill a destiny aimed at providing hope and help to suffering millions.

A preference for qualitative research All in all, I remained unwilling to change my own clinical research directions and speed. And I easily resisted changing my preference for publishing medical books and papers based on qualitative anecdotal content offered by patients vs. statistically based double-blind controlled quantitative studies, at least until after I solved the many, many remaining scientific issues in hand.

Why this preference, you may be wondering, considering my math background? Because it likely takes several costly and time-consuming years, often requiring a team effort, to adequately complete a study dealing with one or a few variables and publish it in a peer-reviewed journal—even longer if initially rejected; and where statistics as well as control groups, rather than patients' verbalized content, are most often required.

[3] http://dyslexiaonline.com/media/patents.html/

By contrast, in that time period, I was often able to discover and publish hundreds of new dots/insights alone and integrate them all into fascinating concepts within a book like this where I had time and words as well as the clinical patient-based content needed to easily and naturally explain my discoveries as I best thought. And besides, given my circumstances and ongoing attempt to clarify dyslexia's final image and exact CVS and related mechanisms, I did not have the time, team, or funding to find and objectively verify, via extensive testing, both normal and non-dyslexic controls.

So being overloaded with new, important, and escalating insights as well as feeling an urgent need to share this life-improving, qualitatively derived information with both professionals and suffering patients, my choice was a mathematical no-brainer. This was especially so since others with a more quantitative bent could better complete the required independent validation of my CVS insights and portrait after shown to them in full clinical/scientific daylight—triple-blind free.

Although justifiably challenged for not conducting controlled double-blind studies, especially for meds, my answer was as simple as my research method: Since I've provided the clinical groundwork for these objective studies to be viably and accurately conducted by those best trained to perform them, I challenge my challengers to personally conduct the studies they deem needed! After all, this is my hobby. And research is their full-time paid job.

Justification So if the end justifies my means, then my choice was proven correct—having only one determined and stubborn master guiding me from within. And a helpful, stabilizing and encouraging angel I lived with who also managed my office and tested patients when our kids were in school. And who also willingly typed and continually retyped all of my initial manuscripts the old fashioned, hard, time-consuming and frustrating way. But only after her day of super-mothering was over, and our two lovely girls were fast and comfortably asleep. And via identification with their parent's ideals, they became wonderful women, wives, mothers and healers. Thus, my Dr. Rose inspired destiny will continue.

A Prediction

Based on my neuroanalytic method's amazing unmasking success, I can once again assuredly predict that all readers will learn vastly more about the 4-D portrait characterizing the dyslexia/CVS syndrome from listening to my many patients than reading all relevant published individual studies to date, my own included.[4]

[4] My qualitative neuroanalytic listening and eyes-open method, illuminating very large and key CVS-determined symptomatic dots, led to a clear scattergram or 4-D dyslexia portrait. So to attain objectivity, all that was needed was to independently validate these illuminated crucial symptomatic dots and determining mechanisms via double-blind studies.

By contrast, most quantitative double-blind dyslexia studies are primarily focused on statistically validating single variables of a complex unseen puzzle mistakenly believed to be derived

Thus, I will now present many more patients in the chapters that follow. They will naturally and convincingly provide you with all the vital clinically obtained "dots" needed to better see, and discover for yourselves, the previously hidden face and many profiles of this one multidimensional and dynamically changing impairment called the dyslexia/CVS syndrome, just the way I did. And how best to treat it.

Validating neuroimaging studies Thankfully, a new generation of researchers and neuroscientists (e.g., Alan and Henrietta Leiner, Robert Dow, and outstanding others), utilizing highly sophisticated neuroimaging and related techniques, have made significant super-scientific advances in the past few decades. They have belatedly explored and independently validated many of my clinically determined "highly original and challenging" dyslexia and cerebellar concepts and solutions—to the benefit of suffering dyslexics (refer to References-A—Independent Validation—Typical of Thousands).

Accordingly, I will specifically highlight and review this amazing content in the following chapters, while also providing all the information about dyslexia that you were originally seeking, and much, much more than you ever anticipated.

---

from incorrect alexia-like or related images. So the resulting scattergram of seemingly infinite dots, if formed, will never correlate with its theoretical concept/image—since the latter is a false illusion or fantasy (refer to Chaps. 8 and 9 for further clarification). This triple-blind fantasy was independently rejected by the APA and DSM-V, thus, belatedly validating my clinically based concepts and definition.

Thus, most of the collective double-blind results so far obtained illuminate nothing tangible about dyslexia's image since they are significantly based on unwittingly mistaken premises/beliefs/definitions. Hence, my tongue-in-cheek term for most double-blind dyslexia studies is "triple-blind."

Chapter 6
Kathy: The Intriguing Complexity of Dyslexia

One Invaluable Portrait Is Worth Countless Studies

Of the thousands of patients' self-descriptions I have encountered, few illustrate the intriguing complexity and multidimensionality of the dyslexia or CVS syndrome with the breadth, depth, and detail of Kathy's. Her astonishing words will vividly demonstrate to you:

- That reading difficulties are often only a small part of the total dyslexia syndrome
- That reading scores are all but irrelevant to the understanding and diagnosis of this complex syndrome
- That major personal—cerebral—compensatory determination is often needed to survive and navigate this disorder, especially when medically untreated
- That dyslexia is truly a medical impairment at its core—and that the term "learning disability" does not even come close to explaining this disorder's overall medical/psychological scope and depth and how it affects most aspects of a person's life, especially impairing self-esteem
- That the disorder called dyslexia does not completely disappear with age, even though many of the surface manifestations (e.g., reading scores) may change or improve
- That the brain damage or developmental lag reading processor theories of dyslexia and their theorists—especially those attempting to explain only the severe reading score impairments—are unwittingly perpetrating a vast oversimplification of the complex disorder they attempt to define

H. N. Levinson, *Feeling Smarter and Smarter*,
https://doi.org/10.1007/978-3-030-16208-5_6

- That the vast majority of dyslexics—even gifted athletes[1]—manifest clear and obvious balance/coordination/rhythmic impairments as well as related symptoms triggering motion sickness and direction/spatial orientation difficulties
- That adults with dyslexia, like Kathy, have a retrospective insight that children have not yet gained and are better able to express their symptoms and feelings with greater understanding, depth, clarity, and even humor

Kathy

Kathy is a 40-year-old healthcare professional who has battled the dyslexia syndrome her entire life. Had experts previously listened to similar dyslexics—rather than "testing them to death"—they might well have solved all the riddles posed by this syndrome before Kathy was even born.

As you read on, notice the categories Kathy uses to label her symptoms. Although these follow the general ones that I provided for her and all new patients, and that serve as the basis of the Self-Diagnostic Test you'll see next in Chap. 7, it is noteworthy that Kathy *began* her report with *balance and coordination rather than reading, writing,* etc. Based on my psychoanalytic experience, I believe this choice was no accident. She intuitively and experientially recognized what you too will soon more clearly see: that the balance and coordination center of the brain—or inner-ear/cerebellar-vestibular system (CVS)—is primarily responsible for all of the many and varied symptoms characterizing the dyslexia syndrome— and specifically, *her* dyslexia syndrome.

Kathy's Amazing Description of Her Dyslexia-Related Symptoms and Experiences

Her self-self-description follows, albeit somewhat abridged:

> ***Balance and Coordination***— *have always been "different," even as a baby. Mom says she could just set me in the middle of a room with toys within arm's length and I'd stay there. My four sisters all crawled everywhere at that same stage.*
>
> *I did finally crawl, then walk and run, but coordination was still a problem. Hated the swing's back-and-forth, up-and-down movement but loved to twist the chain so it could twirl me.*[2]

---

[1]As previously mentioned, even Bruce (now Caitlyn) Jenner, an Olympic gold medalist in the decathlon, likely had severe eye coordination difficulties when he read, and severe fine-motor coordination difficulties when he wrote. He might even have had impaired speech coordination—which he obviously did not. However, none of these inner-ear/cerebellar-determined impairments affected his amazing athletic performance. Nor were they tested in the Olympics.

[2]Twirling triggers motion sickness in many with inner-ear dysfunctioning. However, gifted clinicians have discovered that some patients with inner-ear impairments are actually motion-*seeking* and, thus, love to twirl. Indeed, these two opposites—motion sensitivity and insensitivity—are both considered diagnostic inner-ear signs. Such paradoxes prove over and over again how circuit-specific and complex this inner-ear disorder really is. Black-and-white, binary concepts are too simplistic to describe humanity's complexity.

Throwing and catching, and even following the movement of the ball between other children, were challenges.

I hated kindergarten. I couldn't tie my shoes, put on my own coat, manage zippers or buttons, comb my hair, or even begin to manage over-the-shoe boots. Scissors were a puzzle, as was staying within the lines and then writing.

Every day seemed to bring new injuries. Mom says my legs looked mostly like rotten potatoes. I couldn't judge curbs or steps and fell up a lot. I'd sprain my ankle on the single step into my house. I walked through a glass door with no knowledge that it was there. I kept trying to ride a bike, constantly filling my knees with the gravel of the neighborhood driveways.

My parents had my eyesight checked—better than normal.

Nothing helped my coordination, including the exercises I did for my scoliosis. I nearly drowned, lost as to which way was up after diving. In dance class I kept moving in the wrong direction. I was the mirror image of what was supposed to happen, and couldn't get the tap patterns up to speed.

Direction/Space—*My sense of direction and comprehension of where I am in space is compromised. I lack depth perception. I can close my eyes and just float without reference. I usually forget which way is right or left. But worse than that, I can lose up and down. Example: When painting the eaves of a roof, I grabbed it for fear of falling—falling up, into the clear blue sky just beyond the edge of my paint job.*

I still have trouble with clocks and was probably in sixth grade before I was brave enough to tell someone the time. Both directions, clockwise and counterclockwise, and the sizes of the clock hands, cause me trouble. I keep forgetting which is which.

I never did master skating. By eleven, I was fairly adept at bike riding with a refresher period each spring.

For college, I had to learn to drive. At first I would turn the car in the wrong direction. So the instructor put a glove on one hand and called out directions as "glove" or "hand." I had great difficulty using the side and rear-view mirrors. The first time I saw a semi-truck in the rear-view, I jammed on the brakes. I was ready for a head-on collision.

I sometimes read in the wrong direction—from right to left—and can't find my mistake, as in misreading "step on" rather than "no pets." I also sometimes drive in the wrong direction.

Size is hard for me to estimate. I can't take shorthand because the same symbol means different things according to its size. Measurements mean little to me.

Phobias and Related Moods—*As a child, I was afraid of the dark and was very imaginative about what lurked in it—ghosts, escaped zoo animals, the alligators that lived under the bed, or the lion that lived in my parents' room (my dad snored).*

I was afraid of school because so little went well there at first. It was one giant frustration. I was even afraid of my kindergarten teacher, the one the other kids hugged good-bye. I begged and cried to stay home with my sisters.

I was afraid of both stairs and escalators because I fell on them. I was carsick on drives through the rolling hills of Pennsylvania, and on far lesser excursions.

I used to fear getting lost… because I do get lost—on foot, on bicycle, on mass transit, and in traffic. I still get lost inside buildings, on and between floors.

I am still afraid of diving into a pool head first, even though I love the water.

I am uncomfortable in new places. It is sometimes overwhelming to deal with where I am in space. I need time to become oriented.

I used to be afraid of public speaking. However, as a volunteer docent at the Museum of Natural History, I am getting over this fear.

One thing I am not afraid of is asking questions. If I hadn't asked plenty of them up to this point, I would not be able to effectively deal with the world. So many people are willing to be of help, if only you ask.

Moods and Anxiety— *When I'd had a hard day at school, I'd come home "with my head dragging and a scowl on my face." I have experienced panic attacks and may exhibit some aspects of post-traumatic stress disorder.*

Self-Esteem— *As a kid, I felt I was both smart and stupid at the same time—smart because I seemed to know more than my peers, stupid because I got lost in the numbers, the letters, and the timing and spacing of things.*

Psychosomatic— *As a child, I had motion sickness in cars and boats. Reading would trigger headaches. My biggest complaint was the glare of the sun on the printed page. I was always squinting. And sometimes my light-sensitivity would upset my stomach. As a result, I was a shade-seeker and often wore sunglasses, even indoors.*

Concentration and Activity—*When fatigued I can't eliminate the distractions. And everything is a distraction to me in one way or another: the movements in my peripheral vision, the monotone sounds of fans, ventilation systems kicking on and off, other conversations, appliances, traffic sounds, temperature changes, bodily needs, and, if I'm quiet enough, my own breathing and heartbeat.*

Speech—*I tend to misarticulate words. Sometimes, pleased by the rearrangements, I use them purposely. I prefer flutterby to butterfly. I named our dog Aminal. Sometimes words just won't stop as I'd like, such as banana-nanananana or Christmas-mas-mas-mas.*

In conversations, I find myself checking with a speaker to make sure that I understand their meaning. And I can't recall their original wording. I also have difficulty memorizing dialogue or poetry, and I have difficulty recalling names, even minutes after our introduction.

Spelling, Math, Memory, and Grammar— *It took me all of kindergarten to learn to count from 1 to 100. Thousands of repetitions were needed. It was all verbal. I couldn't make sense of the written format that I viewed.*

The months of the year and the alphabet were learned by singsong rote. I still sing the song in my head when finding or filing information alphabetically.

Spelling was a childhood nightmare. I still don't spell well and so find it hard to look up information.

As far as grammar goes, I was queen of the run-on sentence, or simply run-on phrases. These days I still struggle with the rules of punctuation.

Math is a subject near and dear to my heart. It allowed me to study the sciences, which brought me to my career in physical therapy.

As a young child I did not do well with the numerical calculations of addition, subtraction, multiplication, and division. And I still have to be careful in paying bills and making change. The invention of calculators and computers simplified those numerical calculations which I never conquered.

What a shock it was when we came to algebra, and suddenly I was doing well in math class. I understood the concepts of mathematics and continued on through calculus and statistics.

Memorizing was an almost impossible task. In school plays I was not always faithful to the exact words of the author, but the meaning was there. I could not remember music for my piano recitals. Besides the times tables, I still do not recall the state capitols, most historic dates.... Somehow I manage.

Writing—*I first wrote my name in kindergarten. It looked fine to me, but it was only readable to others in a mirror. Eventually I got the print turned around. My script was huge, though. I couldn't sign a birthday card without a ruler and making lines.*

When they introduced handwriting, everything fell apart. An "in" was a line with two bumps, but the written version had three bumps. Capital letters had extraneous loops and some looked quite different from the printed version. (Refer to Kathy's more specific difficulties in Chap. 10. pp. 88–89.)

*I had great difficulty keeping letters on a proper slant, adjusting size, and remembering which appendages went above or below the line. I made mistakes as to whether loops should be open or closed. I usually missed crossing **t's** and dotting **i's**. I was in sixth grade and still practicing handwriting after school. My right third finger bent as a result of all that drilling.*

***Reading—** My problem was keeping numbers or letters separate—the spaces between them disappeared. It was a spatial orientation nightmare.*

At first I tended to read in the wrong direction and wrote that way too. I couldn't keep letters in order either. There was no discernible difference between: 90, 60, do, and go; wow, mom, and 303; B and 13; spot, tops, pots, and stop.

My first writing was mirror writing. In time I just reversed or inverted some of the letters and learned to write from left to right and read that way too. Phonic classes added a layer of confusion around verbal cues: f and v; hard g and k; soft g and j; w and r; t and d; p and b.

Meanwhile, as a first grader, the nuns wanted me to catch the bus myself. I couldn't deal with the number identifications and kept taking the wrong bus.

Then they introduced the concept of spacing to separate words and sentences. I could not seem to find the spaces they wanted me to see, nor distinguish similar letter shapes. Mathematics went from horizontal to vertical. For a while we folded the paper to help us keep the columns. When that ended, I was working with zigzag columns and not happy with the results.

My days followed the pattern: phonics, reading, and math in school, and then endless repetition at home. I did finally sort out the numbers for math and the letters for reading. However, I was not a fan of Roman numerals and even less so on a clock face.

I did my best to sound out words, with a finger under each sound, until I succeeded. When a whole line appeared, I worked on knowing where a word stopped so I could sound it out. Things worsened when the print came in multiple lines. The letters seemed to blink off and on and wiggled on the page. When I looked at a word, it glowed and the surrounding letters seemed to swirl down a drain. I kept my finger under the word as if I were gluing it to the page. I ran my ruler under the line to keep from adding words from above or below. I read out loud to compensate.

I was in the middle of second grade when I could finally read. The teacher gave me a reader and all summer long I happily read those stories over and over again to my sisters—but out loud. The following year they wanted me to learn to read silently. First I went to whispering, then just moving my lips, and finally to hearing the words in my head. I still use these three methods, and when given the option will read out loud. As a result, I have never finished a timed test. However, I never miss a single word of an author's thoughts. And I am still a lover of books despite all my difficulties.

I needed frequent breaks while reading. As I tired, I often couldn't find the beginning of the next line of print and would reread a line. The word-movement on the page worsened and I'd get a headache. The letters shifted from their dominant black shapes and merged with the white background. By college this fatigue factor could leave me word blind.

Since third grade I have been in choir and playing the piano. The difficulties are the same, but even worse. Changing key signatures and reading more than one line at a time makes reading music complicated. I am still unable to memorize my piano music.

When the time came for me to read to my own sweet children, my finger followed each sound and word. By three and four they had learned to read on their own.

Summary: Dyslexia—A Complex and Functionally Pervasive Disorder

After reading Kathy's self-description, I feel certain that you must be as amazed by her remarkable dyslexia insights as I initially was—and still am. Chances are great that you have never read anything as informative as this, regardless of your professional background and expertise, despite it being abridged. Nor is it likely that another Kathy-like CVS/dyslexia description will soon appear, especially since it took me 50 years to find her.

And I'm more certain than ever that all readers will now better understand dyslexia and its complex CVS syndrome than they would have by reading all of the uncanny results obtained by neuroimaging (refer to the book's section titled, *Independently Validating References*). I also believe you will now be better able to independently judge the astounding merits of my "simple" Q&A clinical research method.

Upon digesting Kathy's amazing portrait of dyslexia as well as neuroanalyzing the mechanisms triggering her symptoms—many of which she clearly reveals herself—you will have arrived at an understanding of this complex disorder more than sufficient to independently critique and compare the traditionalist and neotraditionalist theories vs. my own CVS concepts. Therefore, all of these theories will be presented in Chaps. 8, 9, and 10 so that you can evaluate for yourselves their encompassing and explanatory capabilities. But to do so most effectively, it became important to first review the complete list of symptoms I was able to assemble after listening to, successfully treating, and neuroanalyzing thousands of dyslexics like Kathy. And as chance—really design— would have it, this list became an invaluable diagnostic/screening test for those suspected of having the dyslexia or CVS syndromes.

Chapter 7
The Self-Diagnostic Test: Evaluating Patients and Theories

Evaluating patients After recording and analyzing the symptomatic characteristics and favorable CVS-triggered med responses of over 35,000 CVS-dysfunctioning, Kathy-like dyslexics, I arrived at a detailed outline of the functions and symptoms characterizing the dyslexia syndrome. As a result, this amazing outline now serves as (1) the best holistic, scientifically derived 4-D portrait of the CVS/dyslexia syndrome available today and (2) the best and only comprehensive screening test for those suspected of manifesting this complex CVS syndrome.[1]

Evaluating dyslexia theories So why have I included this detailed sketch of the dyslexia syndrome here—rather than in a later diagnostic section where it truly belongs? *Because this sketch also serves as a unique means of testing the efficacy and value of the various dyslexia theories.*

Thus, I will soon demonstrate in several crucial follow-up chapters that only my CVS theory of the dyslexia syndrome is capable of both explaining and encompassing all of the many and diverse impaired functions and symptoms characterizing Kathy and all other examined dyslexics.

How is that possible, you may wonder? Elementary—since the CVS concept of dyslexia is the only theory conceived and continually expanded so as to fully explain and encompass all of the many reading and non-reading functions, symptoms and mechanisms found characterizing over 35,000 CVS-dysfunctioning dyslexics responding favorably to CVS enhancing meds—and so also resulting in the content within the Self-Diagnostic Test!

By contrast, you will soon learn in the very next chapter that all older and newer dyslexia theories, based on the *dyslexia = alexia = severe reading-score impairment*, explain and encompass little to nothing about Kathy and most other dyslexics

[1] Recall how Kathy used the test's outline and symptoms to illuminate her own CVS/dyslexia syndrome and how some of Kathy's symptoms were then used to further update the Self-Diagnostic Test—to be shortly discussed. This reciprocity was, and is, used for all patients—resulting in the best diagnostic questionnaire possible.

H. N. Levinson, *Feeling Smarter and Smarter*,
https://doi.org/10.1007/978-3-030-16208-5_7

as well as little to nothing about the functions and symptoms within the following test. And the reason is simple: *most other theories are unwittingly geared to explain only alexia—not dyslexia.*

The Self-Diagnostic Test

Sir William Osler, a great clinician, brilliantly stated over a hundred years ago: *History is 90 percent of diagnosis*—that is if you're not given the exact questions to ask beforehand. However, if you know *exactly* what questions to ask—by using the following highly reliable self-diagnostic test—your accuracy will approach 100 percent. That's because this test is derived from, and so based on, the presence of the vital symptoms and functions defining the dyslexia or inner-ear/CVS syndrome in thousands of favorably responding patients.

If many, or even a diagnostically important few, of the following symptoms coexist in an individual believed to have learning, concentration, phobic, or related issues, then the presence of an underlying CVS or dyslexia syndrome is strongly suspected.

1. Reading

- Poor memory for letters, words, sentences, or numbers
- A tendency to skip over letters or words or mix up the order or sequence of letters, words, and sentences (e.g., reading g-o-d and seeing d-o-g, abc = acb, the cat = that)
- A poor, slow, and/or fatiguing reading ability that is accompanied by head tilting, near or far focusing, and/or reading with fingers or a marker so that the poorly tracking eyes can find the correct spot on the page
- Reversals of letters such as b and d, words such as saw and was, and numbers such as 6 and 9 or 16 and 61, reading backward easier than forward
- Word blurring, word and/or letter movement, double images, and flickering, as well as changing letter and word sizes—micropsia or macropsia
- Headaches, dizziness, stomach aches, or nausea brought on by reading
- Light sensitivity (photophobia) that often makes sunglasses helpful even for indoor reading or when shopping in crowded stores or while watching TV (also rapid visual overloading, especially in response to fluorescent or flickering lights)
- Phonic/phonological disturbances (e.g., difficulty recalling the sounds of letters as well as integrating letter sounds into words), "phonetic blurring," and scrambling, as well as disjointed timing of visuals and corresponding phonemes

- Tunnel vision or visual decomposition of words into letter fragments, requiring conscious recomposition of letters into words so as to be able to read
- Reversal or oscillation of foreground and background visuals and sounds
- Condensation or squishing together of letter and word sequences and phonemes
- Delayed and distorted visual processing of read content, lasting seconds or longer

2. Writing

- Messy, poorly directed, or drifting handwriting, involving size, spacing, letter-sequencing errors, including reversals and writing backward

3–6. Spelling, Math, Memory, and Grammar

- Impaired memory for spelling, grammar, math, names, dates, and lists; and for sequences such as the alphabet, the days of the week, and months of the year; and for following directions

7. Speech

- Speech delays and disorders such as slurring, stuttering, minor articulation errors, and poor word recall
- Delayed and distorted recognition/processing of spoken words and sentences. When the sounds are scrambled and so poorly heard, this results in misperceptions by the ear and a compensatory need for frequent repetition. Often a person might say "What?" and then belatedly know what was said before repetition occurs. They need extra time to process the "blurred" sounds.
- Delayed expression of thoughts resulting in slow enunciation and a tendency to experience word scrambling or sequencing errors and slips of the tongue

8. Direction

- Right/left and related directional uncertainty, such as difficulty knowing or remembering east or west and north or south
- Poor sense of direction, which leads to frequently getting lost and the consequent fear of traveling alone to new or even familiar places

9. Time

- Childhood delay in learning to tell time, as well as a host of time-related symptoms, including lateness, compulsive or rigid scheduling, and even procrastination or difficulty starting things on time
- Difficulty with minute and hour hands on clock dials
- Poor understanding of before and after

10–11. Concentration and Activity

- Impaired concentration, distractibility, hyperactivity, or restlessness
- Temper or impulse disturbances such as fighting, stealing, lying, biting, cursing, etc.
- Oppositional tendencies beyond the "normal" range

12. Balance, Coordination, Rhythm, Timing, and Reflexes

- Difficulties with balance and coordination functions, such as walking, running, skipping, hopping, tying shoelaces, and buttoning buttons
- Difficulty in learning karate, gymnastics, etc., due to impaired balance, coordination, timing, and concentration
- Poor eye-hand coordination when catching, throwing, and batting a ball
- Poor eye-foot coordination when kicking a ball
- Poor or delayed reflexes involving swallowing, blowing one's nose, sucking through a straw, etc.—even with rhythmic breathing
- Retention of primitive reflexes that should have disappeared with development—for example, awkward grasp of pencil/eating utensil
- Accident proneness: falling, tripping, bumping, dropping, etc.
- Difficulty walking a straight line, thus bumping into adjacent pedestrians
- Delays in bladder and bowel training as well as frequent "accidents" later on

13. Psychosomatics

- Headaches, dizziness, nausea, abdominal complaints, and motion sickness
- Cyclic vomiting syndrome[2]

---

[2] Perhaps this insight will be as interesting to you as it was important to a very young child with ASD whom I treated. Shortly after birth, he continued to have repeated multiple daily bouts of vomiting—defying all remedial efforts, although diagnosed as cyclic vomiting syndrome (CVS). Amazingly, he rapidly responded to a simple inner-ear enhancer. And although referred to as CVS (cyclic vomiting syndrome), no one to date has recognized its CVS (cerebellar-vestibular system) origin!

- Excessive sweating, cold hands and feet, eating disorders, and possible potency disorders in adults
- Fine motor tremor of the fingers and hands

14. Phobias and Related Mood, Social, and Obsessive/ Compulsive Disorders

- Fears of the dark, heights, bridges, tunnels, crowds, getting lost, and going to school (sometimes resulting in truancy and dropout)
- Fear or avoidance of various balance, coordination, and motion-related activities and sports
- Mood disturbances such as depression, irritability, and even excessive elation mimicking bipolar disorder
- Minor/intermittent anxiety-intensified or-caused difficulty reading one's own feelings and those of others, not as severe or persisting as in Asperger's syndrome, which is now included as part of autistic spectrum disorder or ASD
- Obsessions and compulsions such as repetitive, inescapable thoughts and actions (e.g., preoccupation with germs, excessive hand-washing, rechecking, eating binges [bulimia], and avoidance of eating [anorexia])

15. Self-Esteem and Body Image

- Feeling dumb, "retarded," and brainless—bad
- Feeling ugly—too short, too thin, too fat, etc.
- Feeling klutzy, deformed, etc.

16. Pseudo-autistic Social Delays and Shyness

- Social awkwardness due to sensor-motor and related speech delays and/or insecurity
- Restricted facial and body expressions stemming from motor issues, "klutziness," and/or anxiety
- Poor eye contact in order to avoid sensory overloading (not for ASD avoidance)
- Minimal speech communications due to delayed input/output speech processing

---

I similarly helped a middle-aged woman with dyslexia who experienced chronic nausea and regurgitation (a likely variant of CVS) which eroded her front teeth. Despite extensive GI testing, nothing specific was found. Additional case material is needed before a CVS dysfunction is deemed responsible for all such cases, or just a subsection.

17. Cognition and Thinking

- Slow cognitive or thinking speeds—in otherwise normal or high IQ individuals
- Impaired/delayed sequencing of words, thoughts, and their expression
- Fuzzy or cloudy—blurred—mentation

18. Atypical Sensory Reception and Processing

- Difficulty with gravitational up/down signals
- Difficulty with electromagnetic directional, orientation signals
- Difficulty with full moon signals and related anxiety, depressive, and behavioral seasonal affective disorder (SAD) symptoms
- Difficulty with altitude and barometric signals
- Sensory visual and auditory illusions and/or pseudo-hallucinations (e.g., hearing voices), including hearing the words while reading them

Summary

All of the above-listed symptoms were found to characterize and/or coexist in individuals with CVS dysfunctioning, although the SAD symptoms in the eighteenth category require additional validation since they are likely multi-determined.[3] Importantly, all of these symptoms often improved when CVS-impaired individuals were treated with inner-ear/CVS-enhancing medications. Moreover, upon neuroanalysis, all of the above symptoms had CVS-mechanisms, although other major co-determinants were sometimes present and even dominant.[4]

Because the CVS diagnostic screening power of these varied symptoms may vary from almost 100 percent certain to non-specific, the greater the number of symptoms revealed per patient, the more statistically reliable the CVS screening diagnosis is. Even more important, the better each symptom is qualitatively evaluated as to its causation and even overdetermination, the greater its diagnostic certainty. Needless to emphasize, only medical testing such as that described in Chap. 19 will provide a certain diagnosis.

[3] For those who may not know, I've had two patients with SAD who become depressed in Spring/Summer. And the literature suggests that 20 percent do.

[4] By alleviating primary CVS determinants with the CVS enhancers, there may also result secondary improvements in stress and so also in non-CVS-based symptoms. Thus, symptomatic improvements alone do not justify the conviction that there preexisted a primary or major CVS origin—unless also confirmed by neuroanalysis and neurological testing.

Independent Diagnostic Validation

Many years after deriving the above list, I stumbled upon the website for the *Vestibular Disorders Association* (*VEDA*). And to my amazement, the list of impaired functions and symptoms gathered from thousands of patients complaining primarily of dizziness, disorientation, and imbalance—and exhibiting vestibular dysfunction on testing—was similar to those dysfunctional categories and symptoms listed within the Self-Diagnostic Test. Upon reviewing the VEDA's list (http://vestibular.org/understanding-vestibular-disorder/symptoms), you will likely be as amazed as I was. Thus, you might view the VEDA list as *an independent and unbiased corroboration of my CVS-dyslexia-related findings as well as the clinical methodology I used to illuminate and unmask its content.*

Chapter 8
Kathy and the Mistaken Theories of Dyslexia

The Value of a Theory

Clearly, the value of any theory—dyslexia or otherwise—depends entirely on its encompassing and explanatory powers as well as its ability to lead to new insights and discoveries.

So let's see here just how the traditionalist and neotraditionalist dyslexia concepts might explain—*or not explain*—Kathy's many and diverse reading and non-reading symptoms and determining mechanisms as well as similar characteristics within the Self-Diagnostic Test. Let's also determine whether these theories have led to new scientific insights and breakthroughs, especially involving successful treatments. These determinations are vital toward evaluating their respective efficacies.

And in the next two chapters, I will put my own cerebellar (CVS) theory to the very same value test.

The Traditionalist Views of Kathy and Dyslexia

The Cerebral Reading Processor Damage Theory of Dyslexia

The traditionalists remained irreversibly stuck to a theory that dates back to when dyslexia was recognized by an English clinician in 1896. We've looked at their reasoning already, so I won't describe it again here in detail. The central concept of this initial traditionalist *dyslexia = alexia* reading theory mandates that Kathy *must* have damage to the reading processor in her dominant left thinking brain and so *must* also have a reading comprehension impairment:

- Even if there is no clinical or neurological evidence of damage/impairment in her thinking brain
- Even if she displays intellectual evidence of superior thinking brain functioning

H. N. Levinson, *Feeling Smarter and Smarter*,
https://doi.org/10.1007/978-3-030-16208-5_8

- Even if her superior thinking brain abilities and related determination to succeed enabled her to compensate significantly for her dyslexia syndrome—consisting of both reading and non-reading symptoms
- Even if her reading disorder is not of a primary alexic incomprehension nature
- Even if her reading impairment is characterized by the presence of *only inner-ear/cerebellar-related* symptoms and mechanisms, such as tracking errors, word blurring, word movement, word reversals, light sensitivity, tunnel vision, memory instability, and phonic difficulties (refer to Chap. 16)
- Even if the abovementioned CVS symptoms and related mechanisms are shown to have resulted in her complex dyslexic reading difficulties (refer also to Chap. 17)
- Even if her reading capability eventually soared—further suggesting that her thinking brain's reading processor was compensating, rather than damaged as in alexia
- Even if Kathy and just about all other dyslexics manifest many non-reading symptoms affecting writing, spelling, math, etc., whereas alexics do not
- Even if upon neurological testing Kathy and all other dyslexics show only signs and symptoms absolutely diagnostic of CVS dysfunctioning
- Even if inner-ear-enhancing meds were shown to be helpful—often dramatically so—in improving Kathy's inner-ear-determined symptoms as well as 75–85 percent of those diagnosed with the dyslexia syndrome (refer to Chap. 23), yet are completely ineffective for alexia
- *Even if the traditionalists' brain damage theories can't explain any of Kathy's symptoms/mechanisms—absolutely none—nor her improvements*

In Retrospect

The traditionalists were unwittingly half right about one thing: the importance of the thinking brain in dyslexia. As you've previously read, they just got things substantially reversed. Although the thinking brain does not *primarily* cause the dyslexia syndrome, as I eventually discovered, it does play a vital *secondary* role in compensating for this CVS disorder through its cognitive, descrambling-related, and other neuroplastic capabilities.

The alexia theory explains nothing worthwhile about dyslexia Sadly, the explanatory and predictive powers of the thinking brain damage reading processor theory of dyslexia for Kathy, and all other known dyslexics summarized within the Self-Diagnostic Test, are virtually zero. And yet this theory has survived for over a century—with virtually no criticism other than mine.

So why did/does it persist? Some of the reasons for this theory's survival are probably obvious to you by now. But let me toss out just a few. If no one really knows what dyslexia is all about, any simplistic or easily understandable theory will do, especially if supported by bright, distinguished, and persuasive professionals from leading medical centers. Also, why change a theory that has never been challenged on its own merits and shortcomings or that has never been contrasted with an infinitely more powerful explanatory hypothesis? Until now!

In further attempting to explain the persistence of this fallacious cerebral reading processor theory—as well as its later modifications—I was led to also reason that most dyslexia professionals simply did not spend enough quality time listening to a sufficient number of dyslexics like Kathy. And the gifted clinicians who did appeared unable to cast aside their repeatedly reinforced and thus biased alexia-related views, and so were not psychologically and cognitively free to listen and think independently—objectively.

Take it from a past "believer," the task of switching from a traditionalist *dyslexia = alexia* "expert" to a paradigm challenger is harder than it seems, primarily because of two interrelated reasons: (1) The established "dyslexia monopoly" resists independently minded *scientific entrepreneurs*. Why? Because on a basic psychological level, challengers represent a threat to both the entrenched majority order and groupthink. (2) On a deeper biological level, nature attempts to maintain homeostasis and the status quo—resisting change and changers from both within and without. So it's two strikes and challengers are almost out. And most certainly, they are significantly delayed in implementing new and exciting insights—even life-changing ones, exceptions aside.

The Cerebral Developmental Reading Processor Lag Theory of Dyslexia and Kathy

Although there were no significant challenges to the traditionalists from within their midsts, there was one minor theory modifier worthy of once again mentioning,[1] despite having previously discussed his irresistible concept way back in Chap. 1.

In an attempt to explain the complete absence of *any* of the expected neurological signs diagnostic of a cerebral impairment in dyslexia, as well as the favorable reading outcomes—even "reading cures"—that many dyslexics achieved, a well-recognized and accepted neurological traditionalist, MacDonald Critchley, came up with a slightly more explanatory variation of the thinking brain damage reading processor theory. He suggested in 1969 that dyslexia was due to a *developmental lag within the cerebral reading processor localized within the dominant left brain*,

[1] Although there have been some who recognized the limitations of the *dyslexia = alexia* brain damage theory of dyslexia, and a few have offered diverse versions—including Orton's 1920 impaired dominance concept—no one else has proposed a concept that completely refutes all hypotheses that rely on the above *dyslexia = alexia = "dyslexia"* concept, even when partially modified. And for the sake of keeping a valid discussion simple, I have used my analysis of Critchley's theory's positives and negatives to highlight the dynamics applying to just about all other theorists and their resulting concepts.

as opposed to *damage*. Although this modification was a step in the right direction, it was still very much alexia-tinged. Critchley still believed that: *dyslexia = a cerebral alexia-like reading comprehension disorder or "dyslexia."*

Another strikeout Accordingly, even his updated theory still left the overwhelming majority of Kathy's symptoms and those within the Self-Diagnostic Test—as well as those characterizing the vast majority of Critchley's own dyslexic patients—completely unexplained. In retrospect, the reason for this glaring explanatory failure seems obvious: he remained unable to even entertain the notion that the thinking brain might *not* be the primary *cause* of dyslexia—and so likely overlooked the fact that it may, instead, be its major *compensator*. However, Kathy's cerebral compensating function—involving a conscious determination to succeed and the use of effective decoding methods illustrated in greater detail within the next chapter—is clearly the way many other dyslexics explained their improvements had the professionals simply listened to them.

Sadly, despite his vast clinical experience, Critchley could not escape his traditionalist roots—and alexic theoretical cage—although he did peek out. For reasons now likely obvious to you, he never could also contemplate how his *cerebral lag reading processing theory* might possibly explain—or fail to explain—all the *diverse non-alexia reading and non-reading Kathy-described dyslexic symptoms* he observed in his patients and magnificently presented in his exceptionally written book, *The Dyslexic Child*. Nor did this distinguished neurological clinician recognize the diagnostic significance of the CVS imbalance and discoordination signs that his, and all other Kathy-like, dyslexics invariably manifested or that a possible *CVS developmental lag* might be crucial—not necessarily the cerebral lag he proposed. Only denial could explain Critchley's apparent oversights.

In many ways, denial appears as powerful as Superman and so has disarmed a century-plus of outstanding, dedicated, and brilliant traditionalist super-scientists and super-clinicians.

Thus, Critchley *totally* believed that dyslexia is just a reading comprehension disorder of cerebral origin akin to alexia—as did all of his colleagues. And so if he also wanted to account for *all* the non-reading symptoms he described characterizing dyslexics, he would have had to postulate an absurdity: that bright, gifted, and self-compensating dyslexics like Kathy had *numerous*, non-dyslexia-related sites of persisting developmental delays throughout their brains—one site per one or a few of many symptoms.

And this absurd alternative hypothesis just wouldn't have made sense to him. So he never even entertained it. Had he not sidestepped this consideration, Critchley would have been forced to completely abandon the original irresistible *dyslexia = alexia* cerebral damage theory as well as his improved cerebral developmental delay one—just as I was eventually forced to do. And so he really, really couldn't go there! Thus, he unwittingly settled for a theoretically inadequate status quo instead of contemplating a dramatically different but highly successful alternative CVS-related hypothesis such as that fully described within the next chapter.

One can only wonder if Critchley would have discarded or modified his theory suggesting a developmental lag within the left dominant brain's reading processor had he known about and/or observed the rapidly favorable reading and non-reading improvements of CVS-dysfunctioning dyslexics to inner-ear-enhancing meds as presented here and in my many publications since 1973?

Clearly, these meds can't reverse a primary cerebral brain lag—let alone brain damage! Nor can rotation-triggered and space-induced transient dyslexia create this assumed cerebral processing lag—especially multiple lags! Neither can a vast array of later-acquired inner-ear (infectious, toxic, degenerative, traumatic, etc.) impairments, which may cause or intensify dyslexia—rather its CVS syndrome.

In summary, Critchley's cerebral developmental lag theory—impairment of the reading processor—could generally explain or account for *only two* of Kathy's numerous dyslexic characteristics, and nothing more:

1. Improved reading
2. The absence of cerebral neurological signs

Orton's Cerebral Dominance Theory of Dyslexia

Although I initially intended to head straight for discussing the neotraditionalist theories of dyslexia, I was reminded about Orton's 1920 ingenious concept and so could not skip over it. He hypothesized that dyslexia/strephosymbolia resulted from a failure of the left cerebral brain to functionally dominate the right hemisphere. And that this impairment in left brain dominance led to an inability to connect the visual word forms with their spoken equivalents and also triggered mirror reading and writing.

Why Orton was different Before explaining why Orton was wrong—at least partially—let me first convey that his theory reflected a brilliant *partial attempt to explain* what he believed to be a cerebrally determined alexia-like reading impairment without localizing cerebral neurological signs, while also trying to account for reversals. Interestingly, no other traditionalist concept attempted to explain reversals—because they couldn't.

Therefore, to better integrate and normalize the left brain dominance functioning, Orton reasoned that a multisensory teaching/learning/conditioning approach would be most effective in correcting this "hemispheric conflict." Thus, he advised using kinesthetic (movement-related), tactile, as well as visual and auditory reading strategies. This significantly effective multisensory reading method was later solidified by Anna Gillingham and became well known by their combined names. However, in my opinion, its efficacy resulted from enhancing CVS mechanisms—not improving hemispheric dominance.

Orton's mistaken assumptions Now to explain why I believe the basis of Orton's theory was incorrect. Since the left thinking brain or cerebral cortex also normally controls speech/language and right handedness, the apparent increased frequency of speech issues as well as left and mixed handedness in dyslexics initially reported by Orton suggested to him that the left hemisphere was insufficiently dominant.

This made perfect sense except for a few mistaken facts and misassumptions. To his credit, Orton later acknowledged that there were not any handedness differences in dyslexics vs. non-dyslexics, as did I. And even more important, I recognized that the speech disturbances in dyslexics were not cerebrally determined.

Rather, the speech issues manifested by dyslexics, such as stuttering, articulation errors, and other minor impairments, were found due to dysfunctioning timing and motor and delayed processing mechanisms of a CVS origin. Thus, these symptoms often responded well to CVS enhancers—as did the reading and reversal problems. Sadly, the dual clinical observations supporting Orton's dominance theory were shown incorrect. And his many other assumptions could not be validated—nor were they ever specifically and sufficiently explained.

In summary, Orton's dyslexia theory attempted, but failed, to adequately explain the reading disorder in dyslexia as well as the presence of mirror reading and writing—and so also failed to explain most all of Kathy's symptoms. But he did arrive at a very helpful multisensory reading method—even if the latter did not validate his cerebral dominance concept. And if indeed there are cerebral dominance issues in dyslexia, as some still claim, might they be secondary to asymmetric cerebellar determinants? This assumption would be in line with Occam's razor—use the simplest explanation possible.

The Neotraditionalist Theoretical Views of Dyslexia and Kathy

Although there are many neurophysiological dyslexia theories, I've decided to just summarize two of the most popular scientifically proposed ones. In short, the "neo-traditionalists" tried to scientifically explain *dyslexia as a reading disorder, not a syndrome*, by reasoning in one of two main theoretical ways.

The Phonological Theory

According to this theory, Kathy's dyslexia, and dyslexia in general, is *a reading disorder* due to a defect within a phonological processor in the thinking-linguistic brain.[2] This theory is capable of explaining or accounting for *only*

[2] Quite recently, a neuroimaging study reported differing patterns of thinking brain functioning in dyslexics vs. normal individuals. Accordingly, the authors reasoned that the differences measured in the thinking brain support a cerebral cause. However, these theorists failed to take cognizance of a simple alternative explanation: If dyslexics' inner-ear/cerebellar systems send scrambled signals to their thinking brains, isn't it reasonable to consider that an initially normal thinking brain, via compensatory adaptations, will handle these abnormal signals differently from normal ones? Perhaps there may even be impaired cerebellar-cerebral circuits? So further testing is vital.

two of Kathy's many reading characteristics, and nothing more, except for a few of her speech issues:

- The presence of a phonological dysfunction (i.e., a problem related to manipulating the sounds of language), which was just one of Kathy's many dysfunctioning reading mechanisms
- A corresponding reading improvement when utilizing phonologically enhancing tutoring and cognitive conditioning techniques, e.g., Fast ForWord (FFW)

The Magnocellular (Cerebellar) Theory of Dyslexia

Based on this theory, Kathy's dyslexia, and dyslexia in general, is a *reading disorder* resulting from a defect within the visual, auditory, and tactile magnocellular systems in the lower nonthinking brain where the cerebellum reigns supreme, as well as a possible coexisting cerebral impairment.[3] This theory, as proposed, attempts to explain or account for:

As will be discussed in Chap. 18, neuroscientist Paula Tallal and colleagues who developed Fast ForWord may have made a couple of unwitting assumptions—and errors: (1) believing this linguistic phonological defect was of a cerebral vs. CVS origin, and (2) possibly confusing the efficacy of their Fast ForWord reading method to remedy the one rapid word-processing defect they found in speech and reading disorders. Improving just one of many mechanisms may not significantly improve the total reading disorder as simply as Tallal assumed.

[3] The magnocellular theory of dyslexia, especially as eloquently explained by Professor John Stein, appears to be a modified, albeit significantly incomplete, replica of my CVS concept. Thus, Stein recognizes that the cerebellum is the head ganglion of the magnocellular systems. He cites the visual and auditory systems to be smaller in dyslexics and so likely assumes it contributes to timing difficulties with binocular fixation and to inner speech for sounding out words. Both these impairments decrease orthographic skills and so explain the reading impairment—mistakenly equated with the dyslexia syndrome. In other words, *dyslexia* = *"dyslexia."* He also cites the language areas of the right and left dyslexic thinking brains to be abnormally symmetrical—suggesting a primary linguistic component to the dyslexic reading impairment. If proven valid, might this finding be secondary to the CVS impairment? The latter assumption of mine is supported by two considerations: (1) Were this abnormal symmetry primary to determining the dyslexic reading symptom, then CVS enhancers couldn't be helpful since they can't reverse this stated defect. (2) Nor would rotation, vertigo, and other CVS triggers be able to intensify dyslexic symptoms, reading included. And as you will read in the paragraph below, the abnormal embryonic cells found by Galaburda within this lower brain area were also found wherever the assumed cause of the alexia-like reading disorder was traditionally assumed to be.

Thus, for example, Galaburda and colleagues initially found atypical embryonic cells in the thinking brain's reading processor of one dyslexic adult many years ago, mistakenly believing this proved the alexia theory of dyslexia, e.g., *dyslexia= alexia*. Then these large abnormal cells, referred to as brain "warts " (ectopias) by Stein and others, were found in the brain's language centers and then later on within the visual and auditory magnocellular systems (and elsewhere) in others. These cells, and the assumed impairment they represent, were then also mistakenly assumed—believed—to cause linguistic and later visual and auditory processing defects in dyslexia.

- Two main dysfunctioning *reading symptoms*, e.g., impaired binocular visual fixation triggering word blurring and movement [oscillopsia] as well as decreased phonological skills and perhaps a few more characteristics
- Two existing helpful non-tutorial therapies: tinted lenses and Fast ForWord (FFW)—perhaps also the efficacy of a multisensory reading method

Why the Neotraditionalist Theories Fail the Kathy Explanatory Test

If you take another glance at Kathy's many symptoms and those of the other dyslexics presented so far, as well as the scores of dyslexic manifestations within the Self-Diagnostic Test, it should be readily apparent that these "newer" theories are still substantially deficient. They can only collectively account for a very small set of reading symptoms and/or mechanisms, as well as a few

---

According to my critique within *A Scientific Watergate—Dyslexia*, Chapter 18, pages 341–355, I reasoned that these and all other neotraditionlist theories insufficiently and/or incorrectly explained only one or two of many reading mechanisms and absolutely none of the other non-reading symptoms characterizing dyslexics and their complex syndrome. So I initially reasoned that the brain "warts" may be secondary or even irrelevant phenomena since they do not correlate with, nor explain, the symptoms and mechanisms that dyslexics voice. Rather, they seemed erroneously used to support the mistaken traditionalist theory "du jour."

Because of its importance, allow me to repeat what was just said above, but in a slightly different way: *The CVS-enhancing meds can improve all known reading symptoms and mechanisms in dyslexia but can't remove/dissolve Galaburda's embryonic cells nor grow Stein's missing magnocellular cells nor normalize the cerebral language asymmetry within the right and left brains. So clearly, the phonological and magnocellular theories are seriously deficient—especially since stopping the meds cannot restore these structural abnormalities once dyslexic symptoms return!*

Unfortunately, these brilliant theorists and their fascinating experimental findings were never reconciled and so never integrated with my CVS theory of the dyslexia syndrome and clinical findings. Had these academic researchers used my clinical findings to devise objective experiments, their resulting concepts would have better explained the reading disorder as well as all other dyslexic symptoms in a valid, solidly grounded and holistic context. In other words, their research would have been far more productive had it been directed to further elaborate and/or modify my CVS theory, rather than mistakenly used to prove the mistaken neotraditionalist ones. And had these gifted researchers properly referenced my clinical research—as just explained—I believe follow-up investigators would have likely avoided needless similar dead ends and thus more significantly and rapidly advanced their altruistic aims.

On later thinking, perhaps Galaburda's embryonic cells support one of my long-held concepts described at the end of Chapter 9: that dyslexia may result from delayed and/or abnormal embryonic development. Do not all very young children normally manifest all the symptoms characterizing the dyslexia or CVS syndromes? Thus these cells may likely be non-specific embryonic markers, explaining their appearance throughout the CNS. Accordingly, Galaburda was correct, albeit partially so. And I was wrong, although partially so. This is the zigzagging needed to advance. Hopefully, the above back-and-forth reasoning illustrates that discoveries do not often occur in straight lines and that mistakes are a dime-a-dozen. Yet their admission and correction—rather than denial—are vital.

corresponding reading-related therapies—and nothing or little more. None of the theories have led to any new scientific breakthroughs in terms of medical diagnosis, treatment, etc. And all have been justifiably challenged by other investigators.

The reasons for these theories' failures are simple. They all lack sufficient clinical foundations similar to that provided within this book by Kathy and others—and by a very long shot. And they are all replete with mistaken alexia-related assumptions and convictions of their own as well as those taken from other well-respected and cited theorists and researchers.

Had these theoretically based misassumptions been modified and/or corrected by the invaluable anecdotal content provided by Kathy-like patients, I believe the resulting hypotheses would have become infinitely more valid. Perhaps they then might have independently led to a CVS theory of the dyslexia syndrome similar to mine, although several of the more recent cerebellar/inner-ear lookalikes left much to be desired.[4]

---

[4]Developing a holistic theory of dyslexia dependent on expertise in multiple complex medical/scientific disciplines is infinitely more difficult than it might seem. Thus, for example, apparently considering dyslexia to be primarily a reading disorder—as most do—neurotologist Tapani Rahko independently validated the presence of benign paroxysmal positional vertigo (BPPV) in dyslexics. So he recognized that the resulting increase in involuntary rapid eye movements caused impaired focusing and thus "dyslexia." And by treating the BPPV and by increasing the reading speed of dyslexics, he apparently also found improvements in visual (increased visual span during reading), auditory processing, "ADHD," and "dyscalculia"—postulating that this vestibular mechanism interferes with other brain functions. So he apparently hadn't read of all, or perhaps any, of the other reading and non-reading mechanisms I described resolving and defining the dyslexia syndrome. And I never previously read of his fascinating research—or I would have added it to mine, albeit in modified form.

Although Rahko did propose an important inner-ear theory and treatment for dyslexics, he apparently failed to comprehensively explain and encompass most of Kathy's symptoms and mechanisms, albeit he appeared far better in doing so than all the non-CVS theorists.

Accordingly, Rahko's important research also highlights the difficulties gifted clinicians and investigators have in properly integrating their findings with those of others. And the reason is simple. As a neurotologist, Rahko does not really understand dyslexia as I do. And as a psychiatrist, I do not really understand neurotology, especially as he does. And no doubt, this same difficulty holds for all attempting to solve the dyslexia riddle. In retrospect, I was forced to become a jack of all trades, sacrificing true expertise in most. But it took me 50 years to do it imperfectly, but sufficiently. Thus, I'm a slow learner! But there was lots to learn about dyslexia—including neurotology—and even more mistaken assumptions and convictions to unlearn. And nature holds onto her secret insights, using kryptonite to help out.

Because I could not obtain an English translation of Rahko's research, only a summary, it was difficult to be sure of his concepts or what exactly he knew of my prior research, albeit I was referenced. And he failed to respond to my communications. Thus I footnoted his theory and therapy here until I understood them more accurately, rather than discussing this content within the main text.

(Tapani Rahko (2003). "Alleviating dyslexia by treating benign positional vertigo and eye movement disturbances, saccades." *Finnish Medical Journal*. 39: 3883–3886.)

Three Changes Eventually Made

In all fairness, the neotraditionalists did eventually make three beneficial changes—two of their own accord and one forced on them by the American Psychiatric Association's (diagnostic criteria) researchers and their DSM-V manual:

1. *Severe reading scores alone are non-diagnostic*—Several years ago, the neotraditionalists finally dropped the nonsensical criterion that in order to be officially "blessed" with a diagnosis of dyslexia, you had to be intellectually, neurologically, and otherwise *normal* and *also* be two-or-more years behind your peers and/or your potential in reading. (An oxymoron? You decide.)

   And it took them four decades to appreciate Critchley's finding that "reading-cured" dyslexics existed—and so inadvertently highlighted the fallacy of defining this complex disorder on the sole alexia-like basis of *severe* reading score impairments. And it took them only three decades to partially understand my concept of *reading-compensated* dyslexics—resisting this rather obvious clinical insight every step along the way for decades. No doubt, my synonymous but more challenging-appearing paradox *dyslexics without 'dyslexia'* is still difficult to accept for all those equating dyslexia with only its severe reading score characteristic, e.g., *dyslexia = "dyslexia."* Was not kryptonite in play?
2. *Phonological deficits are also not absolutely diagnostic*—Based on important findings indicating a phonological impairment in the reading of dyslexics, it is now traditionally mandatory to include this dysfunction in all current dyslexia definitions. However, this phonologically focused definition unwittingly excludes—or completely fails to encompass: (A) many of Kathy's visual and other sensory-motor reading difficulties, (B) all her many other non-reading symptoms, as well as (C) the compensatory mechanisms affecting all her reading and non-reading symptoms, not counting her favorable response to the CVS enhancers, as you will later observe in Chap. 23.

   It also fails to account for the many avid readers with phonological deficits (refer to Jenny in Chap. 20) as well as typical dyslexics with normal phonological skills. *After reading Kathy's self-description, would anyone believe that she wasn't dyslexic, even if she were either phonologically normal or even gifted?*

   Also, my many dyslexic patients with reading, speech/language, phonological, and significant sound and auditory processing deficits were found to have only CVS dysfunctioning as well as CVS-related mechanisms. And all the abovementioned symptoms responded favorably to CVS-enhancing meds—clearly suggesting that all are likely of a primary CVS origin. Accordingly, the primary cerebral basis of phonological deficits is also probably mistaken.

   In fact, one of my patient's impairments in speech, sound/word perception, and auditory processing so improved on CVS enhancers, as did his reading and other more typical dyslexic symptoms, that he became a competent ventriloquist (refer to Chap. 24).
3. *Dyslexia does not exist as a disorder when defined as a pure reading impairment*—the DSM-V "recently" *refuted* the existence of traditionally defined dys-

lexia as a discrete diagnostic entity. Instead, the DSM-V *justifiably* reclassified this one-symptom-defined reading disorder as merely *one neurodynamically caused symptom among many* within the specific learning disability (SLD) diagnostic category—thus recognizing the presence of a dyslexia or SLD syndrome. And by so doing, *the* DSM-V has *also justifiably refuted all of the traditionalist and neotraditionalist theories based on their flawed, single-symptom, "alexia-like" reading concept and mistaken definition.*[5]

The APA also considered—but did not apparently implement—an alternative definition as a compromise to satisfy dyslexia foundations and their researchers. This compromise definition is now used and also required by many dyslexia experts in order to continue much needed research and publications. It mentions dyslexia by name, defines it as phonologically based, but also indicates that it should be regarded as part of SLD.

So where do I differ from the APA? *I maintain that both the reading disorder called "dyslexia" and SLD are both part of a still larger CVS syndrome!*

"Then what is the value of all these dyslexia theories," you may be wondering at this point, "if they explain little to nothing about dyslexics, led nowhere scientifically with respect to medical treatment, and were just *rejected* by the APA?" I can only echo your doubts. But there may be a very important lesson to be learned here: *The theoretically gifted cannot succeed by following the clinically blind!*

Conclusions

Dyslexia theories require clinical validation In my research experience, missteps are easy when you are operating theoretically and so relying mainly on assumptions and untested prior convictions, especially those that appear too obvious and irresistible to challenge, e.g., *dyslexia = alexia = "dyslexia."*

Clearly, no researcher, alone or as part of a gifted team, could have accurately conceptualized a holistic and fully explanatory 4-D portrait of the dyslexia syndrome without the combined clinical insights provided by thousands of Kathy-like dyslexics. Relying on theory alone, *even when formulated by the best and brightest*

---

[5] Because the reading scores in dyslexics may vary from one extreme to another, two brilliant and productive dyslexia researchers at Yale (Sally E. Shaywitz, M.D., and Bennett A. Shaywitz, M.D.) questioned dyslexia's existence. Similarly, this observation led many laymen to believe that dyslexia is a fiction—representing just the severe end of a normal bell curve distribution of reading capabilities in otherwise normal individuals. However, both groups failed to recognize that dyslexia is a CVS syndrome of many reading and non-reading symptoms. And both failed to fully realize that the quality vs. severity of the reading impairment in dyslexia is diagnostically significant. Yet this concept may have merit, since it is explained by my embryonic CVS dyslexia theory.

minds and agreed upon by a vast like-minded consensus, can result in convictions based largely on illusions and/or our normally limited conceptual abilities.

Why else has there been only one Einstein? And even he was mistaken about quantum mechanics. And only one Freud, who was initially theoretically misled by a few of his clinical findings. So, these required his later corrections and a better concept. Why has dyslexia remained an unsolved mystery for well over a century, despite the dedicated and altruistic scientific efforts of countless researchers?

The influence of bias in science For those who may still have difficulty believing the scope and influence of bias and misjudgments in science, I ask you to also explain why Einstein was repeatedly refused the Nobel Prize in physics for his theory of relativity by the super-distinguished Nobel science committee, which reluctantly—begrudgingly—awarded him one for his "relatively minor" photoelectric research after many years of debate and external pressure? And similarly, why was Freud refused this very same elegant prize for medicine 13 times, never receiving it?

Believe it or not, the three of us have at least one thing in common. No, Einstein and Freud were not born or raised in Brooklyn. But they may have passed thru.

In summary, gifted traditionalists misapplied theories proven valid for *alexia* to explain a completely different disorder called *dyslexia*. Despite being shown that their theories explained nothing much about dyslexics and led nowhere scientifically, many still resisted believing, by analogy, that the Earth is round and not the center of the universe.

So, traditionalists repeatedly proposed and pursued varied theories without completely abandoning mistaken *dyslexia* = *alexia* convictions. And instead of benefitting from the invaluable anecdotal insights revealed by dyslexics about their disorder, the traditionalists often defensively rejected the value of these clinically based clarifications. Thus, they remained lost in theoretical space for over a century—without knowing and/or acknowledging it. And they often unknowingly projected their confusion and errors onto others.

Perhaps a Brooklyn truism and analogy may be helpful here. Just as you can leave Brooklyn, yet be unable to remove the Brooklyn from within—it appears that many dyslexia professionals had a similar problem. Despite untiring and admirable scientific efforts, the traditionalists appeared unable to remove their alexia convictions from within. No doubt, it was an intuitive understanding of the above bias-led errors that guided my research to significantly rely on data and insights derived primarily from patients such as Kathy, rather than from experts and their mistaken theories. As a result of a different non-groupthink scientific approach, my clinically based efforts eventually hit gold and resulted in the CVS theory of dyslexia and its breakthrough medical treatment.

This CVS theory, which will be discussed in the very next chapter, is now fully capable of encompassing and explaining 100 percent of Kathy's symptoms as well as those of all known dyslexics and so also those summarized within the Self-

Diagnostic-Test. Also, this repeatedly updated hypothesis has led to new diagnostic insights as well as a groundbreaking and successful medical treatment and much more while also helping to clarify both the value and shortcomings of all other proposed dyslexia concepts. Since seeing is understanding and so believing, just turn the page.

Chapter 9
The CVS Theory of Dyslexia: A Theory's Value Is Entirely Dependent on Its Explanatory and Predictive Capabilities

Science progresses not by convincing the adherents of old theories that they are wrong but by allowing enough time to pass so that a new generation can arise unencumbered by the old errors.

—Max Plank, Nobel Laureate in Physics

When in the grip of false scientific convictions, our perception of reality inevitably becomes distorted and narrowed to fit expectations. As a result, even the more recent highly sophisticated traditionalist investigatory efforts in dyslexia were often as unwittingly distorted by false *dyslexia=alexia=severe reading impairment* assumptions, as were the older theories dating back to 1896. Sadly, they all lacked sufficient explanatory and predictive capabilities to justify their existence. And the reason is simple, as many of you may now realize.

As repeatedly clarified, alexia and dyslexia were shown by me to be completely separate disorders—having absolutely nothing in common besides differently caused and so completely distinct reading disorders. As a result, the varied alexia-based theories explained absolutely nothing about dyslexics and their complex syndrome—0 percent. By analogy, would a theory designed to explain a fish—a bass—be confidently used to explain my now familiar zebra, based on the fact that both animals are striped?

Fortunately, every once in a while breakthrough discoveries are made, seemingly by chance. Suddenly, previously denied and disparate data that have been long before one's eyes are seen in an entirely new, panoramic light—and make perfect sense. Suddenly *all* the seemingly random pieces to a previously vexing puzzle fly together and become integrated into a fresh portrait and then into a new, holistically encompassing and explanatory theory. This is the nature of scientific awakenings.

The process of recognizing the fallacies of the varied *dyslexia=alexia* concepts and then understanding the inner-ear/cerebellar (CVS) cause of dyslexia—utilizing a large number of diversely obtained patient-based insights—was *my* awakening. Following this CVS theory's initial formulation, I repeatedly modified it to both encompass and explain all the symptoms and determining mechanisms I'd

H. N. Levinson, *Feeling Smarter and Smarter*,
https://doi.org/10.1007/978-3-030-16208-5_9

obtained directly from over 35,000 CVS dysfunctioning dyslexic children and adults who responded favorably to inner-ear/CVS-enhancing meds. So, it shouldn't surprise anyone that this CVS theory then proved capable of fully explaining all other dyslexics—the total "clinical 4-D dyslexic picture," Kathy included.

So, in order to best appreciate my CVS theory's amazing capacity for explaining 100 percent of the characteristics encompassing dyslexia and its entire syndrome as well as leading to new diagnostic and therapeutic discoveries, it's important for readers to review and thoroughly understand this unique, dynamic, and multidimensional concept as well as a new definition of the dyslexia disorder.

The CVS Theory of Dyslexia

A TV analogy Let's start with a simple analogy: The inner-ear/cerebellar system (CVS) acts like the fine-tuners on a TV set. However, instead of working in two dimensions with mechanical antennas, the CVS uses super-advanced four-dimensional temporal and spatial fine-tuners and super-enhanced Bluetooth-like signal technology. In other words, for signals to be clear and effective, their timing and organization in space must be perfectly fine-tuned.

Any dysfunction of these CVS tuners and transmitters results in (1) the distorting of sensory signals entering the thinking brain (as well as other brain centers) and/or (2) the scrambling of motor (balance/coordination/rhythmic) signals leaving it. As a result of this signal scrambling, a previously normal thinking brain, even a gifted one like Kathy's, will have *secondary* difficulty processing the distorted information it receives—just as you or I might have trouble watching, listening to, and understanding a scrambled TV channel.

If we assume a separate "channel" for each of the hundreds, likely thousands, of functions and sub-functions that are found to be impaired in dyslexia, then all of the diverse reading and non-reading symptoms and mechanisms affecting writing, spelling, math, memory, etc. that characterize dyslexic individuals—including Kathy—can be holistically explained as *a syndrome rather than just a severe reading impairment.*

The resultant symptoms and their severity will then depend on:

- The specific inner-ear and cerebellar sites radiating the drifting signals to varying brain destinations, including to other destinations within the CVS
- The specific internal CVS and external brain sites receiving, processing, and further transmitting the scrambled signals
- The degree of signal drift or distortion
- The genetic and learned ability of the thinking brain and other CNS (central nervous system) processors—including the higher cerebellum—to descramble, decode, or otherwise compensate for the distorted or misperceived input and output

The CVS Theory Encompasses and Explains the Entire Dyslexia Syndrome

Perhaps you may now better understand the challenging novelty of this all-encompassing and all-explanatory "simple" CVS theory of the dyslexia syndrome. It represents a radical departure from earlier, and all other, concepts because it requires only *one* basic clinically verified and dynamically interactive CVS impairment to explain the scores of reading and non-reading symptoms and disorders characterizing dyslexics like Kathy as well as all the manifestation within the Self-Diagnostic Test. *And this impairment was reasoned to be a primary fine-tuning dysfunction within the inner-ear/cerebellum, resulting in a diverse array of secondary signal scrambling and related transmission "errors"—dyslexic (or CVS) symptoms, depending on the cerebral/higher-cerebellar descrambling/compensatory capability.*

The CVS and related overlapping disorders Additionally, the CVS theory easily resolves a major traditionalist paradox: how bright and even gifted dyslexics like Kathy invariably manifest many overlapping or "comorbid" non-reading disorders—mistakenly assumed to result from multiple diverse *primary* brain impairment sites. As discussed before, this misassumption leads to a dead end—unless you're willing to conclude that Kathy's brain is diffusely and severely impaired, which would place her IQ at close to 0 vs. gifted and her prognosis poor vs. favorable.

The CVS concept restated in a slightly different way *According to my CVS theory, these differing reading, writing, math disorders co-occur or overlap in dyslexics because they share a common CVS dysfunctional origin. And the resulting disorders are qualitatively different from one another because their scrambled signals target different brain destinations, which have differing functions and appearances, and perhaps distinct descrambling and perceptual capabilities.*

Each initially normal brain destination gives rise to quality-unique SLD, ADHD, phobic, mood-related, and many other disorders after it secondarily fails to properly descramble or compensate for the received "dizzy" signals, not counting the tertiary emotional and behavioral fallout as well as their circular complications.

Perhaps due to the sensory, motor, and related signals being distorted in space and time by a dysfunctioning CVS fine-tuner, there results a "rapid processing deficit"—more detectable before compensatory mechanisms kick in. Hence, I designed and patented 3-D optical, auditory, and tactile scanners to detect these delayed processing deficits when present. Needless to say, rapid motor and related speech and recall tasks (really delayed processing) may be similarly affected, including rapid naming, etc.

Dyslexia and IQ Because the CVS has little to do with IQ, and since there are not multiple distinct sites of brain dysfunction as the traditionalists believe, it's now easy to understand how even geniuses such as Einstein and Edison can be dyslexic—

even severely so. Gifted brains—like Kathy's—remain gifted, even in the presence of dyslexia. Indeed, gifted brains can more readily decode and descramble the drifting CVS signals—and so better compensate for them.

The gift of dyslexia "Dreamers" who believe dyslexia is a gift, rather than the opposite, are likely misled by wishful thinking, exceptions aside.[1] And the exceptions are due to those who are fortunate enough to have compensated and overcompensated—thus maximizing capabilities that might never have otherwise occurred. Sadly, this so-called gift does not apply to the many dyslexics who forever fail, remain frustrated, drop out of school and the mainstream, etc.—unless diagnosed and successfully treated early.

Acquired dyslexia This simple inner-ear/cerebellar theory can also readily explain why ear infections, spinning, and zero gravity may result in transient or permanently acquired dyslexic or ADHD—even phobic—symptoms at any age, or serve as symptomatic intensifiers. All of these disparate conditions may destabilize the inner-ear/CVS fine-tuners and transmitters and thus intensify signal scrambling.

Different reading and non-reading symptoms, mechanism, impairments, and severities In fact, the inner-ear/cerebellar theory can also account for why dyslexics have *differently appearing reading disorders*—depending on the specific overlapping combination of their CVS-determined vs. compensatory reading mechanisms (refer to Chap. 16).

By contrast, the traditionalists/neotraditionalists maintained the mistaken illusion that there was *only one* dyslexic reading impairment—either an alexia-like visual reading incomprehension one or now a phonologically based reading deficit. Both concepts are way too simplistic—and misleading! Only bias, denial, and/or inadequate experience keeps them afloat.

Similarly, all the traditionalist dyslexia concepts proved just as incapable of specifically explaining all of the diverse non-reading symptoms, mechanisms, and severities characterizing those with the Kathy-like dyslexia syndrome. However, the magnocellular concept significantly resembles mine, and so potentially has greater explanatory capabilities.

CVS deficits plus major brain impairments As previously mentioned, many major brain disorders, such as cerebral palsy, traumatic brain injuries, ASD,

[1] Speaking of exceptions—which I enjoy exploring and making sense of—it is likely that the dyslexic impairment may secondarily trigger compensatory brain "islets," resulting in exceptional or "gifted" functioning in a lucky few, especially in those predisposed to it. That's like one arm becoming exceptionally stronger—hypertrophied—to compensate for a weaker atrophied one. However, there's another idea I had that may make sense of the above "dream/fantasy," perhaps also explaining the exceptional splinter capabilities seen in Asperger's. *Might a failure in brain inhibition result in the release or escape of previously suppressed exceptional talented functions?* Thus, every dream or fantasy may have a grain of truth worth exploring.

Down's syndrome, mental deficiencies, schizophrenia, etc. are frequently complicated by CVS dysfunctioning. Thus, these patients really have two disorders. And by treating the CVS signal scrambling, the severity of the overall impairment is often improved.

The Brain's Autonomous Descrambling Capability

Before proceeding any further, I would like to provide you once again with a tangible example of the brain's *autonomous descrambling capability*. This simple exercise may do more to illustrate how those suffering from the dyslexia syndrome often compensate for the scrambled signals they receive than all other non-CVS explanations combined. Thus, it will enable you to better understand my CVS theory of the dyslexia syndrome and so also how dyslexia and alexia are completely different.

What do you see when you look at the following four scrambled sentences?[2]

7H15 M3554G3 53RV35 7O PR0V3 H0W 0UR M1ND5 C4N D0 4M4Z1NG 7H1NG5!

C4N U R34D 7H13?

1MPR3551V3! 1N 7H3 B3G1NN1NG 17 WA5 H4RD BU7 N0W, 0N 7H15 LIN3, Y0UR M1ND 1S R34D1NG 17 4U70M471C4LLY W17H0U7 3V3N 7H1NK1NG 4B0U7 17.

B3 PR0UD! 0NLY C3R741N P30PL3 C4N R3AD 7H15

Decoding capability Amazingly, although the above input is "scrambled," your normal brain was able to *somewhat rapidly and automatically*—subconsciously—compensate and thereby read and understand it. Similarly, the various normal non-reading brain centers of dyslexics also receive scrambled signals due to a dysfunctioning CVS. And so, they also must similarly and autonomously compensate for these distorted signals—with varying degrees of success. Failure invariably results in symptoms. And the sudden appearance of successful descrambling over time appears synonymous with terms such as late-blooming, spurting, etc.

I'm certain that after some re-reading of the above scrambled sentences, your decoding ability increased without even *consciously* thinking about it. The same increase in decoding capability likely explains why dyslexics such as Kathy often improve as well. And this seemingly innate—perhaps genetically determined—compensatory characteristic, which no doubt varies among individuals and likely resides in the thinking brain and/or related higher cerebellar circuitry, may also explain Critchley's "cured" dyslexic readers, and also why time, repetition, tutoring, determination, and therapeutic methods help, depending also upon the degree of scrambling.

[2] These examples of scrambled sentences illustrating our innate and learned abilities to spontaneously decode them were taken from an internet site: http://www.relativelyinteresting.com/7h15-m3554g3-53rv35-7o-pr0v3-h0w-0ur-m1nd5-c4n-d0-4m4z1ng-7h1ng5//

Interestingly, a failure of this higher descrambling capability may play an important co-determining role in the final symptoms and outcomes of dyslexics—indirectly supporting those believing dyslexia is of a cerebral origin, albeit the higher cerebellum may be significantly or even entirely involved. Future neuroimaging research will likely clarify this issue as it will many others.

I will further explain some of these, and other, compensatory methods and therapies later in the book. But keep this key observation in mind: the scrambled signals—symptoms—may persist even when properly interpreted or decoded. And this seeming paradox will later be more fully clarified.

Redefining Dyslexia

This "challenging" CVS theory naturally led me to a new definition of the dyslexia syndrome, which I believe further highlights the absurdity of both: (1) the arbitrary two-or-more-years behind in reading one belatedly dropped by dyslexia experts after a century and the mistaken or over-simplistic traditionalist definition and concept—that dyslexia is a pure reading incomprehension impairment—more recently and justifiably refuted by the APA's (American Psychiatric Association's) diagnostic manual, DSM-V.

My concept also suggests that (3) we ought to replace the latest accepted traditionalist assertion/requirement that dyslexia is due to a cerebral phonological deficit. As I noted earlier, a phonological deficit is now an *official requirement* by traditionalists in order to be diagnosed dyslexic—meaning someone with a reading impairment. And the scientific basis for this new, single-variable definition is over-simplistic, especially so since a phonological deficit cannot explain the vast majority of non-reading symptoms—nor even most of the reading symptoms—characterizing dyslexics. (Refer to Kathy's reading symptoms.)

Many dysfunctioning reading mechanisms Most professionals failed to consider that there are more than 20 reading-determining mechanisms in dyslexia (presented in Chap. 16). Thus, Kathy described many of these reading symptoms and impaired determinants which I further clarified in the next chapter using my CVS hypothesis. And most readers will by now have realized the error made by those defining this highly complex Kathy-like dyslexia syndrome, which consists of many reading and non-reading symptoms, by only one dysfunctioning reading mechanism—even if phonological impairment is indeed *one significant determinant* of reading failure. Such a narrow definition doesn't come close to describing and encompassing all of Kathy's many and diverse dyslexia symptoms or those of the vast majority of dyslexics.

And as repeatedly mentioned, there are dyslexics with normal phonological mechanisms, and avid-reading dyslexics with severely impaired phonological processing—the latter best exemplified by Jenny in Chap. 20.

Re-explaining the Total Dyslexia Syndrome

To re-explain the total dyslexic syndrome in which reading symptoms are only a segment, I propose the following all-explanatory concept—which is scientifically compatible with the APA's new diagnostic criteria:

> *Dyslexia and/or Specific Learning Disability (SLD) are merely subsets of a far larger and more complex CVS syndrome. These subsets occur when initially normal (and/or genetically predisposed) reading and related writing, spelling, math, and other processors within the brain fail to descramble, decode, or otherwise compensate for the distorted signals—impaired in space and time—radiating to their sites from a fine-tuning dysfunction within the inner ear and its supercomputing CVS.*
>
> *The diverse pattern, quality, and changing severities of the resulting symptoms are co-determined by the brain processors receiving, and then further transmitting, distorted signals, as well as by the degree of signal distortion and compensation (descrambling, decoding, etc.) that takes place.*
>
> *Decompensating factors, such as medical, psychological, environmental and other destabilizing problems, may also play an important tertiary role—one often overlooked by over-simplifiers.*

A Simple Formula

Importantly, I decided to condense *all* the above CVS/dyslexia concepts into the following simple formula, which also includes decompensatory factors:

> *Dyslexia Syndrome = CVS Dysfunction + Compensatory (cerebral, higher cerebellar, and other) Decoding + Decompensatory Negative Factors (anxiety, depression, medical, family, environmental-social problems, etc.)*

By comparison, the *dyslexia = severe alexia-like reading comprehension impairment* formula represented a century-plus-old over-simplistic fantasy that encompassed and explained nothing worthwhile about dyslexics. In fact, among the very many dysfunctioning reading mechanisms characterizing dyslexics, *the one they don't have is primary reading incomprehension, perhaps an atypical exception aside!* And adding a phonological deficit was insightful but did not meet the criteria for a valid definition, as previously discussed.

Enhancing the CVS Theory of Dyslexia

Although the CVS fine-tuning theory of the dyslexia syndrome just described is the best and simplest general overall description of this 4-D impairment to date, your understanding of this syndrome as well as an enhanced concept will be immeasurably expanded once you add on the reading insights within Chap. 16

and, more importantly, the super-ten all-clarifying CVS determining mechanisms within Chap. 17. When merged, these concepts provide an explanatory synergy second to none.

The Embryonic Origins of the CVS/Dyslexia Syndrome

Finally, to complete my CVS theory and chapter, I'd like to add a rather unique insight into the likely origins of the CVS/dyslexia syndrome. Hopefully, you'll find it as fascinating as I did when this concept initially hit me one morning upon awakening. Although simple and even obvious, the details were slowly and belatedly arrived at—suggesting an unwitting resistance at its clarification. Clearly, it was crucial to explain how and why Kathy and most other dyslexics were seemingly born with this disorder.

Embryonic dyslexia Before continuing, I'd like to ask you a simple question: Why is it that most very young children *normally manifest* dyslexic-like reading, writing, spelling difficulties, reversals, etc. as well as imbalance, dyscoordination, impaired rhythm, etc.? Is this the reason why some believe that dyslexia is normal? Or that we all have/had dyslexia?

I had provided answers to these questions in my medical text, *A Solution to the Riddle—Dyslexia* way back in 1980. My reasoning at that time—which also speculated about dyslexia's embryonic origin—was surprisingly simple, albeit I've now further clarified it. Accordingly, I reasoned:

- All very young children manifest the CVS/dyslexia syndrome—but normally so—and then most outgrow it.
- As a result, the CVS/dyslexia syndrome is considered to be developmental in origin.
- The sequence of transitioning from a non-to-quasi pre-reading stage to a normal reading state follows the well-known biological principle that the developing human embryo, extending into late childhood—and likely longer—repeats the stages of evolution, a phenomenon called *ontogeny recapitulates phylogeny*.
- When this transition is delayed or fails, due to genetic or acquired embryonic considerations and/or abnormalities, then the CVS/dyslexia syndrome may often persist into adulthood.[3]
- Since the (embryonic) developmental CVS/dyslexia syndrome manifests differently among individuals, I was led to assume that the original evolutionary transitions to a reading state were likely multiple and spectral in both degree and characteristics vs. one-shot and pure.

[3] Might Galaburda's findings of abnormal embryonic cells within the dominant cerebral reading processor, and throughout the dyslexic brain, support my rather novel evolutionary CVS concept, albeit he mistakenly believed they initially validated traditionalist dyslexia theories and later on the neotraditonalist concepts? Thus, Galaburda's microscopic data may have been correct, even if his varied interpretations of their significance as to dyslexia's causation were likely not. However, to better understand both the specifics and context of these important insights, you will have to refer back to my prior discussion within Chap. 8, footnote 3.

- Normal, late, or even real-late CVS "blooming" often spontaneously occur clinically and may likely signify the pre-reading-to-reading spurts characterizing evolutionary development—eventually resulting in man's normal reading and related CVS-cerebral functioning.
- Dyslexia, when acquired embryonically or thereafter, may reflect similar phylogenetic setbacks during evolution.

The embryonic dyslexia state persists subconsciously As noted, we've all had the "embryonic dyslexia syndrome" when very young. But this state normally disappears with continued maturational development. And most of us mistakenly assumed that it was entirely eradicated—completely replaced. However, this "embryonic CVS syndrome" appears to have been suppressed and layered over, remaining subconsciously active rather than lost.

Why do I believe this? Because we all tend to lapse into momentary or transient "dyslexia states"—evidenced by the so-called Freudian, really dyslexic, slips mentioned in prior chapters.[4] Clearly, we couldn't lapse into this momentary "dyslexic state," manifesting characteristic "slips and other OCD-related thought intrusions" as well as dreaming, if this state didn't continue to exist. And it similarly explains the presence of universal phobias where previously inhibited evolutionary adaptive responses suddenly leak into consciousness—seemingly from nowhere.

Accordingly, subconscious dyslexia-related "embryonic intrusions" or slips are facilitated or pop up more readily into consciousness when the efficacy of higher cerebral/cerebellar mechanisms is minimized and/or when CVS signal scrambling is intensified via spinning or acquired injuries. Thus, for example, stress and anxiety, fatigue, day- and night-dreaming, distractions, sleep deprivation, etc. tend to transiently decrease concentration as well as conscious logical thinking and related inhibitory/filtering mechanisms. And CVS signal scrambling is temporarily intensified during rotation, and chronically so during acquired CVS impairments. Needless to say, there may be genetic and/or acquired impairments as well.

Answering puzzling assertions So, as initially promised, I believe that the above content may help answer the seemingly confusing and conflicting assertions about dyslexia made

[4] I long ago discovered that the very same mechanisms that Freud used to explain dream content and slips as well as neurotic symptoms were similar to those I found characterizing dyslexic errors. These include omissions, insertions, displacements, condensations, reversals, opposites, etc. Refer to the Reading Error Diagram within my medical text, *A Solution to the Riddle—Dyslexia*, as well as here in Chap. 19, Fig. A. It thus appeared likely that Freud's unconscious or primary (primitive) process "language" or thinking mechanisms were also derived from the CVS—especially the higher cerebellum. And just as we all tended to deny Freud's discovery of subconscious activity and motivation, we similarly denied the amazing functions of the higher cerebellum which likely modulates this activity!

It's also worth mentioning that this subconscious thinking is, like a young child's, pictorial, concrete, and 2-D or linear.

By contrast, there likely is also significant cerebral subconscious functioning akin to a fast computer. This might explain how I, and many others too, often go to sleep puzzled and wake up with solutions. Or insights spontaneously arise while we are busy with unrelated activities. Might this computer be continually active—printing out solutions when the timing is right? Perhaps, conscious thinking, which is slow and tedious, is the exception to man's overall thinking capabilities?

by some in the first chapter: *that dyslexia is normal... it exists... and that everyone has it.* However, if this is so, then one might also reason alternatively *that no one has a dyslexia disorder and so that dyslexia does not exist—since its manifestations are considered normal.* And also dyslexia, when traditionally misdefined as a pure alexia-like reading disorder, does not exist—according to diagnostic APA experts and their official DSM-V manual. Thus, it appears that there is a hidden basis or significance for all the varied dyslexia theories—even those proposed and verbalized by laymen (refer to Appendix 9).

The amazing value of anecdotal content Perhaps readers will now better understand Freud's ingenious recognition that *all* expressed content, including all the *qualitative anecdotal verbalizations* derived from patients like Kathy as well as dreams and neurotic/psychotic manifestations, have significant meaning and value *once properly listened to, questioned, analyzed, reconciled—and so really understood.*

As a result, the analysis of the anecdotal content derived from well over 35,000 successfully treated CVS dysfunctioning patients has led to a unique CVS theory of dyslexia fully capable of explaining and encompassing all known dyslexia phenomena while leading to new and fascinating insights and discoveries. And as you will soon read within the next chapter, this CVS theory can now explain all of Kathy's many and diverse symptoms, and so much more.

In fact, this very same CVS concept—significantly derived from patients via Q&As—even proved capable of explaining all of the abovementioned atypical and paradoxical dyslexia ideas proposed by both professionals and laymen and even additional contradictory and nonsensical appearing ones, e.g., *we all have dyslexia, no-one has dyslexia*, etc. And after repeated modifications, this CVS theory evolved into the best "kryptonite-free" hypothesis about dyslexia to-date.[5]

I also wondered if my many spontaneous insights—many occurring soon after awakening—came from the very same subconscious brain?[6]

[5]And via a Freudian analysis, the very opposite was shown true about anecdotal content: It is scientifically meaningless, as some traditionalist critics maintain, *when improperly listened to, questioned, analyzed, reconciled, and so never really understood. Or when never listened to at all due to bias and so denied altogether.*

Thus, when properly analyzed, all verbalizations can be eventually understood and so have scientific value—even opposites and seemingly nonsensical expressions.

[6]Another Zag

In writing this chapter and discussing how insights just pop into consciousness after sleep, I suddenly wondered: Might these occurrences result due to decreased conscious inhibition of subconscious processes akin to dream content or what Freud called primary process thinking surfacing? Seems likely. And suddenly I had a probable "validation" for how dyslexics like Michael Shultz and Meg Fex began reading content they previously did not consciously know once medically treated (refer back to Chap. 3). Might med treatment have lessened over-inhibitory memory mechanisms? Or simply enabled suppressed normal reading mechanisms—which would explain how gifted readers just spontaneously function from the start, without prior learning.

Clearly, there are many latent thoughts and insights roaming about our subconscious—otherwise they couldn't suddenly enter consciousness—just like dreams. So, might most be normally or adaptively held in check by cerebellar/cerebral inhibitory mechanisms? Might the latter prevent flooding and/or dreams and dream-like delusional and hallucinatory content from becoming conscious and interfering with normal conscious, logical, or secondary thinking processes and functioning?

Chapter 10
Only the CVS Theory Can Explain All of Kathy's Dyslexic Symptoms and Mechanisms

Now that I've updated and clarified my "synergistic" CVS theory of the dyslexia syndrome, I can more easily explain *all* of dyslexia's—Kathy's—specific symptoms and dysfunctioning vs. compensatory mechanisms. However, were I to do so here completely, this chapter would become book-sized. So, I'll compromise. I'll clarify a convincing array of Kathy's CVS-determined dyslexic characteristics here and use subsequent Chaps. 16 and 17 to elaborate significantly further. But I can assure you: *My CVS theory, especially when supercharged, and its defining formula explains and encompasses all known dyslexic manifestations, including those within the Self-Diagnostic Test—100 percent of them.*

So, let's get started with specifically clarifying Kathy's CVS-determined dyslexia symptoms:

Dysfunctioning vs. Compensatory Reading Mechanisms

Dysfunctioning reading symptoms and mechanisms Kathy experienced reading difficulties because of *primary CVS problems* with memory, ocular fixation and tracking, perception, spacing, orientation/direction/sequencing, letter/word reversals, word blurring, shifting foregrounds and backgrounds, word movement and scrambling (sometimes even flying off the page), inadequate and/or delayed phonetic discrimination, light and glare sensitivity, tunnel vision, difficulty integrating or connecting letter/word sequences—including visual and phonetic counterparts—in both space and time, visual overloading, impaired concentration and distractibility, as well as corresponding auditory or phonetic/phonological symptoms similar to the visual ones.

Once again, the CVS mechanisms responsible for all of Kathy's abovementioned reading symptoms—including her non-reading symptoms—will be further discussed in Chaps. 16 and especially 17.

H. N. Levinson, *Feeling Smarter and Smarter*,
https://doi.org/10.1007/978-3-030-16208-5_10

To reemphasize—Owing to all of the above-stated *primary reading* symptoms resulting from a CVS-determined signal impairment as well as the more specific super-ten mechanisms, dyslexics like Kathy then also experience additional difficulty in properly perceiving, remembering, and thus understanding some of what they read. By contrast and analogy, alexics clearly see letters and words—and so have no signal or perception distortion. However, they just can't process the meaning of the clear words they're looking at—thus manifesting a *primary reading comprehension impairment*.

Perhaps another simple illustration here will help. Dyslexics see and so must decode scrambled reading signals such as C4N U R34D 7H13? to understand them. By sharp contrast, alexics clearly see CAN YOU READ THIS? but don't know what these symbols mean.

Delayed processing* vs. *incomprehension It's likely that Kathy also experienced delayed word recognition or processing in her attempt to descramble the "dizzy" signal input while reading. Because these durations lasted from seconds to perhaps minutes, a therapist and/or theorist without proper clinical experience might mistake these compensatory delays and resulting errors for a primary alexia-like reading incomprehension. But the distinguishing factor, diagnostically speaking, is that delayed processing may lead to only belated recognition, whereas true alexic incomprehension remains complete—and forever. And even applies to single letters.

Some reading symptoms/mechanisms appear entirely intra-CVS Since many of Kathy's reading symptoms and mechanisms appeared to be *entirely* inner-ear/CVS-determined and modulated, it's probable that their signals' origins and destinations were entirely confined within the inner-ear and its related CVS. Thus, to more completely explain all of Kathy's reading, and even non-reading symptoms, it is crucial to combine the general scrambling/descrambling mechanism described above with the ten super-mechanisms presented within Chap. 17—resulting in what I call an explanatory synergy.

Compensatory reading symptoms and mechanisms Bright dyslexics like Kathy eventually have a very favorable reading outcome by virtue of their normal or superior thinking brain's—and likely higher cerebellar—ability to compensate for the "dizzy" signals received from a lower CVS dysfunction. As a result of reading-score compensation, the quality vs. severity of reading capability in Kathy-like dyslexics is considered more diagnostically important.

A compensatory reading miracle Can anyone believe that Kathy learned to read despite the following spatial disorientation or scrambling of letters and numbers as well as her related misperceptions of the heights, spaces, depth, etc. of letters and words? She described her visual difficulty as follows:

"***Reading***—*I arrived in kindergarten ... My problem was keeping numbers or letters separate. It was a spatial orientation nightmare. There were:*

- *lots of circles with straight lines attached: 6, 9, a, d, b, p, g, q, Q*
- *double bumps: 3, m*
- *three pointers: MWE*

- *single bumps: S, 2, 5, u, U, n, h, r*
- *cut circles: C, c, e, G, Q*
- *check marks: V, v, 7, L*
- *biplanes: K, I*
- *crosses: 4, t, and x*

At first I tended to read in the wrong direction and wrote that way too. I couldn't keep letters in order either. There was no discernible difference between: 90, 60, do, and go; wow, mom, and 303; B and 13; spot, tops, pots, and stop."

Considering this was only one of Kathy's many reading symptoms/mechanisms, can anyone postulate how she compensated sufficiently to complete graduate school—although she did somehow learn to distinguish many compressed words by the shape of their tops? And so, we might ask: What were her other compensatory mechanisms? And where in the CNS were the interacting dysfunctioning vs. compensatory vectors located?

Was her misperception a primary co-existing impairment or secondary to a more generalized fine-tuning disorder? Was her misperception of a lower CVS, higher cerebellar, and/or cerebral origin? Wouldn't Kathy have been considered dyslexic even without phonological difficulties—supporting my conviction that impaired phonological processing alone is too simplistic for properly defining this complex 4-D syndrome?

Unfortunately, I did not have an opportunity to question Kathy sufficiently to obtain further insights. However, it's likely that Q&As as well as neuroanalyses with other Kathy-like dyslexics will provide us with answers to most of the above questions.

Symptomatic complexity and variations in dyslexia In any large sample of dyslexics—and also in the Kathy-like cases presented within this book—there is always both quantitative and qualitative diversity in the reading and non-reading symptoms and mechanisms characterizing those clinically examined as well as in their decoding and other compensatory mechanisms—and also characterizing their unique responses to med and non-med therapies. Hence, I realized that the dyslexia in every dyslexic was very different; yet, they were all diagnostically united by a common CVS dysfunction—which also seemed to significantly vary among dyslexics, as did compensation. And a valid dyslexia theory must account for all these variations.

Explaining Kathy's seeming atypical symptomatic panorama To additionally explain all the complex variations rendering Kathy-like dyslexics both unique and typical as well as paradoxical, I was belatedly forced to recognize the co-existing and overdetermined presence of a large number of dynamically interacting lower/older and higher/newer CVS vs. CNS multidimensional variables and vectors that were certainly too complex for the 2-D linear explanations characterizing all other theories of dyslexia—the latter based significantly on *dyslexia = alexia*. So, higher and more complex reasoning and insights were needed to eventually understand the dyslexia syndrome as a 4-D hologram.

Fortunately, all of Kathy's many and complex symptoms and mechanisms—many seemingly atypical— became readily explainable only when viewed retrospectively, after fully conceptualizing my 4-D theory of the dyslexia syndrome. But it's taken 50-plus years of continuously updated and upgraded research and 3-D to 4-D thinking to succeed—no doubt hampered all the way by kryptonite's resistance and/or a baseline need to think 2-D.

Understanding alexia vs. dyslexia was easy By comparison to dyslexia, there are few, if any, unexpected and paradoxical findings in alexia for an obvious reason. Alexia is a relatively "simple" linear disorder: There is only one cerebral reading processor impaired in alexics and only one resulting severe reading comprehension symptom. Although alexic improvements are very unlikely, those occurring would probably involve the very same impaired reading processor, exceptions aside, since there is no compensatory super-cerebral reading processor to help out. And this very same simplistic 2-D thinking level was then likely responsible for theorists creating the mistaken *dyslexia* = *alexia* = *"dyslexia"* concepts—while simultaneously denying Kathy's 4-D multi-symptomatic complexity.

The CVS origin of Kathy's non-reading coexisting dyslexic symptoms As previously postulated and later further demonstrated, all of Kathy's many non-reading symptoms and overlapping disorders characterizing the dyslexia syndrome result when initially normal cerebral and related writing, spelling, math, etc. processors fail to descramble the dizzy signals received from a fine-tuning impairment within the inner-ear/CVS. Moreover, the CVS theory becomes significantly more explanatory—synergistically so—when the super-ten CVS mechanisms discussed in Chap. 17 are added to the existing and more general CVS theory of dyslexia. By contrast, no other dyslexia theory comes close in explanatory capability.

Kathy's favorable response to the CVS enhancers Most importantly, Kathy and her CVS impairment responded amazingly well to CVS meds, as noted in Chap. 23. This response can only be explained by the CVS theory of the dyslexia syndrome, especially when viewed in the context of all of Kathy's other CVS manifestations!

Summary

Needless to say, I could go on and on and explain each of Kathy's many and diverse non-reading symptoms and mechanisms as I did for her dyslexic reading issues. But I believe it is obvious by now that all of Kathy's symptoms are encompassed and clarified by my latest CVS concept of dyslexia and its syndrome. However, for those who would benefit from additional explanatory capability—and synergy—I've added, as previously mentioned, two chapters later in the book. Chapter 16 specifically describes and explains *all* of the CVS-determined reading mechanisms and symptoms in dyslexia that I've thus far discovered. And Chap. 17 provides ten general CVS-determined super-mechanisms formulated to describe and encompass not only *all* of Kathy's symptoms but also those characterizing *all* dyslexics so far examined—more than 35,000 of them. In addition, Kathy's neuroanalysis led me to many other unique insights, which I will additionally discuss in the very next chapter.

And don't forget that my CVS theory also led to an amazing medical treatment for Kathy and 75–85 percent of all dyslexics as well as new medical means of diagnosis and screening. Importantly, this hypothesis also enabled an in-depth understanding of a wide range of previously overlooked puzzling, atypical, and even paradoxical phenomena. So, the CVS concept—especially when "synergized"—most certainly satisfies the criteria used to justify a theory's capability and validity.

Now I will leave it to you readers to decide which of the theories best describes Kathy and all other known dyslexics—and which has the greatest value. However, you may have important questions to ask at this point. So, I will address them in the very next chapter.

Chapter 11
Some Important Q&As: Especially About the Higher Cerebellum and Kathy

Since we are a few chapters short of the halfway point within a book replete with a great deal of new and often complex information to digest, I believe this may be a good time to "pause" and answer a few important questions that might be on your mind.

Important Q&As

1. ***Question:*** You might still be wondering, for example, *How in the world can a dysfunctioning cerebellar-vestibular system (CVS)—man's lower brain—be capable of determining all of the cerebral higher-brain-type speech-linguistic, phonological, memory, and other cognitive symptoms comprising the dyslexia syndrome?*

Answer: I've already explained the basic signal-scrambling and descrambling mechanisms. But there's another highly important angle to the cerebellum that needs to be clarified in order to answer this question. I believe the following neurophysiological insights will shed greater light (refer also to Appendix 1):

The higher cerebellum modulates cerebral-like functions For over a century, most neuroscientists mistakenly believed that the cerebellum or "little brain," the supercomputer for the inner-ear system, controls mainly balance/coordination/rhythm. As a result, all higher functioning/dysfunctioning was naturally, but erroneously, attributed *exclusively* to the thinking brain. And there wasn't a distinguished neurologist or neurophysiologist I could convince otherwise—for decades. This included a colleague on the famed Nobel Scientific Committee that I attempted, but completely failed, to convert while trapped on a Swedish ferry during a dyslexia convention. I feared—justifiably—that he might jump overboard rather than continue listening.

H. N. Levinson, *Feeling Smarter and Smarter*,
https://doi.org/10.1007/978-3-030-16208-5_11

Nevertheless, since only CVS dysfunctioning was found in those with the dyslexia syndrome, I reasoned that *all* observed/reported dyslexia symptoms were CVS determined—certainly those responding favorably to CVS enhancers, unless proven otherwise.

Carrying my reasoning one step further, it seemed very likely to me that the cerebellum must also be performing higher cerebral-like functions.

Background support This novel and "highly original" idea seemed consistent with the fact that the cerebellum is the *highest* brain of many animals and therefore must process all of their sensory motor, memory, and communications as well as some primitive emotional and mental/cognitive functions. And needless to say, via evolution, we retained these "animal capabilities" while growing an even larger cerebellum and higher brain: the cerebral cortex. Because the newest/highest functioning cerebellum and the cerebral cortex simultaneously enlarged together over time, I further reasoned that both brain areas must also be significantly interconnected via feedback circuits—since they have to "talk to" one another in order to maximize their overall functioning.

A similar cerebellar concept was long ago independently arrived at and proposed by several outstanding cerebellar neurophysiologists. For example, Ray Snyder and Averill Stowell at John Hopkins University published *Receiving Areas of the Tactile, Auditory, and Visual Systems in the Cerebellum* (Journal of Neurophysiology, 1944). Although these and other brilliant researchers continued to amplify their highly convincing concepts, it appears that their studies could not be validated until 50 years later. And so, their insights were ignored—denied.

Belated neuroimaging validation Consistent with the slow march of science, independent and highly sophisticated neuroimaging and related neurophysiological research by such outstanding neuroscientists as Leiner, Leiner, and Dow (1991, *Behavioral Brain Research*), quoted below, belatedly verified my deductions, and those of Snyder and Stowell:

> *The role of the cerebellum in these (cognitive and language) human functions has tended to be obscured by the traditional preoccupation with the motor functions of the cerebellum which have been widely observed in other vertebrates as well ... Anatomical evidence and behavioral evidence combine to suggest that this enlarged cerebellum (in the human brain) contributes not only to motor function but also to some sensory, cognitive, linguistic, and emotional aspects of behavior.*

And in a later publication (*The Lancet*, 1998), Rae and colleagues—as well as many, many others—reported, via highly sophisticated magnetic resonance spectroscopy testing, that the cerebellum was directly implicated in dyslexia[1]:

> *Dyslexic people are often uncoordinated with poor balance and delayed motor milestones such as crawling, walking, and learning to ride a bike. Anti-motion sickness medications,*

[1] Since a wide range of neuroimaging publications—thousands—have validated almost all of my clinically derived data thus far presented, as well as the insights to follow, I have included many of these within a special reference category called, Independent Validation—Typical of Thousands.

which may be considered "cerebellar-vestibular stabilizers," have been shown to improve reading performance in dyslexia. The present study has shown significant metabolic abnormalities in the cerebellum in dyslexia.

Importantly, the recognition that the higher cerebellum also modulates linguistic functions further supports my assumption that even phonological processing is likely of a primary CVS vs. cerebral origin, especially since the latter also frequently improves in Kathy-like dyslexics treated with inner-ear/CVS enhancers.

2. ***Question:*** "If what you say and publish is valid, Dr. Levinson, why haven't interested colleagues joined your CVS-determined dyslexia 'bandwagon'? And why has it taken so long?"

Answer: Bias and denial I've already offered my partial answer to this question by pointing out that the traditionalists have been fixated on an oversimplified equation: *dyslexia = alexia = "dyslexia" (or impaired reading comprehension)*. And the reason they couldn't shake free from it was that they never sufficiently studied or listened to dyslexics like Kathy, especially those successfully treated, who would have pointed them in my direction.

I've also frequently alluded to the negative power of "scientific kryptonite"—*bias*. In addition, there's a basic human tendency to resist letting go of older, more familiar, and previously ingrained beliefs, especially those formed in early childhood or early in our careers. Might not this tendency be related to my prior discussion of nature's need for homeostasis? No doubt, it's probably a combination of all of the above, and much more.

However, I have a few additional insights as to why many experts have ignored or rejected my well-documented and validated work, while a few of them just borrowed it and made it their own via improper referencing. If your curiosity is piqued about such matters, I suggest, once again, that you take a look at one of my prior works, *A Scientific Watergate—Dyslexia* and also follow-up content within the Appendices of my latest revision of *Smart But Feeling Dumb*.

And applying an insight related to *embryonic dyslexia*, I arrived at a new understanding as to why some professionals may "neurotically" or defensively resist and/or refute the CVS theory of dyslexia—without providing reasonable scientific cause and/or a more valid alternative hypothesis: Might many need to defensively resist and deny the inhibited but active embryonic CVS/dyslexia syndrome within themselves that *all* definitely still have subconsciously, some even clinically? This would then also explain the otherwise unexplainable *need* for really gifted and dedicated researchers to maintain farfetched—obviously mistaken—cerebral alexia diagnostic criteria for dyslexia so as to define themselves out of the definition and disorder.

If, indeed, the above Freudian-based reasoning has validity, then this "mild" psychological variant of denial—subconsciously refuting an impairment—likely stems from a more primitive biological need called *organic denial*, where, in its initially recognized severe delusional form, lost limbs, for example, are absolutely believed present. (Refer to Q&A # 5, later in this chapter.)

3. ***Question:*** I now hear another valid question clamoring for a response: "Dr. Levinson, what did you learn from Kathy?"

Answer: My short answer: *humility*. I won't quote Goethe again, but I will tell you that I was astounded by the amazing complexity of her disorder which I had studied for many decades and thought I knew thoroughly—but obviously didn't. I was also especially impressed by Kathy's uncanny ability to compensate for her disorder, as well as her magnificent self-reflections and writing style. In fact, her insights led me to add an eighteenth diagnostic category to the self-diagnostic test.

These new Kathy-related insights include the following.

Atypical Sensory Reception and Processing This new eighteenth diagnostic category includes symptoms seemingly related to a dysfunction of gravitational and electromagnetic reception and processing. This category helps explain Kathy's severely impaired sense of direction as well as her occasional inability to instinctively tell up from down—as evidenced by her heading *up* a ladder when she intended to climb *down* and doing the reverse while underwater. Perhaps she was also unable to properly sense upward water displacement and downward pressure. And these symptoms may also explain claustrophobic anxiety or the fear of being trapped in enclosed or shielding environments where predisposed individuals are deprived, or fear deprivation, of vitally needed external stimuli.

While developing this new Kathy-inspired category, which is likely overdetermined, I also added barometric pressure and other sensory inputs and responses that may be *part* of dyslexic or CVS dysregulation, including full-moon-triggered depressive, anxiety, and behavioral dysfunctioning.

Because most of the above symptoms in this category occasionally improved in some of my successfully treated dyslexics, I came to suspect that their determining mechanisms may be, in some possible way, part of the CVS or dyslexia syndrome—or just secondarily related. However, much more research is needed before I feel comfortable with some of these assumptions.

But you might be interested and reassured to learn that Paul Schilder, a brilliant neuropsychiatrist, had postulated a vestibular role in modulating gravity—as well as contributing to mental symptoms—way back in the 1930s. However, he had overlooked the crucial role of the cerebellum, as did most others, leading me to ponder: Why did this *cerebellar denial* exist and persist—a question which I previously discussed in my medical text?

So, as promised, I have also provided you with some fascinating insights into how we, our brain, and especially the CVS, interact with the cosmos and its signals—thanks to Kathy's help and the insights conveyed and/or triggered by many of my other patients, as well.

Freud, Einstein, Kathy, and anecdotal content Perhaps you may now better understand my frequently discussing both Freud and Einstein in a book allegedly having nothing to do with them. Clearly, their contributions were subconsciously linked to both the above paragraphs' content and Kathy's insights as well as the role of bias and its analysis in science, especially dyslexia—themes that run throughout these pages. And this seemingly random, really subconsciously directed, linkage further demonstrates the amazing value of carefully listening to and analyzing Kathy-related anecdotal content. Sadly, some critics refuted this anecdotal content's value and so missed a God-given opportunity to solve the many dyslexia riddles—and so help suffering Kathy-like dyslexics long before I did.

Visual and auditory illusions or pseudo-hallucinations As you might recall, Kathy could hear the words she read, as did many dyslexics I examined. And two of my adult dyslexic patients who heard "voices" were incredibly *relieved* when these psychotic-like symptoms rapidly disappeared on inner-ear enhancers. So, I included these symptoms here, whereas these patients will be presented in a follow-up text.

And another one of my adult patients named Bonnie, in psychotherapy many years ago, *regrettably* lost "hearing" her deceased mother's voice. This hysterical symptom had two determinants: An intense *psychological need* to regain/maintain her lost mother who died during childbirth and a *CVS somatic facilitator* similar to that enabling Kathy-like dyslexics to hear what they are reading and sometimes thinking. I published her psychodynamics in 1966 ("Auditory hallucinations in a case of hysteria," BJP). And her later-diagnosed and treated dyslexia is discussed in my medical text *A Solution to the Riddle—Dyslexia (1980, p. 274).*

Understanding a reading paradox I've already presented this Kathy-inspired insight in the prior chapter, so I will omit duplicating it here. But I did want to remind readers that my understanding of many atypical and seemingly paradoxical findings might not have occurred had I not been supercharged—inspired—by reading Kath's amazingly written self-description.

Better understanding normal reading mechanisms I also arrived at yet another overlooked vital insight after listening to Kathy: By recognizing defective reading mechanisms in dyslexics, we gain an *invaluable mirror-type insight into the many and diverse hidden mechanisms vital for normal reading.* I don't believe this 4-D idea was ever so well understood or clarified before, although Orton and Gullingham came close. And the reason is simple. No one else really ever listened to Kathy-like dyslexics sufficiently enough to overcome their *own hidden instinctive oversimplification or denial mechanisms.*

No doubt, this same oversimplification or 2-D thinking/reasoning mechanism misled me, and all others, way back in 1973. Thus, we viewed dyslexia as if it were merely a severe alexia-like reading impairment of visual origin, albeit characterized by reversals and currently as just a phonological impairment. Fortunately, listening to Kathy-like patients forced me to think in 3-D or 4-D, at least more often.

Clinical research is faster, panoramic As you may have surmised by now, especially after listening to Kathy, clinically based dyslexia research rapidly continues to advance in unpredictable directions, adding new and fascinating insights at every scientific twist and turn. And one can "easily" attempt to verify any new speculation by just listening to, examining, and successfully treating more patients before implementing complex and time consuming, but absolutely necessary, double-blind validating experiments, as thoroughly described in Chap. 5.

Too complex to fully understand Having studied dyslexics and dyslexia for over 50 years, I can emphatically assure you of one thing: There will never be enough Kathy-like patients to render the highly complex dyslexia syndrome completely understood. In fact, this very idea is yet another 2-D illusion fostered upon us by a dyslexic-like oversimplification mechanism. Thus, I concluded my medical text, and this one also with a final line: *The end is just a new beginning!*

Also, you may now better understand my comparing dyslexia research to endlessly peeling an onion, since every layer turns into yet another onion. And so also my other opening statement indicating that understanding the dyslexia syndrome is equivalent to comprehending humanity.

4. ***Question:*** The next question is an obvious corollary to the previous one: "What do you think the traditionalists will derive from Kathy's detailed self-description?"

Answer: Obviously, I can't speak for anyone else. However, if past is prologue, I would have to bet against some hardcore traditionalists ever seeing Kathy the same way I do—and as you may now see her too—especially since her content refutes all their century-old *dyslexia* = *alexia* concepts while supporting my CVS theory.

Sadly, I can hear them saying, "She's just *atypical*" and also that "The verbalizations of patient content is *merely anecdotal* and so has no scientific merit." Well, perhaps it's only her uncanny ability to describe her symptoms that's atypical. And bias may have misled those I've previously referred to as "triple blind" to deny the obvious: that the invaluable clinical anecdotal insights provided by Kathy-like dyslexics have not only led to solutions to all the known dyslexia riddles—they've led to thousands of neuroimaging studies validating all of Kathy's cerebellar-related content (refer to Independent Validating References—Typical of Thousands).

So, I'm optimistic that Max Planck's quote, with which we opened the prior chapter, was right: that a new generation of clinicians and researchers unencumbered by old errors and biased views will continue to benefit from reading Kathy's words and my interpretation of them. And even more importantly, both dyslexics and their dedicated healers will similarly benefit once these insights have sunk in—thus overcoming prior resistance barriers.

5. ***Question:*** And here's a somewhat personal question that also merits a response: "Why do you seem so hard on the dyslexia experts and traditionalists—those you call triple-blind?"

Answer: A great question! I've attempted to answer it previously, in part. But let me try to do so more completely here. My reasons are multifaceted:

Needing a foil By far, the most important reason for being hard on the "experts" in this book is that I sometimes find it useful to create a foil, akin to Superman and kryptonite, so that I can better illustrate contrasting points. In the end, my criticism of the mistaken theorists and traditionalists or experts wasn't any more personal than their criticism of me. And so, my own self-criticism and the analysis of my own limitations and bias also proved highly informative—since it was similarly "impersonal."

Take Critchley, for example. The fact is that I sincerely respected his neurological talents and erudition—and definitely harbored him no ill will. Indeed, I read all of his brilliant neurological works, and he taught me a great deal. I believe the reverse may have been possible, too, had most of my research appeared before or shortly after his.

Accordingly, I was able to use Critchley in good conscience as an example of a highly qualified and universally admired neurologist and dyslexia expert who was nonetheless vulnerable to hidden scientific bias mechanisms—similar to those just reviewed, despite all his "sweated lore." And as repeatedly mentioned, I was a typical traditionalist expert early on who completely agreed with him.

However, were it not for the recognition, analysis, and resolution of my own bias mechanisms and self-criticism—which continues daily—as well as my independent "outsider" nature and psychoanalytic training, I would never have advanced. Indeed, if the famed and erudite Critchley could be so scientifically misled by kryptonite, likely having biological roots (as illustrated here and described in the below footnote),[2] so must we all. Perhaps you now better understand why I credited my Freudian background and training for enabling me to solve the dyslexia riddles.

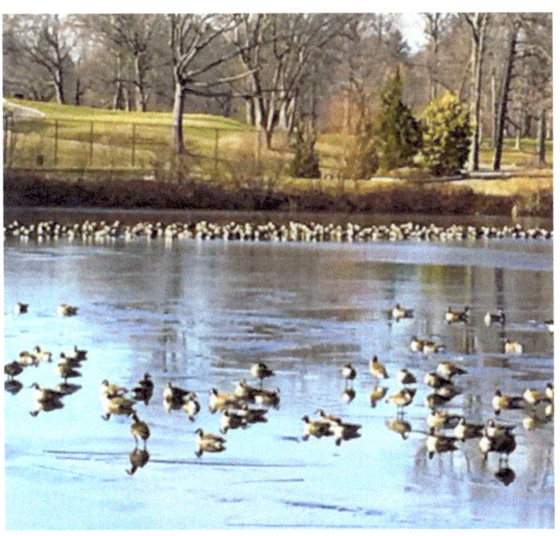

Biological Roots of Bias

[2] ***Possible instinctive origins of bias***—I've repeatedly observed how two species of geese and seagulls seldom, if ever, mingle while shifting across the ice on a nearby lake. Each species maintains its respective territories and herds together. So, I wondered: Might there be an instinctive origin to bias in man—so explaining our varied hardwired prejudices—continuing to resurface and shift, despite pauses? Could these instincts direct us to create and herd in small clubs and even large ones—societies. And also rigidly determine our mental and physical territories which remain susceptible to group-think? Might these herding and territoriality instincts best explain man's resistance to accept alternative ideas and customs—others? Strangers? Do not these very same instincts exist in scientists too—despite their efforts at objectivity? Might these deeply subconscious determinants be denied by man and rationalized—so as to preserve the illusion that he is master in his own house—psyche? Have we not encountered some of these manifestations during this dyslexia research effort? Might we not have discovered, in part, the origins of kryptonite?

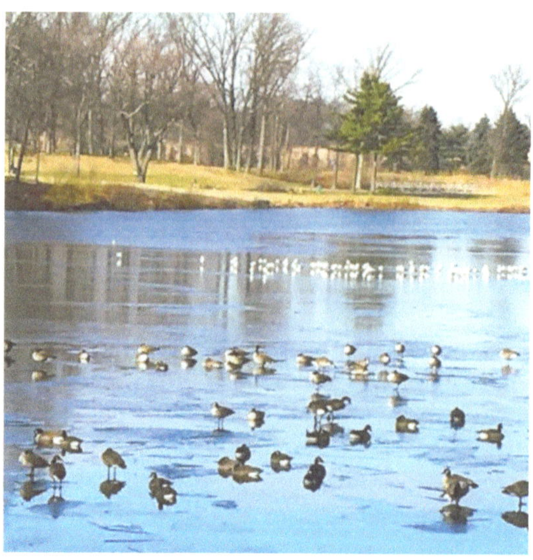

Analyzing critical content and critics During the first two decades of my challenging CVS research effort, it became vital to understand, expose, and so rechallenge the really subjective anecdotal content of many defensive and even offensive traditionalist critics so as to clarify their resistance toward accepting a better clinical and theoretical CVS reality. This process illuminated the hidden—subconscious—motivation and defensive bias mechanism within my critics just as this very same analytic method unmasked the dyslexia syndrome within dyslexics. And among the traditionalists' many motives, as above noted, there was a likely need to deny the embryonic and/or clinical dyslexia within their psyches—previously referred to as organic denial.

All in all: My vigorous response to *negative critics and criticism* refueled my energy to succeed scientifically while also exposing the traditionalists, mistaken assumptions and convictions—and/or defensive rationalizations. And the *positive or justified criticism* of many—including the insights exposed by my self-analysis—enabled me to better clarify my own errors. Thus, criticism and its analysis served to further catalyze my scientific efforts to a successful conclusion.

Although criticism can be harsh and deeply felt, especially to those most altruistic and passionate, its anecdotal content invariably illuminates crucial insights when dealt with scientifically vs. personally. And the success of my Freudian-like analytic method and process inadvertently validates, yet again, the value of objectively using and understanding similar anecdotal content in dyslexia research—with both patients and researchers.

So, in the end, understanding dyslexia was akin to successfully and sufficiently peeling an onion and also simultaneously eliminating—really minimizing—the derailing role of bias. Needless to say, both processes are never-ending and so require super vigilance and determination.

Truth be told, I feel fortunate to have walked a unique scientific dyslexia path never similarly traveled. And also to have analyzed and so transformed negative criticism and its energy—kryptonite—into positive super fuel for further research and an eventual solution to the many dyslexia riddles. So, I do owe the traditionalist dyslexia critics something, perhaps honorable mention.

Benefitting from supporters I must emphasize that not everyone in the "establishment" was resistant to, and so opposed, my challenging research. In fact, I had well-known and gifted clinicians and neurophysiologists who supported my clinically derived CVS concepts and whom I've also mentioned in my prior works. And believe it or not, I even successfully treated the children of establishment experts and executives from opposing—political-like—dyslexia "clubs" who privately agreed with my concepts but were reticent to "go public" out of fear for their positions. And sadly, their reticence was well-founded several decades ago. It's often difficult to believe just how offensive defensive resistance can be. Clearly, the history of man, politics, and science would have been clear sailing were it not for the storms, shipwrecks, and dead ends brought on by nature's negative forces, included within the term kryptonite.

My Second Hippocrates Then there was Sir John Eccles, Nobel Laureate in cerebellar neurophysiology. He became a valued and inspirational ally. His Nobel-winning insights into *cerebellar signal inhibition, regulation, and cerebellar learning* led me to unique understandings that were crucial to my evolving research and resulting dyslexia and also phobia concepts (refer to Chaps. 13 and 15).

After our initial personal contact at The Rockefeller University, this brilliant, kind, and generous scientist supported my cerebellar-based dyslexia and phobia research professionally and personally. Perhaps most significantly, he inspired me to continue moving dispassionately forward, despite entrenched initial opposition.

And he helped, despite his own well-justified skepticism about my original speculations of higher cerebellar functioning—which could not be proven at the time we first became friendly. The neuroimaging and related techniques needed to find the hidden cerebellar-cerebral circuits, postulated to exist based on my dyslexia research and that of Snyder and Stowell, were not yet available—not for another decade or two. Nevertheless, Eccles really helped and inspired me over the years—as I tried to do for my students and patients. And in doing so, he became my second Hippocrates.

6. ***Questions:*** And now before moving on, I'd like to turn the tables and ask *you* a couple of questions that are important to me: "What do you think of Kathy and her dyslexic symptoms? Were these last few chapters helpful to you in better understanding this complex, previously misunderstood disorder that may have devastated you or someone you love? Or patients of yours? And are you now more hopeful of a successful treatment and overall outcome than ever before?"

Your responses will reach me at dyslexiaonline.com. And I assure you that I will read them with care and interest. After you finish this book, of course!

7. ***Question:*** Perhaps you're wondering: "What ever happened to Kathy? How did she respond to treatment?"

Answer: Don't worry; you'll read about her feedback later on in the book, in fact, within Chap. 23. But I can promise you one thing: that Kathy's favorable treatment responses to CVS enhancers, which were achieved rapidly and effortlessly, will inspire you as they did me. And they further support and explain the validity of my dyslexia theory and the CVS syndrome it encompasses. In fact, no other dyslexia theory has led to such an amazing med treatment. Nor can any other dyslexia theory explain Kathy's beneficial response.

8. ***Question:*** One last question: "Dr. L, you've been contrasting alexia with dyslexia from the very beginning of this book in order to prove that the traditionalist equation *dyslexia* = *alexia* is completely mistaken. Yet the concept you use about alexia is over-simplistic— incomplete. Doesn't that mean that the concluding differences you've drawn about dyslexia and alexia are possibly incorrect?"

Answer: Your question is very logical. Thus, I had already answered it within the Preface, footnote 1. I will, however, reemphasize that the mistaken alexia influence on dyslexia research persists—despite the growing understanding of alexia since Dejerine's initial descriptions in 1891 and 1892, as well as my repeated distinctions between these two disorders since 1973.

As this answer was short, I'll allow one additional question.

9. ***Question:*** "How is it that no other dyslexia expert significantly factored into their theories and definitions the role of compensation and the fact that the dyslexia in dyslexics is characteristically different?"

Answer: Clearly, the reading impairment in alexia is dramatically less complex and diverse as well as infinitely more severe than that in dyslexia and rarely compensates. So, if *dyslexia* = *alexia* is mistakenly believed by traditionalist researchers, then there is only one impaired reading mechanism in dyslexia—a reading incomprehension deficit which is always severe. Thus, why would experts build multiple CVS reading and non-reading mechanisms and compensatory concepts into their dyslexia theories and definitions that do not apply to alexia?

Chapter 12
Another Remarkable Case: Highlighting the Dyslexia/ADD/ADHD/Phobia Connection

All parents are primarily interested in helping their reading- or learning-disabled and ADHD children, especially those who are also anxiety ridden—and as quickly as possible. That's *their* bottom line. With that in mind, let's get back to looking at some real, successfully treated cases, as these patients provide the greatest understanding and hope to all other suffering dyslexics and their parents.

John Whitney's symptoms, as you'll see, clearly illustrate the vital—but previously unknown—connection between CVS dysfunction and dyslexia, ADD/ADHD, and phobias. Also, the dramatic favorable responses of his three seemingly different CVS-related disorders to inner-ear-/CVS-enhancing medications serve to further validate this link, especially when his symptomatic triad is echoed loudly, clearly, and repeatedly by thousands of other patients such as those we have seen—and will continue to see in this book.

H. N. Levinson, *Feeling Smarter and Smarter*,
https://doi.org/10.1007/978-3-030-16208-5_12

John Whitney

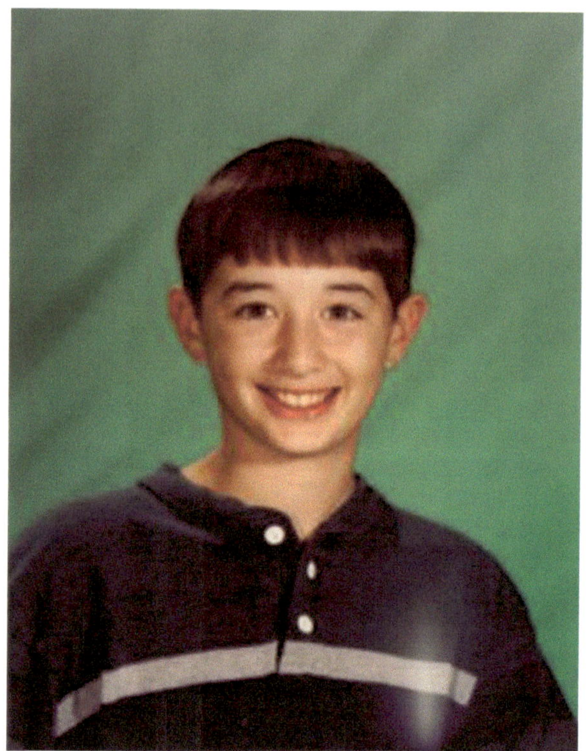

Overlapping Disorders: Dyslexia, ADD/ADHD, Phobias

Before we read Mrs. Whitney's detailed description of her son, I believe you will benefit from my briefly reviewing his overlapping dyslexia, ADD/ADHD, and phobic symptoms.

Dyslexia-Related Symptoms When I first examined and treated John, he was almost 11 years old and about to enter sixth grade. His sight-reading was on a late fourth grade level, and his writing and spelling were severely impaired. Worst of all, he felt dumb.

ADD-/ADHD-Related Symptoms His attention span was short, and he was very restless, easily distracted, and frustrated.

Fears/Phobias/Anxiety Disorder Symptoms John demonstrated a fear of heights when confronting elevators, bridges, and amusement park rides. And he was fearful—even panicky—about facing new, unfamiliar, and unanticipated situations.

Mrs. Whitney's Description of John

Since John's mother is a gifted teacher with LD experience, she is the most capable of describing her son's symptoms—both educationally and clinically, as well as his improvements on inner-ear-/CVS-improving medications.

> ***Background information:*** *John was verbal very early—by 18 months he talked in sentences, fluently by age two. He was a bright and well-adjusted preschool child and had no apparent problems in junior or senior kindergarten. However, by the start of first grade he could not remember or recognize the simple word combinations of the "-it" words (i.e., sit, fit, hit, bit, etc.). And he could not tell the difference between the letters "b" and "d." He reversed "on" for "no" and "saw" for "was." He did not read endings of words like "-ed" or "-ing" or "-s." He memorized small storybooks but could not read the actual words. And he had difficulty tracking the words down a page without using a ruler or his finger. He often reread the same words as he lost his place. And he would often substitute another word with a similar meaning for a word he was reading. All of the above are classic manifestations of dyslexia.*
>
> *His grade 2 teacher did not believe he had a learning disability or reading problem and said he would outgrow his [letter and spelling] reversals by age 8. But I knew or felt otherwise—although I did not know what was wrong with him.*
>
> *John had a fantastic third-grade teacher. After the first week and half of school, she showed my husband and I that John could not recognize the word "the." She recommended a tutor who worked with John for the next three years. Despite tutoring, he still could not recognize many words or word endings. And he read only from the contextual clues provided by meanings and pictures. He read better silently than orally—but remained behind despite all our efforts.*
>
> *He wrote good story ideas and dialogues but his mechanical errors and spelling were awful. His handwriting was large with irregular spacing. And he evidenced trouble maintaining an even margin or straight columns.*
>
> *John's spelling was his version of phonics. He did not get many letters correct in a word and so seldom got a word spelled correctly. (He could not spell or read small words.)*
>
> *In grade 4, John complained about headaches if he were asked to read for more than ten minutes. At first I thought that he just did not want to read. Eventually we took him to an optometrist who said he had a visual-perceptual problem and needed prism lenses, despite 20/20 vision. With the use of these prisms, his headaches disappeared and his tracking improved. However, his reversals with letters and poor writing and spelling, as well as concentration/distractibility symptoms, remained.*
>
> *Additionally, I had John tested by a psychologist in fourth grade. She also said that he had a visual-perceptual problem but diagnosed him as learning-disabled—definitely not dyslexic. Why? Because his silent reading level was appropriate for his age despite the fact that his oral level was on a 2.2 grade level. I watched Dr. Levinson on the Canadian National Television Show,* CBC News World, *with Pamela Wallin as host. His inner-ear dyslexic theory made sense to me because it explained John's brightness and how the information he received did not always go into his brain and come out correctly and that John felt just like the title of Dr. Levinson's book, Smart But Feeling Dumb.*
>
> *Coincidentally, I met three other parents who had taken their children to see Dr. Levinson. All the children had improved to differing degrees. Thank God I decided to consult with Dr. Levinson. His treatment has given John a completely new and positive life. John's improvements in self-esteem, reading, writing, spelling, concentration, anxiety, coordination, and overall school performance have been miraculous.*

Our Visit to Dr. Levinson

Mrs. Whitney's Account Continues

Following his exam with Dr. Levinson, my husband and I were relieved to learn that John had dyslexia with slight degrees of ADD as well as phobias. His specific phobias included fears of heights, elevators, bridges, and amusement rides, as well as a fear of new situations. A medical treatment plan was formulated.

And to psychologically help John's poor self-esteem, we were advised to read with him two books written by Dr. L. to help children better understand themselves and all their symptoms: The Upside-Down Kids and Turning Around the Upside-Down Kids.

John loved these books and said throughout, "See, I told you I felt like this." Clearly, these books were written from inside a dyslexic child's head. And so, they helped us truly understand dyslexics and what caused their many and differing symptoms. This understanding enabled all of us to bond with John's symptoms and feelings and enabled John to recognize that his disorder was not his own fault—and was not due to the fact that he was stupid.

Just as Dr. Levinson had predicted, John never responded to our compliments. He did not believe how smart he really was—until he listened to and understood the content and symptoms described within these books.

Responses to Treatment

John's response to medication treatment was truly revealing.

His Mom's Initial Observations

As advised, John started with a quarter of the first pill. He then went to a large amusement park with his friends. He came home that night and said, "It's kinda weird. I went on all the rides today and even walked on the outside of the steps to the tall slide. And I was not even frightened. It couldn't be that pill I took did it?" He had been to this park two weeks before with his cousins and would not ride the large twisted water slide because it was too high. He was only on the first quarter pill. Our whole family was doubtful. But it was *the pill! And as he continued to take his medications over the next few weeks, he continued to amaze us with such unsolicited comments as, "My eyes stay stuck to the Nintendo," "I can do puzzles I could not do last week," "I can listen more clearly," "The words and letters do not move on the page." He also started to read word endings and lost his place less frequently. His tutor and his Special Education teacher both were amazed at the positive changes in his memory and concentration, as well as at his reading and spelling improvements. The most amazing change was his handwriting. It shrunk in size and spacing dramatically over the next three months and continued to improve over the rest of the year.*

Improved Grade Scores: After Treatment – By January, after only 3½ months on the medications, his BRIGANCE test scores went up two to three grade levels. His special education teacher was amazed. We all watched him grow and blossom in leaps and bounds. One day John became very excited: "I can see the whole word and page in my head instead of only parts. And I can track the whole word and sentence without losing my place as before."

His BRIGANCE scores for March continued to improve: Sight Reading – grade six, Oral Reading – grade six, and Silent Comprehension – grade seven. All scores at grade level. His spelling scores are also amazing. If he studies the words for a couple of minutes each week, he can get twenty out of twenty correct. And even his free-written spelling has dramatically improved. Before treatment, he could not get more than two to three words correct on a page and made several errors in a single word. After treatment, he'll make only three or four very simple errors on a page of writing (and the errors are only one-letter omissions).

John's Fearless Television Debut

Among John's many improvements, none were more dramatic than the reduction—and disappearance—of his fears and anxiety:

John and I were asked by Dr. Levinson to appear with him on the TV show we had watched the previous year, CBC News World. *When I told John I would like to talk about him on national television, his immediate reaction was, "Why am* I *not going to talk about myself on TV? I know more about how I feel than you do." He and I appeared on the TV show together and John was terrific. The producer said, "The kid's a star. (Refer to "It's a true miracle!"* http://www.dyslexiaonline.com/media/media.html*) John was a shy eleven-year-old boy who would never have had the confidence to appear on television. On the way home from the TV station he confirmed this by stating, "I'd never have gone on the show if it weren't for the medications. I'm not as shy or fearful of new situations as before."*

The television opportunity was a wonderful experience for my son. John also said after the show, "I don't care who knows I have a learning disability. Because I hope their parents will listen to me and get their kids the same help I got." I have since received, on average, about two to three phone calls per week from strangers who have been referred to me as a result of John's television appearance.

The next evening John and I went to a lecture given by Dr. Levinson—where John talked to several parents who were concerned about their children's learning. He would never have had the confidence to talk freely about himself to adult strangers—or any stranger—before.

Mrs. Whitney's Summary

The most visually dramatic external change can be seen in John's handwriting. Before Dr. Levinson's treatment, John's handwriting was large and dysgraphic: it had irregular spaces, the margins were on an angle, he crowded work into the corners of a page, and it was generally hard to decipher and very messy. It is now neat, controlled, and very small in size. He starts at a margin and keeps it aligned. There are no large irregular spaces. It is easy to read and neat on the page. He also does not have large black eraser marks throughout the writing. And John remarked that he does not grind his pencil or eraser into the desk anymore. He claims to listen more clearly and is driven to do neater work and takes pride in it. He even wants to come in from recess early to finish his work properly.

Seeing Is Believing: Writing Samples Before and After Treatment

Med-triggered writing improvements No doubt, seeing is believing. So, here is an actual before and after treatment sample of John's writing. Although I've frequently seen med-triggered improvements such as these—as have you by recalling Meg Fex in Chap. 2—each and every such rapid, dramatic, and effortless treatment response appears miraculous, especially since there were no other factors influencing this change. And all prior repetitive attempts to help his writing and spelling were merely frustrating failures. In most cases, cessation of meds after a short trial results in regression, although this wasn't tried with John for obvious reasons. He came for help—not experimentation. However, I have many cases where meds were stopped prior to surgery and for other reasons and where regression in the patients' drawings and in other med-triggered improvements rapidly occurred.

Dysgraphia is diagnostic The first *dysgraphic* writing sample prior to medications is typically diagnostic of dyslexics, or rather those with CVS-determined grapho-motor dyscoordination, although there are significant exceptions for nearly all of the symptoms found characterizing the dyslexia syndrome.

Overdetermined and compensatory mechanisms I have, as patients, dyslexic artists who can draw their writing, and so their *cerebrally determined calligraphy* is magnificent, whereas their uncompensated *CVS-determined reflex* writing dysfunctioning remains illegible.[1]

In other words, most dyslexic symptoms are overdetermined. And compensatory cerebral and higher cerebellar vectors often strengthen over time—even in the untreated. So, their writing and Goodenough figure drawing samples often slowly improve with age, despite the subclinical persistence of the CVS impairment. This is similar to what may also happen to their initial reading and spelling and just about all the other symptoms that characterize this fascinating syndrome. Accordingly, those professionals predicting gloom and doom based on early impairments—before compensatory mechanisms kick in—are betting in the dark. And sadly, the same is sometimes true for unfounded optimism—although significant improvements are far likelier than stagnation or regression due to maturational factors. However, the following improvements often occur in treated cases.

Importantly, the ensuing simple visual writing samples, when neuroanalyzed, dramatically highlight the quality and essence of the dyslexic disorder as well as the therapeutic benefits often obtained for all dyslexic-related symptoms, not only those affecting writing and spelling.

[1] To be crystal clear: The reflex writing involving script, print, and drawing appear to have differing determining and overdetermining mechanisms and circuits among dyslexics, explaining why these functions are separately impaired and respond differently to the CVS enhancers. And the same complex and dynamic considerations hold for many of the other symptoms and characteristics found among dyslexics. Thus, for example, it is quite common that dyslexics have difficulty with algebra and yet are gifted in geometry, and vice versa, and even good with the multiplication tables, except for 7 × 6 or recalling the 6s. And I even have a gifted mathematician who can't perform simple addition, subtraction, and multiplication without a calculator. So, one must assume the presence of distinct circuits for each of these many functions and sub-functions.

John's Dysgraphic Writing and Spelling: Prior to Med Treatment

John's Writing and Spelling Dramatically Improved: After Only Several Months on a Simple Inner-Ear-Enhancing Antihistamine

The door creaked as it opened, and I felt a cold, stale gust of wind.

Never again will I have such a birthday party

Mrs. Whitney Continues

John's Special Education teacher said she has noted improvements in his organizational skills, his spelling strategies, his tracking of words on a page, and his attitude and self-esteem in general. He also does not panic when he is frustrated or lost in his work or a new situation. And he tries to correct his work on his own.

John has said that his eyes read the whole word, he likes to read, he can spell, the letters and words do not move around, he concentrates and listens better, he has a new pride in his work, and he does not fear heights associated with elevators or bridges anymore. Amusement park rides and swings do not frighten or nauseate him anymore. New situations no longer panic him, and he is willing to take more risks with a new sense of personal self-confidence. He is also amazed by his new controlled handwriting style. His Nintendo game-playing skills have also improved dramatically. He told me that in one baseball game he now gets twenty-three out of thirty hits, whereas he used to get only three out of thirty hits. And he says that since treatment his eyes are stuck to the game, unlike before where his eyes wandered away from the screen.

Thanks to Dr. Levinson's research and dedication, John is a whole new child. And he is happier with his newfound abilities and confidence.

Sincerely,

Mrs. Janice Whitney

Final Thoughts

John's many and diverse symptoms and their favorable responses to inner-ear/CVS-improving medications clearly support the inner-ear or CVS origins of *dyslexia—the syndrome*—that I've been describing throughout this book. In addition, an analysis of John's varied improvements simultaneously highlights and validates a hidden scientific connection never before clearly recognized and reported: *that dyslexia, ADD/ADHD, and phobias or anxiety disorders are all interrelated reflections of this very same CVS dysfunction.* And because of its vital importance, this correlation will be examined further and clarified in the chapters to follow.

Chapter 13
Making the Connections: An Introductory Overview

Were it not for the invaluable insights provided by dyslexic patients like John Whitney as well as those offered by his mom's detailed observations, who would have initially thought that there was a neurophysiological connection between *dyslexia*, *attention-deficit hyperactivity/impulsivity*, and *phobias/anxieties*? And who would have thought that all three of these differently named symptom clusters or disorders were determined by inner-ear/CVS dysfunctioning?

Certainly not I! And certainly no other clinical researcher made this connection! Indeed, most experts viewed and defined these three separately named impairments quite differently, though many did belatedly recognize them as often overlapping or comorbid. And most experts were, and unfortunately still are, convinced that these disorders stem from completely different origins and so must likely respond to completely different therapies.

Because this linkage is as important as it is surprising and challenging, I decided to provide a brief introductory overview of these disorders before going into further details in the chapters to follow.

Traditional Definitions and Hypothesized Sites of Origin: Dyslexia vs. ADD/ADHD vs. Phobias/Anxiety Disorder

Dyslexia Dyslexia, as I've repeatedly stated, was misdefined by traditionalists as a severe alexia-like reading comprehension disorder of cerebral origin in which otherwise normal individuals were required, until recently, to be two or more years behind their peers or their potential in order to "qualify" for a diagnosis. And the traditionally accepted treatment of choice was, and still is, referral for Special Ed. In other words, the traditionalists had, and have, no way of medically treating dyslexia. So, after examinations or testing, they refer these patients away. More recently, dyslexia has been redefined by some neotraditionalists as a phonologically caused reading

H. N. Levinson, *Feeling Smarter and Smarter*,
https://doi.org/10.1007/978-3-030-16208-5_13

disorder of cerebral linguistic origin—with a corresponding conditioning treatment. We've already reviewed these mistaken or limited concepts in previous chapters and will further elaborate on them in Chap. 18 dealing with many helpful therapies.

ADD/ADHD ADD/ADHD is traditionally defined as a cluster of concentration, distractibility, impulsivity, and activity symptoms. And to qualify for this diagnosis, a child must exhibit six out of the nine symptoms listed in the DSM-V. Since this definition is primarily quantitatively or statistically determined, it suffers from a similar drawback to the dyslexia definition. Thus, the current ADHD/ADHD diagnosis also significantly excludes all mildly and even some moderately suffering patients—and so requires urgent reworking.

Fortunately, individuals diagnosed with ADD/ADHD, as well as the milder cases failing to qualify for this diagnosis, often respond rapidly and favorably to stimulant medications (e.g., Ritalin, Dexedrine/Adderall/Vyvanse, etc.). Although there have been as many hypothesized causes for ADD/ADHD as dyslexia, traditionally directed research now suggests a dysfunction within the front part of the thinking brain and/or corresponding neurotransmitter/receptor difficulties at this site (refer to Chap. 14 for significant and new insights).

Phobias and related anxiety disorders Phobias and related anxiety disorders were, and are, defined as exaggerated anxiety states without obvious *realistic* causes or triggers. These include fears of heights, elevators, crowds, snakes, leaving home, and other triggers, as well as panic states and even repetitive thoughts and actions called obsessive-compulsive disorder (OCD).

Although these mental symptoms were considered primarily emotional or psychological in origin years ago, many researchers now believe that these disorders are significantly due to neurochemical dysfunctioning. And more recent pharmacological data indicate a favorable response of anxiety to the antidepressant/anti-panic selective serotonin reuptake inhibitors (SSRIs)—of which Prozac is the most widely known and prescribed—as well as other meds to be later described, including the serotonin-norepinephrine reuptake inhibitors (SNRIs).

Finding a Common Link

As you can imagine, it required considerable clinical efforts to initially discover a previously unsuspected connection between dyslexia, ADD/ADHD, phobias, and CVS deficits. Once again, the credit for this discovery must be given to my patients. All I did was initially listen to, observe, examine, and belatedly treat them.

After successfully treating large numbers of dyslexics like John Whitney for their reading and related learning difficulties by using CVS-enhancing antihistamines, many of these CVS-dysfunctioning individuals began revealing to me all the vital insights required to make the abovementioned connections. And the inner-ear/CVS link "suddenly" materialized—as you will now see for yourself in many other cases. Only recently have neuroimaging studies independently validated this linkage (refer to References A-Independent Validating References—Typical of Thousands).

Four Cases that Validate the Connection

Here are summarized reports about four SLD (specific learning disability) patients of mine who responded favorably to medication. They are representative of the thousands of cases that prompted—forced—me to "make the connection" between the inner-ear/CVS and the triad of dyslexia, ADD/ADHD, and phobias.

John Wood

An adult patient of mine, John Wood, wrote:

> *Dr. Levinson, my reading and writing are better. But so is my concentration. I can read for much longer without burning out. Distractions are not as bothersome. I don't get as frustrated easily. And I'm not so impulsive. I feel calmer, not as restless.*
>
> *My balance is better. I'm no longer accident-prone. In fact, my golf is significantly improved—it's easier to concentrate and coordinate.*
>
> *A funny thing happened. I'm no longer afraid of heights and carnival rides. And I don't get so overloaded and panicky in crowded/noisy places. Now I can be in a crowded supermarket or a library crowded with books and even a crowded noisy party without becoming anxious. Are these improvements related? Are they due to chance? Or are my fears improving because I don't feel as klutzy, inept, and stupid as before? In fact, I was just asked to present a report at work. And I did—without notes and without panic. I could never do that before.*

Andrew

His mother writes:

> *Dr. Levinson, since starting my son Andrew on your non-stimulant meds, his reading didn't improve as much as I expected. But he's no longer as restless or distracted as before. He can sit still in class and pay attention to the teacher without squirming, getting-up, or falling out of his chair.*
>
> *He's not fighting with everyone as much—especially his siblings. He's less sensitive than before. And spontaneously he told me, "Mom, now I feel I have a brain."*
>
> *There's something else too. He falls asleep—and is no longer afraid of the dark or being alone. Before, we'd find him in our bed or sleeping with his brother. Now he is comfortable sleeping alone. His nightmares and sleepwalking are gone and he no longer bed-wets.*
>
> *Also, he's not afraid of getting on the school bus. Before, he'd delay and stall, so we'd have to drive him. Now he says he's no longer dizzy and nauseated on the bus.*

And the same is true in the car. Before, he'd fight us and absolutely refuse to go in the back seat. Now he tells us that he used to get dizzy and anxious in the back and felt much better in the front seat when he would look out the window.

Another thing. He now goes up and down escalators. Before, he'd panic coming down. So, we had to either walk or take the elevator.

He's also much more assertive now. He'll speak up for himself without being merely argumentative as before. It's as if he's no longer fearful of sounding stupid as before.

Linda

Her mother observes:

Since starting Linda on your antihistamine medication, we had to reduce the Ritalin she was previously given by another physician for her concentration, distractibility, and hyperactivity. It's like the two medications were working together.

But now she's reading and writing so much better. This didn't happen on the Ritalin, even though Ritalin really helped her ADHD.

After raising the antihistamine dose, as you requested, in order to see if we could give her more help academically, two things happened that shocked us. We no longer needed the Ritalin as before—and still had the same results. She claimed to feel more comfortable on elevators and escalators. And she said the fluorescent lights in the school and other places were no longer "driving me crazy." Are all these things related?

Sheila

Sheila is an adult who had difficulty reading and writing. Her balance was severely impaired, even when she wasn't feeling terribly dizzy. After responding favorably to medication, she reported:

Dr. Levinson, I'm no longer fearful of leaving my house alone. Before, I'd panic when having to cross a street by myself. Now I do so unassisted. It's like I'm no longer fearful of losing my balance... losing control... fainting with cars coming and going and no one there to assist me should this happen. Now I can walk anywhere instead of having to walk next to buildings or use a walker or umbrella or even an empty cart to hold on to so as to prevent falling in the middle of oncoming traffic. I never told you this—and you never asked—but I've been in therapy for years for agoraphobia. Your simple medications cured me of my agoraphobia... Is this an accident?

Questions I Initially Asked Myself

Is it just an atypical coincidence that ADD/ADHD and phobic/anxiety symptoms improved in CVS-impaired dyslexics or learning disabled who were given inner-ear/CVS-improving medications or that for a few patients, the anti-motion sickness meds worked similarly to, or even better than, stimulants for their ADD/ADHD symptoms? Is it merely by chance that balance, coordination, motion, and sensory-motor-determined fears similarly improved, together with ADD/ADHD symptoms, in inner-ear/CVS-dysfunctioning dyslexics?

At first I didn't really know the answers to these questions. But the coincidence was just too significant to ignore. And the possible linkage was too tantalizing for a clinical researcher like me to resist over time and in the face of ever-accumulating patient-based experiences.

Eventually I demonstrated that inner-ear/CVS-dysfunctioning mechanisms similar to the ones responsible for the "typical" dyslexic symptoms also triggered ADD/ADHD and phobias. And there existed a very significant overlap (70–90 percent) of dyslexia, ADD/ADHD, and phobic manifestations in *referred*, and so likely more severely impaired, patients when their stringent diagnostic criteria were lessened. Importantly, the overlap is less in milder non-referred cases.

We'll discuss and clarify these fascinating CVS connections as well as the corresponding ADD/ADHD and phobic disorders over the next few chapters. Needless to say, there were many cases where this triad did not occur—and their analysis proved just as insightful. Thus, I was led to conclude for patients with the CVS syndrome that only by understanding all the data, especially the diverse exceptions, will the ultimate rule be unmasked. And to a large degree, it has.

Two Independent Validations from Space

Around the time I was initially correlating these previously disconnected "dots," a couple of "messages from outer space" came though loudly and clearly, helping to confirm my suspicions about the wide range of conditions in which the inner-ear/cerebellum played a vital role.

NASA's Neurochemical Confirmation

The National Aeronautics and Space Agency (NASA) scientists tested a whole spectrum of medications many years ago in order to minimize space sickness in the astronauts. They found that, in addition to the anti-motion sickness meds, stimulants used to successfully treat ADD/ADHD, as well as anti-panic medications (e.g., Valium, Xanax) and antidepressants (e.g., Tofranil and probably the SSRIs and SNRIs which were not yet discovered at the time) used to treat anxiety/depressive disorders, are all somewhat *effective in preventing or minimizing motion/space sickness.*

Thus, I reasoned that they all must be considered inner-ear/CVS-enhancing medications to at least some minimal extent, albeit likely using diverse mechanisms and having differing efficacies. And I was again and again forced to wonder: Are these correlations due to chance alone? Or is there also a hidden—but important—

neurochemical supporting link?[1] If all of these very different medications, which were used to treat seemingly different disorders, are targeting the inner-ear/cerebellum in some way, then it was possible that all of these disorders shared a common inner-ear/CVS origin. Maybe these weren't entirely different disorders at all but merely unique manifestations of the same complex syndrome yet to be significantly unmasked.

The French Connection: The Inner-Ear and Space Dyslexia

Either by chance or destiny, I was also sent a correspondence by a medical scientist monitoring the French space program. And to my surprise, he reported that astronauts at zero gravity not infrequently begin reading upside-down and backward—a condition I termed "space dyslexia."

Quite clearly, the anti-motion sickness medications tended to prevent space sickness and "space dyslexia" for many astronauts. Once again, these reported clinical observations both highlighted and further validated the hidden link concerning the inner-ear/CVS origin and treatment of dyslexia and related conditions.

Convictions About the Connections

Over the past several decades, I've studied many, many additional patients with a vast array of dyslexia/ADD/ADHD/phobia symptoms, as well as associated inner-ear/CVS dysfunctioning. And I've explored and described their interrelated connections and links in many research papers and books. As a result, I am confident about the correlations between these seemingly unrelated impairments and their CVS-determined mechanisms—mainly because my patients in the past provided me with the proof, just as they are now doing for you. All of these amazing and startling discoveries—and many more—were ready and waiting to be made. Once again, only one thing was required—listening to patients and asking them some simple questions and, of course, observing and analyzing their favorable responses to inner-ear-/CVS-enhancing meds.

Remember that the value of a theory lies in its ability to encompass and explain all the relevant data—both the typical and atypical—as well as *lead to* new and unexpected insights. As you've also previously read, the simplest explanations are usually the best.

---

[1] Follow-up NASA studies suggest the presence of significant differences between motion and space sickness as well as the medications helpful for these syndromes. In addition, medications appear to have uniquely distinct effects in normal vs. zero-gravity situations.

Fortunately, the inner-ear/CVS theory of dyslexia and related disorders meets *all* of these vital scientific benchmarks. But you will have to read the next chapters for these new understandings to be more fully clarified and better appreciated. Only then will you all likely believe, and even feel, that these uncanny, previously overlooked correlations are true. Perhaps even skeptics will also agree.

Chapter 14
New Insights into ADD/ADHD

The aim of this chapter is to provide you with many new and important insights into ADD/ADHD that go substantially beyond what is traditionally understood about this impairment. In addition to my discussion on an added helpful classification of ADD/ADHD, three successfully treated children will teach you how to best understand and overcome this disorder. And several others will even demonstrate that the inner-ear antihistamines may sometimes—atypically—be more effective than stimulants, and why.

In fact, it's now possible to improve the whole CVS syndrome in patients with this overdetermined ADD/ADHD impairment—including its dyslexic, phobic, psychosomatic and other related segments. As you will see, many patients diagnosed with ADD/ADHD often remain inadequately described and treated, since the rest of their complex CVS syndrome is too often ignored or denied. So let's proceed—since I'm sure all of you will significantly benefit from the following insightful content—much of it novel.

Some ADD/ADHD Characteristics

ADHD* vs. *Dyslexia ADD/ADHD has become the most diagnosed mental disorder in children. In fact, it has all but replaced dyslexia in the minds of most teachers and medical practitioners, despite the fact that dyslexia was in the educational/medical limelight for over a century—long before ADD/ADHD was recognized as a diagnostic entity and given credence.

No doubt, many are wondering, as did I, why this switch occurred, especially since these different appearing, but frequently overlapping, disorders represent two sides of one multifaceted "CVS coin." And as usual, this question triggered a likely explanation: Once the stimulant treatment for ADD/ADHD became accepted, pharmaceutical companies invested large sums toward enhancing the research and education needed to sell their meds. And it worked miracles.

H. N. Levinson, *Feeling Smarter and Smarter*,
https://doi.org/10.1007/978-3-030-16208-5_14

By contrast, dyslexia research remained stagnated by the traditionalist fixation to a mistaken *dyslexia = alexia* theory—leading nowhere insofar as medical advances. And their experts refused to acknowledge my new all-encompassing and fully explanatory CVS theory and its successful med treatment, preferring to stay put and/or reinvent imperfect lookalikes.

Thus, vitally needed independent validating research was resisted until dyslexia, as traditionally understood, was deemed dead in the water by the DSM-V. Hopefully, the insights within this chapter and book will rekindle new advances for both these and other related disorders having common CVS origins—for the well-being of countless millions.

ADHD's likely causation and links Though ADD/ADHD's exact neurophysiological causation remains admittedly unknown by most researchers, many believe that this disorder has genetic and neurochemical cerebral determinants within the brain's frontal lobe. Despite the fact that most clinicians and investigators now understand that learning, anxiety, and mood disorders are very frequently overlapping or comorbid in ADD/ADHD, none of them have scientifically recognized what you have already learned—that ADD/ADHD is part of a far larger and more complex CVS syndrome, exceptions aside.

Since this linkage becomes more apparent when the stringent DSM-V criteria are loosened, it appears that the currently used diagnostic rigidity may distort the population studied, e.g., misleading us to believe that all with dyslexia and/or ADD/ADHD have only moderate to severe impairments.

The current diagnosis of ADHD As I noted earlier, the current diagnosis of ADD/ADHD in children is dependent on their displaying six of nine core symptoms listed in the DSM-V, such as *often fails to give close attention to details*, *often does not follow through on instructions*, and *often has difficulty organizing tasks and activities*. Currently, this disorder, affecting over 11 percent of children, is recognized to comprise three types: (1) inattention or ADD, (2) hyperactivity and impulsivity, and (3) combined. The symptoms within each type include:

- *Inattention or ADD symptoms*: inattentive, daydreaming, distractible, forgetful, as well as having difficulty listening, organizing, and completing tasks
- *Hyperactivity symptoms*: difficulty sitting or staying still or quiet—always moving
- *Impulsivity symptoms*: trouble waiting for others to complete talking and actions—blurting out or interrupting and difficulty inhibiting anger and frustrations

Dr. Paul Wender's Brilliant Clinical Connection

As previously mentioned, in reviewing the scientific literature for validation of my inner-ear/cerebellar theory of dyslexia and ADHD, I discovered that Dr. Paul Wender, the well-recognized ADHD pioneer, had long ago clarified many of the above symptoms.

Two important correlations Wender reported two *statistically correlated* characteristics of ADD/ADHD—*the true significance of which was largely overlooked by all, Wender included:*

- "School difficulties related to dyslexia, Learning Disabilities, or the recently named Specific Developmental Disorder." (They are all basically synonyms.)
- "Impairment in balance and coordination, including fine and gross motor incoordination, often resulting in handwriting and eye-tracking difficulties."

An unwitting discovery Without specifically recognizing the connection of ADD/ADHD and dyslexia (LD/SLD) to a dysfunctioning CVS (impaired balance/coordination), and thus without any *favorable bias* toward my research, Wender reported that among ADD/ADHD patients:

1. 50 percent or more have dyslexia and related learning disabilities.
2. 50 percent or more have balance/coordination disturbances.

Amazingly, he obtained these correlations in hindsight.

This surprising correlation was reminiscent of my unexpectedly demonstrating only CVS dysfunctioning in 75 percent of dyslexics when searching for only cerebral neurological signs. But at the time, Wender, like all other traditionalists, myself included, was under the sway of a cerebral or thinking-brain causation. So, unwitting bias prevented him from recognizing the inner-ear or CVS significance of his imbalance and dyscoordination findings. And thus, he also overlooked their likely causal CVS link to his other two ADHD/dyslexia (or LD/SLD) correlations.

Had Wender specifically searched for these three links in follow-up studies, his correlations would have been significantly higher—likely matching mine. Once again we might wonder: Was nature's need for homeostasis at work, slowing down the rate of progress and preventing Wender from fully recognizing the significance of, and following up on, his newly found, important insights?

Validating the Connection

Having previously and independently recognized that ADD/ADHD was linked to dyslexia/SLD and CVS dysfunctioning, I specifically tested for these connections in patients seeking help. My research showed that among those I diagnosed with ADD/ADHD:

1. More than 90 percent had definitive evidence of inner-ear/CVS dysfunction.
2. 70–90 percent had dyslexia and/or related specific learning disabilities in referred cases.

Clearly, these amazing results strongly supported Wender's findings as well as my growing conviction that both dyslexia/SLD and ADD/ADHD are CVS-determined or CVS-related disorders and so represent two sides to the same complex multi-sided CVS coin—exceptions aside.

The Diagnostic Importance of Symptomatic Quality

After having neurophysiologically examined significant numbers of additional subjects with ADD/ADHD, I was led to conclude that this disorder is CVS-related in the vast majority of patients. And that the *quality* of each of the ADD/ADHD symptoms and their respective determining mechanisms are diagnostically as important, in certain respects, as whether or not individuals have six or more symptoms—as currently required for an official DSM-V diagnosis. However, these stringent criteria may be more helpful for research purposes requiring "overkill statistical certainty."

Adding diagnostic quality to quantity In other words, one or two properly and qualitatively evaluated ADD/ADHD symptoms (e.g., inattention, distractibility, impulsivity, hyperactivity) in a patient are often sufficient for an experienced clinician to make initial therapeutic decisions—provided the symptoms are also supported by diagnostic evidence of CVS dysfunctioning and also coexist with dyslexia-related "clues."

Why is this important? By adding the correlated CVS-related impairments to the DSM-V criteria, we can then properly diagnose patients with milder forms of ADD/ADHD having only a few DSM-V recognized symptoms. Even more important, we can now effectively treat a large number of previously excluded suffering patients with mild ADD/ADHD who were misdiagnosed and possibly mistreated simply because their disorder wasn't severe enough to meet the DSM-V criteria. Perhaps the following diagnostic insights will help change this oversight.

A New Analysis and Classification for ADD/ADHD-like Symptoms/Mechanisms

After studying the various psychological and neurophysiological mechanisms responsible for *ADD/ADHD*-like symptoms, I realized that there are at least four distinct determinants or intensifiers, excluding medical causes such as anemia, thyroid impairments, related endocrinological dysfunctioning, infections, etc. Thus, as with phobic and SLD-based symptoms, I recommend that clinicians consider qualitatively analyzing *ADD/ADHD*-like symptoms and classifying them into four types:

Type I ADD/ADHD-like	Realistic mechanisms
Type II ADD/ADHD-like	Neurotic mechanisms
Type III ADD/ADHD	Inner-ear or CVS dysfunctioning
Type IV ADD/ADHD	Frontal lobe (CNS) dysfunctioning

Type I ADD/ADHD-like mechanisms are what I call "realistic." For example, a recent death or illness or trauma in the family may contribute to distractibility/impaired concentration or agitation-triggered restlessness and impulsive-like symptoms, or may even create them.

Type II ADD/ADHD-like mechanisms result from neurotic conflicts stemming from past subconscious issues dating back to childhood, as well as from mood and personality disorders, etc. These mechanisms may also contribute to, or cause, impaired concentration and distractibility—and even anxiety/agitation-triggered restlessness and irritability—also short fuses. Types I and II both respond best to psychotherapy and/or behavior modification techniques.

Type III true DSM-V ADD/ADHD is related to CVS dysfunctioning, as we've been discussing in this book. Based on my clinical research and inner-ear/cerebellar testing, more than *98 percent of referred patients* with typical concentration, distractibility, activity, and related symptoms of ADD/ADHD are in the Type III category—based on CVS diagnostic validation as well as a qualitative analysis of the symptoms.

Type IV ADD/ADHD There also appears to be a small group of very severe ADD/ADHD cases whose symptoms are significantly more intense than, and appear qualitatively different from, those characterizing Type III ADD/ADHD.

Upon neuroanalytic examination, Type IV ADD/ADHD individuals appear to have greater degrees of primary *frontal lobe* dysfunctional mechanisms and characteristics. They seem significantly more self-focused, instinct-driven, and lacking in empathy, insight, foresight, and planning. They account for approximately 1–2 percent of the DSM-V ADHD cases I examine, and their overall treatment outcomes are significantly less favorable.

An Additional Therapeutic Insight *Needless to say, the above diagnostic insights are also important for therapeutic purposes since Type I—IV ADD/ADHD mechanisms may overlap with one another. And so, for best results, all contributing or overlapping Types I–IV mechanisms must be determined and treated—especially when Type III meds and related therapies fail.*

The Value of a New Classification

In retrospect, the traditionalists were once again partly correct in trying to make sure that everyone they diagnosed with neurologically determined DSM-V Type III ADD/ADHD really had it—just as they were by mandating that dyslexics had to have *severe* reading impairments. Thus, the DSM-V diagnostically separated out the more severe neurologically determined *Types III and IV ADD/ADHD* from the other milder *Types I and II ADD/ADHD* lookalikes by mandating the stringent multi-symptomatic quantitative requirements mentioned above, as well as others. Unfortunately, as I previously emphasized, to obtain greater diagnostic certainty, the DSM-V omitted many patients with milder and fewer Type III symptoms—depriving them of a proper understanding and successful treatment.

Diagnosing milder cases Had the DSM-V recognized Wender's (and my) correlations of ADHD with impaired balance and coordination, CVS dysfunctioning, as well as dyslexia (LD or SLD)-related symptoms, they could have added in these important diagnostic parameters to their final algorithm. And by doing so, fewer typical Type III ADD/ADHD symptoms would have been required for an accurate diagnosis. Thus, milder Type III ADD/ADHD cases with less than six of nine symptoms would have benefitted from a proper understanding and a highly effective med treatment.

ADD/ADHD Medications and Related Insights

Stimulants work best for ADD/ADHD By and large, the proper use of stimulants, which also have inner-ear-enhancing properties according to NASA research and the experience of many clinicians, offers the best results for those with neurologically based ADD/ADHD. By contrast, inner-ear/CVS-enhancing antihistamines better treat the remaining "dyslexic" segment of the CVS syndrome.

Combining stimulants and anti-motion antihistamines When attempting to treat the total dyslexia/CVS syndrome while also trying to reduce individual doses, combinations of both medication groups are often found most helpful. In fact, they may even be somewhat synergistic—meaning, for example, that 1 + 1 = 3. Importantly, this combination of meds often significantly eliminates or minimizes the negative or "rebound" withdrawal-like effects stimulants often trigger when wearing off. And for those who may not know, this rebound negative effect may be severe enough to discontinue an otherwise helpful med.

Atypical responses It is significant that inner-ear/CVS-enhancing antihistamines *atypically* work better with ADHD than do stimulants. This clinical observation—supported by both Andrew and Linda described in prior Chap. 13, and then Joey, whose case we'll see shortly—add further to my growing conviction that there must be a CVS component to ADHD.

But overall, the stimulants work much better more frequently.[1]

[1] Why is the minimum six-symptom requirement helpful for research? you may wonder. Because it prevents diagnosing false positives—patients with concentration and distractibility symptoms due to other causes. But as a *clinician*, this need for quantitative diagnostic certainty creates lots of false negatives—it omits many milder ADD patients deserving of a proper diagnosis and beneficial treatment.

Pseudo-ADD

Because those with dyslexia or SLD require extra concentration to avoid errors while also attempting to compensate for dozens of reading and non-reading symptoms—often resulting in mental fatigue, "typical dyslexics" also benefit from stimulant-enhanced concentration, even when Type III ADD/ADHD is not present or comorbid. It's as if the dyslexic's compensatory struggle triggers a *secondarily acquired pseudo-ADD*, which requires stimulants to minimize burnout and failure.

Also, enhanced interest and concentration plus visual fixation are proven inner-ear/CVS-enhancing mechanisms. Thus, these mechanisms may contribute to overall improvements in most patients with the dyslexia/CVS syndrome, including those with only ADD/ADHD.[2]

Case Demonstration: Ken

To help illustrate the above insights while adding a measure of clinical validation, I decided to present Ken. I initially examined him when he was 8 years old and at the end of third grade. He had been diagnosed by a prior psychiatrist as having ADHD with comorbid dyslexia and anxiety—the latter responding well to Inderal (a beta-blocker). Seroquel (an antipsychotic) helped his frequent, severe verbal outbursts that required substantial recovery times. Prior use of stimulants had been only mildly effective. He'd also been tested and treated since age 5 for expressive speech difficulties as well as central auditory processing impairments.

However, his improvements had plateaued, and his academic issues, ADHD, anxiety, and verbal outbursts still remained troubling. Speech difficulties and related avoidance of social interactions with schoolmates persisted—although he was better controlled behaviorally and related well with relatives of all ages. Behavior modification had recently been introduced.

Summary of My Initial Findings

History: Specific Symptoms Ken manifested a great many typical *ADD/ADHD symptoms* including impaired concentration, distractibility, rapid boredom, procrastination, restlessness, difficulty sitting still, overactivity, low frustration tolerance, impulsivity, oppositional behavior, and severe temper outbursts—especially with siblings.

[2]A few non-stimulant ADD/ADHD meds should be tried when the above fail—although they have less chance of working.

He also had a wide range of symptoms typical of the *dyslexia syndrome*. These included impaired reading, writing, spelling, math, memory, speech, sense of direction and time, and simple grammar. Ken also evidenced *generalized and specific anxiety* (fears of animals, being alone, getting lost, falling asleep). Lastly, he manifested *typical inner-ear/cerebellar-related indicators* such as bumping into others, tripping, difficulty skipping, and motion sickness.

Neurological exam To put it bluntly, Ken would have failed the DWI test. He had difficulty balancing on one foot, rotating arms in opposing directions, walking heel to toe, accurately touching finger to nose, and directing his thumb to the other four fingers in sequence. Ken also had trouble maintaining smooth eye pursuit. (Refer to Chap. 19, Four Steps to a Certain Diagnosis.)

Bender-Gestalt (BG) designs and Goodenough figure drawings The illustrations below reveal severe visual-motor and related spatial difficulties of a CVS origin—especially obvious when the BG copied designs are compared to the normally drawn one on the left.

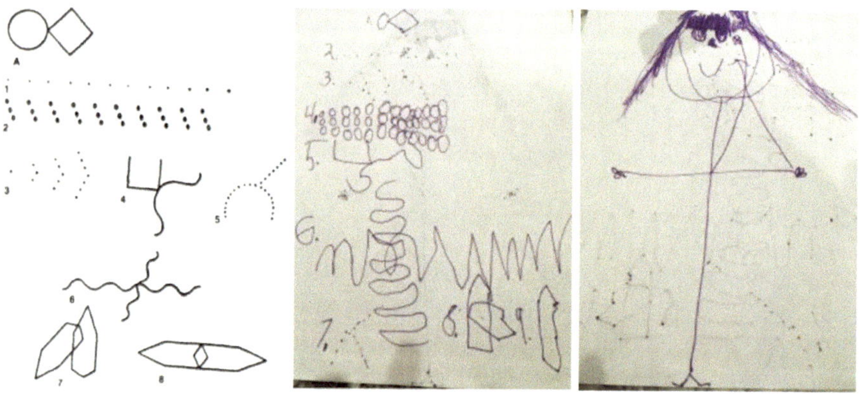

Response to Medical Treatment

- An inner-ear-enhancing antihistamine helped his reading and writing, spelling, math, and speech as well as balance and coordination.
- The stimulant Vyvanse significantly improved his ADD/ADHD symptoms.
- Increased doses of Inderal better reduced his anxiety level.
- All meds together significantly reduced his severe and frequent outbursts, enabling a reduction in dosage of Seroquel.

Ken's Mother's Observations

Overall, Ken has had incredible improvements since starting treatment with Dr. Levinson. This has been most notable in his reading, writing, spelling, math, and speech articulation, and also in his enhanced frustration tolerance, concentration and decreased distractibility. His anxiety, mood and self-image are better—so is his socialization.

Language is still difficult for him. Proper word retrieval and usage is still a challenge. And so are spatial and directional activities.

Although his self-regulation of anger outbursts is better, he still has some difficulty, particularly in competition with his brothers and in unstructured environments.

Summary of Ken's Evaluation and Treatment

Upon reviewing all of Ken's symptoms, his neurological exam, and his other diagnostic indicators, it should be clear to you that he suffers from a CVS syndrome. And although his leading diagnosis was ADD/ADHD, he manifested an array of more typically recognized dyslexia-related symptoms as well as definitive evidence of CVS dysfunctioning. Clearly, ADHD is seldom "pure" in cases referred for treatment, as you might have mistakenly believed before reading this book and listening to my patients. Nor does the use of stimulants *significantly* help with most of the numerous non-ADD/ADHD "dyslexic" and anxiety symptoms, exceptions aside.

As repeatedly noted, the stimulants typically improve the important ADD/ADHD segment—while the remaining aspects of the syndrome are often mistakenly ignored or viewed as simply comorbid by most clinicians. Importantly, the stimulants also help the pseudo-ADD characterizing most dyslexics who secondarily burnout when attempting to cope, forced to use excessive compensatory concentration efforts.

Accordingly, it's likely that in those with both dyslexia and ADD as well as in non-ADD dyslexics, pseudo-ADD coexists and responds favorably to stimulants. And since the anti-motion antihistamines help the dyslexic segment as well as ADD, it should also be combined with the stimulants.

As emphasized above, *all* of Ken's CVS signs and symptoms should be added to the official diagnostic ADD/ADHD criteria. This would enable a better overall understanding and successful treatment of mild cases of ADD/ADHD with less than six well-recognized and defined symptoms.

Joey: Another Case of ADD/ADHD + Other Related Disorders

Joey is a bright, verbal 8-year-old fourth grader referred for ADHD and significant difficulties listening to, and following, instructions. Prior to my referral, he was nonresponsive to four trials of diverse stimulants. There had been minimal, if any, improvements on attempted vitamin therapy. But he very slowly improved somewhat on neurofeedback. Speech therapy helped. And he was about to start CBT.

Initial Examination Joey's ADHD was characterized by severe inattention and distractibility, hyperactivity, impulsivity, short frustration tolerance, difficulty transitioning from task to task, oppositional responses (improving), rapid boredom, disorganization, and severe procrastination as well as deficient working memory.

His difficulty listening to, and following, instructions was in part related to his ADHD and poor short-term memory. But it was also codetermined by a mild bilateral hearing loss, as well as central auditory processing delays and distortions.

Joey also manifested the prior "official" reading severity required to diagnose and define dyslexia: he was two years behind in reading, despite tutoring. And he also manifested writing, spelling, math, memory, and speech difficulties—symptoms typical of those characterizing the dyslexia or CVS syndrome.

Significant generalized anxiety was apparent when Joey first came to my office. Fears of the dark and bugs had decreased, seemingly related to his benefitting from neurofeedback. Joey also showed CVS-related delays affecting his speech, eye-hand and many other fine-motor coordination skills, as well as a reflex inability to blow his nose.

Neurological testing revealed a CVS dysfunction and related imbalance—even with eyes open—as well as other signs corroborating this impairment. Despite this, he proved very adept at riding a bike—highlighting the function-specific nature of CVS functioning, dysfunctioning, and compensation. His Bender-Gestalt designs and Goodenough figure drawings were also diagnostic of a significant visual-spatial-motor impairment of CVS origin.

Medical treatment As noted earlier, Joey failed to respond favorably to four distinct trials of stimulants. After failing to respond to a number of typically effective dyslexia meds, we hit the jackpot with a very low dose of Dramamine. Joey tolerated only his starting test dose of one-eighth to one-quarter of a tab every morning; otherwise fatigue and irritability set in. His mother writes:

> *His teacher reports he's suddenly better—functioning more like any other child. Joey's anxiety levels are now less. He's concentrating and no longer so distracted. He's trying new foods—something he'd never do before. And he no longer needs his prescriptive glasses any more—they were thick. His ophthalmologist was shocked by the sudden improvement.*
>
> *Prior to starting this treatment, after eating something he claimed to dislike, he would sometimes later admit that it really tasted good. But he would put up a fuss at first anyway—because he hated to admit he was wrong. This adversarial behavior has lessened now and he's more cooperative. His reading, writing, and vocabulary have suddenly improved. He's now listening, concentrating, and following instructions more.*

Insights

Most of Joey's improvements occurred after starting on very low doses of Dramamine. By contrast, stimulants and most other anti-motion meds triggered side effects. Importantly, most of his improvements diminished as soon as he was given the same very low Dramamine dose *twice* a day—indicating how dose-sensitive some patients are. Were this a placebo effect, as some understandable skeptics may be wondering, how would you explain his failure to respond to other inner-ear/CVS enhancers as well as to a slightly higher minimal dose of Dramamine that many might mistakenly believe was too low to work in the first place? Or his negative response to all stimulants tried thus far, despite the fact that these were the meds expected by all to work best and fastest?

In summary, Joey's symptoms and favorable response to inner-ear enhancers once again support the linkage between the CVS and the triad of dyslexia, ADD/ADHD, and anxiety/phobia disorders. Also, *similar ocular/refraction improvements detected in Joey were also reported by others.* This important observation suggests that CVS mechanisms not infrequently overlap or codetermine primary ocular impairments, including strabismus. Since Joey's treatment is still a work in progress, he may do markedly better once additional add-ons are tried.

Finally: Checking Back with Michael Shultz

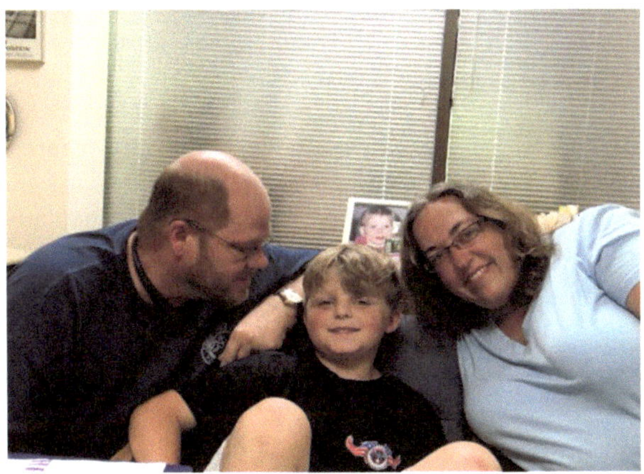

History Michael is a very bright 10-year-old third grader whose amazing and rapid improvements justified his appearance on this book's opening page. However, as promised, I will now reintroduce him here so that you can better understand his dyslexia syndrome and his response to an evolving treatment protocol.

Multiple diagnoses Because Michael had symptoms belonging to *dyslexia, phobias/anxiety, and ADD/ADHD, as well as speech/communication issues*, in which he characteristically used only one-word answers in response to questions, he could have been placed diagnostically in any one of several book chapters. And as you might recall, his initial responses to a test dose of an inner-ear-enhancing med demonstrated a rapid and dramatic improvement in symptoms characteristic of all four of these diagnostic categories, and others as well—further supporting a common CVS origin.

However, because he also later responded very favorably to an added stimulant med, I decided to review his overall symptoms and improvements here in this chapter—in order to demonstrate the amazing benefits possible when both inner-ear-enhancing antihistamines and stimulants are combined. And I also wanted to reemphasize the degree of symptomatic overlapping that frequently occurs in patients, irrespective of the primary neurodynamic diagnosis made. Again, it is crucial to realize that all of these disorders fall into a larger and all-encompassing impairment I called the *CVS syndrome*.

Pre-treatment symptoms Before beginning treatment, Michael's symptoms included difficulties with reading, writing, spelling, math, memory, speech, time, direction, and grammar. They also included *impulsivity*, *frustration tolerance*, *concentration*, *distractibility*, *rapid boredom*, *procrastination*, *disorganization*, anxieties/phobias, and problems with balance and coordination.

Michael also manifested headaches, dizziness, and motion sickness in addition to some CVS-related reflex symptoms, including inability to properly blow his nose and gagging when attempting to swallow even very small pills—symptoms that spontaneously and rapidly improved on meds. He thus demonstrated the amazing complexity characterizing his CVS syndrome—most of which was initially described in the first few paragraphs of the Preface.

Importantly, when Michael was 2 years old, he ran high fevers and required an adenoidectomy and four sets of draining tubes to eliminate febrile convulsions. Might these middle ear difficulties have impaired his inner-ear and so intensified or caused his CVS syndrome? Might this not explain his ear noises and clicking (tinnitus) and why these symptoms rapidly disappeared on an inner-ear-enhancing med?

After a trial dose of an antihistamine Half an hour after being tried on an inner-ear-enhancing antihistamine, Michael had a remarkable improvement—especially in his reading, as briefly described in the first page of this book. His verbal—linguistic—communications also continued to dramatically improve as his doses were slowly increased. He now engages in long conversations rather than one-word responses or mere nods. And his socializing rapidly improved as well—probably related to his enhanced word and thought recall, as well as to his dramatically improved auditory processing.

His enhanced social skills were also aided by his improvements in both input and output verbal communication capability, concentration, distractibility, and the other ADD/ADHD-related symptoms, as well as by his dramatically decreased anxiety and phobic responses. His headaches, dizziness, and motion sickness also disappeared—significantly adding to his overall feeling of well-being and dramatically increased self-esteem.

After a stimulant was added two months later Following the addition of a stimulant medication, Michael's mother reported a second "night-and-day improvement"—as if all his prior favorable changes had suddenly been given a turbo boost.

Michael's Summary

Importantly, upon neurophysiological testing, Michael was diagnosed with only a CVS dysfunction. And a review of his *symptoms* indicated that he evidenced ADD/ADHD, dyslexia, anxiety/phobias, and speech/language issues, suggesting once again that there is significant overlapping among these differently named disorders.

As previously noted, his reading capability rapidly jumped—also revealing, upon analysis, significant improvements in many of his underlying reading-determined mechanisms, including the ability to better hear, discriminate, and remember phonetic sounds and maintain their proper sequence when reading.

Since Michael had only CVS dysfunctioning, and his auditory and phonetic processing improved on CVS enhancers as did his speech/language functioning, is it not reasonable to consider that these latter functions are CVS-determined rather than of a cerebral linguistic origin as some researchers mistakenly ASSUME—or, should I say, erroneously BELIEVE?

How CVS enhancers may help those with ASD Remember, when Michael's speech and auditory processing functioning increased, so did his verbal expression and socialization. In fact, his verbalization and language functioning rapidly improved on test doses of an inner-ear-antihistamine—otherwise he would never have been able to express his emotions and insights so well so fast.

This insight is important to keep in mind when treating these overlapping CVS symptoms in autistic patients. By improving similar speech-related and other crucial CVS-determined functions, it became possible to help autistics better speak and communicate—and hence to better socialize. In fact, these very improvements were shown to occur in patients with ASD when treated with CVS enhancers. No doubt you will be fascinated by the favorable responses of three boys with ASD described in Chap. 22 and of another youngster diagnosed with autistic traits.

The phobia connection Next, we'll be looking in greater depth at the surprising connection between phobias/anxiety disorders and the inner-ear/cerebellar system. But first, let's answer a few questions about ADD/ADHD that you may be thinking about.

Some Q&As About ADD/ADHD

Question 1 "So, why do stimulants work best for those with ADD/ADHD, if this disorder has a CVS origin similar to dyslexia or LD/SLD and phobias?"

Answer Great question, one I've repeatedly asked myself but to which I have no definitive answer. What do we clinically know? The frontal cerebral cortex is presumed to play the most important role in ADD/ADHD—responding best to the stimulants and less so to the CVS-enhancing antihistamines. The other cerebral and related areas which are more important in shaping/determining the typical dyslexic reading and related symptoms best respond to the CVS-enhancing antihistamines and less so to the stimulants. The cerebellum or CVS as a whole, best responding to the CVS-enhancing antihistamines, is interconnected with both the frontal and non-frontal brain areas, although differing parts of the cerebellum appear to be vitally involved with ADD/ADHD and "dyslexia" based on neuroimaging studies.

So what may we tentatively assume? The (frontal) cerebral cortex and its receiving and transmitting fibers may play a different—*perhaps more predisposing and even determining*—role in ADD/ADHD than do the other thinking-brain processors for the remaining segments of the dyslexia syndrome. It's also possible that the specific cerebellar structure involved with ADD/ADHD responds better to stimulants—since neuroimaging studies have shown that different parts of the cerebellum are involved with dyslexia, ADD/ADHD, and even autism?

Question 2 "Do ADD/ADHD and dyslexic Olympians like Bruce (now Caitlyn) Jenner and Greg Louganis really have balance/coordination/rhythmic difficulties? Seems very unlikely. Surely the presence of dyslexic athletes—especially those who also have ADHD—tend to refute your CVS theory of dyslexia/ADD-ADHD!"

Answer Needless to say, these insightful questions, which challenged the paradigm that athletes are perfect models of physical coordination, initially puzzled me too. That is, until I examined scores of gifted dyslexic and ADD/ADHD athletes and nonathletes. And I discovered a simple clinical truth: Upon neurological examination, Bruce (now Caitlyn) Jenner and similar athletes, such as Greg Louganis, may likely show poor eye coordination only when reading and poor hand coordination only when writing.

Gifted and klutzy coordination may coexist Relatively minor inner-ear/CVS impairments, and even speech dyscoordination, are neither tested for, nor relevant to, competing in the Olympics. Athletes are tested for these frequently overlooked non-Olympic impediments only by clinicians like myself. So contrary to our need for over-simplistically believing in absolute athletic purity, it became readily apparent that gifted athletic functioning need not generalize to all motor mechanisms in dyslexics. And in fact, gifted and klutzy athletic (sensory-motor) functioning coexist and are frequently improved by the CVS enhancers.

Klutzy athletes Since recognizing the above insights, *I've tested dyslexic and/or ADD/ADHD athletes who not infrequently tripped when walking up a flight of stairs, yet were gifted on a flat playing field.* Some athletes were good at one sport and mediocre or even poor in other balance, coordination, and rhythm-oriented activities. (Recall that gifted basketball star Charles Barkley was alleged to be klutzy in golf.) And some were best in only one of several team positions—illustrating just how function-specific inner-ear functioning and problems can be. Occasionally, I found athletes who were completely discombobulated neurologically with their eyes closed. But they performed superbly with their eyes open, thanks to their innate *gifted skills and compensatory visual fixation mechanisms.*

Athletes need not be perfect CVS specimens And you don't have to be a complete klutz to have an inner-ear or CVS dysfunction. It's not an all-or-none problem anymore than the reading, writing, spelling, math, etc. disorders have to be complete and hopeless in dyslexics. In fact, these functions may be normal and even exceptional—and yet a CVS impairment may be diagnosed. (Refer to Jenny in Chap. 20.)

Quantitative Variability in all CVS/dyslexia-related functions Nearly all of the typical dyslexic and non-dyslexic functions in patients may vary significantly from one extreme to another —contrary to naive expectations. And the same functional variability holds true for those with ADHD and phobias as well as for their underlying CVS diagnostic parameters.

As a result of this variability, especially when also factoring in the roles of potential compensation vs. destabilization, it should be readily apparent why assumptions and convictions, as well as outcome predictions about highly complex and multidimensional disorders like dyslexia/ADHD, based on small samples, are subject to significant errors.

Qualitative evaluations are significantly more diagnostic Thus, for example, the reading scores among dyslexics may vary from high to low and so are nondiagnostic of dyslexia by themselves. By contrast, the following reading characteristics or qualities have significant diagnostic value: reversals, tracking errors, distractibility, visual overloading, memory and related CVS-determined balance and coordination impairments, etc.

Overfocusing *This mechanism is also a very important, unique and variable compensatory factor that should be emphasized.* Those with dyslexia or ADD/ADHD, both athletes and "absent-minded professors," most often exhibit poor concentration and distractibility unless they are very interested in the sport and/or topic. They then reflexly shift into a state termed *overfocus*—whereby they autonomously tune everything else out and their concentration becomes razor sharp and prolonged—super-normal.

By comparison to normal individuals who have sufficient concentration, even when not interested, those with ADHD manifest adequate concentration *only* when really involved. Accordingly, athletes and professors with ADD when not zoned in are often *zoned out* and thus are predisposed to tripping, falling, cognitive and emotional errors, etc. Hence the existence of absent-minded professors and klutzy athletes as well as an explanation for their seemingly paradoxical behavior.

Question 3 "Why do stimulants decrease hyperactivity?"

Answer This is the most frequently asked question because, in large part, it seems counterintuitive. So, I believe an analogy will be most helpful. When driving a car, for example, if you stimulate the brake, it slows down the speed—thus simply explaining the so-called paradoxical effect of stimulant meds on hyperactivity. And if impaired concentration and filtering mechanisms are simultaneously stimulated by stepping on the accelerator, then brain fog and distractibility disappear. However, in clinical practice, any combination of *positive and/or negative* possibilities occurs when stimulants, or any other meds, are used for ADD/ADHD.

Since no one knows beforehand whether the meds will stimulate the accelerator and/or brake, or how hard—for any mechanism—it's essential to test-dose all patients first.

Hopefully, this "insider" content and corresponding insights have been as helpful to you as they have been to me as a clinician. Needless to say, few if any of these insights were theoretically predictable. Rather the opposite: the syndrome we are dealing with is far too complex for most mortals—however Einstein-brilliant—to have holistically conceptualized in theory before a vast amount of patients with dyslexia and/or ADD/ADHD helped them. So, for now, let's move to the phobia connection.

Chapter 15
The CVS/Phobia Link: Three Steps Toward Conviction

Of all my surprising insights over the past 50-plus years, the one that struck me as the most fascinating was the recognition of a link between dysfunctioning inner-ear/cerebellar mechanisms and phobias. Perhaps the reason for this "shock" had to do with my Freudian psychoanalytic training, which continually reinforced the belief that mental symptoms—especially those related to anxiety and phobias—were primarily due to subconscious mental causes.

On the other hand, I was perhaps more open to this new inner-ear insight than other psychologically trained professionals—partly because I had gained enormous clinical experience during my CVS/dyslexia research and partly because I cognitively and instinctively knew and felt there was a void in our understanding of phobias, similar to the way I had come to recognize the traditionalists' void in understanding dyslexia. Thus, I was subconsciously ready and waiting for the clinching insight to materialize when it did.

So, once I observed fears of heights and bridges, as well as fears of moving elevators, escalators, trains, planes, buses, cars, and even agoraphobic fears, disappearing rapidly in dyslexics responding successfully to inner-ear/CVS enhancers, a solution to the phobia puzzle suddenly materialized. It was akin to a déjà vu experience. However, famed Yankee baseball catcher Yogi Berra said it better and funnier, "It's like déjà vu all over again."

Having already neuroanalyzed the inner-ear-determined balance, motion, and directional/orientation mechanisms affecting dyslexics, I immediately saw, like a eureka flash, that these same mechanisms might trigger all of the above phobias and thus sensibly explain their shape or quality, for the first time. And using the same Q&A techniques that enabled me to solve the dyslexia and ADD/ADHD riddles, I rapidly found myself capable of explaining and successfully treating the vast majority of phobias in patients seeking my help.

H. N. Levinson, *Feeling Smarter and Smarter*,
https://doi.org/10.1007/978-3-030-16208-5_15

The Inner-Ear/Cerebellar Involvement in Phobias

In what seemed like another flash, I rapidly collected, analyzed, and published all of these uncanny insights in a few papers and several of my books, especially *Phobia Free*. Over time, I refined and dramatically expanded my understanding of phobias, primarily by better recognizing just how the cerebellum is likely involved in every step of triggering and regulating the signals in the phobic/anxiety process, including a crucial step that had been eluding me for years:

> ***The phobia process***—*I initially came to recognize that an anxiety response is triggered when the inner-ear fails to properly handle sensory-motor and related functions. However, for the triggered inner-ear-anxiety responses to intensify and stick like glue—and so, lead to persisting phobias rather than be discarded as harmless, the cerebellum must fail to inhibit and/or otherwise cause an underlying perseveration/sticking mechanism. This is similar to the CVS impairment resulting in verbal stuttering or reading stuttering—where the "dyslexic/CVS" tongue or eye sticks to one word when talking or reading, unable to let go and so move on to the next word. These abnormal anxiety mechanisms are also likely related to failures of cerebellar inhibition.*

Why are all these considerations so important? This novel cerebellar concept is crucial because it explains why only some with similar dysfunctioning inner-ear mechanisms develop anxiety, flooding and phobias, and not others! Similarly, not everyone with inner-ear-determined motion sickness will develop motion anxiety/phobias. And also, why only some develop motion sickness. The final outcome likely depends on where specifically these signals originate, radiate to, and how the cerebellum acts or fails to regulate these signals!

I also felt it important to highlight that "severe" anxiety and panic may often result when the cerebellum fails to adaptively modulate or inhibit the degree of excessively released *internal* anxiety signals from a maladaptive CNS (central nervous system) processor—resulting in an escalating overload. This is similar to the way the cerebellum often fails to neutralize/filter-out excessive or even normal *external sensory input signals*, including motion, light, noise, etc., resulting in varied apparent oversensitivities as well as triggering corresponding warning or compensatory responses.

So, why do I believe the cerebellum is involved? The cerebellum must be crucial in the complex anxiety process because the signals connected with phobias often improve on CVS enhancers! More important, the cerebellum vs. the inner-ear is a "little brain" fully capable of regulating these overdetermined signals! Also, as previously stated, Sir John Eccles had brilliantly demonstrated that the cerebellum is involved in signal inhibition at receptor sites—thus preventing/controlling overloading—which I theoretically expanded to include all signal regulation!

Thus, as stated, a cerebellar failure may likely result in overloading and/or sensitivity responses. In other words, I just generalized Eccles' Nobel Prize findings and then applied them to anxiety and phobia signals. And I hoped that other gifted cerebellar neurophysiologists would experimentally validate and expand my clinically derived concepts in vitally needed formal studies.

With these new insights in mind, I will attempt to illustrate and explain my most recent understanding of the causal links between the CVS and phobia. And I will do so in a three-step manner—the last step of which involves the analysis of the CVS mechanisms in real/primarily phobic patients and their favorable response to meds.

The Three Vital Steps

Having already demonstrated the inner-ear or CVS links to ADD/ADHD and dyslexia in the last chapter, I will now attempt to clinically validate the phobia connection in a three-step manner: *Step I*, analyzing previous patients exhibiting CVS dysfunctioning within this book for phobic symptoms; *Step II*, scanning the past scientific literature for possible hidden clues; and *Step III*, demonstrating the CVS/ phobic connection in newly presented patients.

And so here are the three important steps to solving the phobia connection.

Step I: Reviewing Prior Patients' Content for Phobic and Related Clues

Since the primary focus of this chapter is to clarify the phobia/anxiety links to the inner-ear/cerebellum, I will *italicize only the phobia-related symptoms* in all of the referred dyslexia and ADD/ADHD cases thus far presented in order to easily call attention to them.

But remember: most referred phobics also have apparent overlapping manifestations of dyslexia and ADD/ADHD as well as imbalance and dyscoordination. So several phobics will be presented in Step 3. I should also emphasize here that all patients in this book were diagnosed as manifesting *only* inner-ear/cerebellar dysfunctioning on the basis of medical testing.

Michael Schultz, whom we met at the start of the book and again in the last chapter, reported rapid improvements in reading, concentration, and behavior shortly after taking a test dose of an inner-ear enhancer. He also experienced *a sharp decrease in his fear of rain, hail, and tests, and in his overall anxiety level. Maria*, who you also read about at the start, magnificently described *her agoraphobia disappearing when her directional mechanism and dyslexia were significantly treated* (Pre-Preface). Mrs. Paula West (Chap. 2) noted how her son *Ron* surprisingly *lost his fear of amusement rides* while taking non-drowsy Dramamine to prevent motion sickness. Similarly, *John Whitney's* (Chap. 12) handwriting, reading, spelling, and balance/coordination improved, as well as his *fears of public speaking and social fears (i.e., his shyness).* In addition, his *pre-existing fears of heights, elevators, bridges, amusement rides, and new situations* also disappeared together with his academic and ADHD symptoms.

Another powerful demonstration of the above linkage (prior to any medical therapy) was provided by *Kathy* (Chap. 6), who evidenced typical dyslexic and concentration/distractibility symptoms as well as *past and/or present fears of the dark, school, teachers, stairs, escalators, amusement rides, getting lost, losing things, driving, new places, and public speaking.* In addition, she described clear-cut and obvious balance/coordination/ rhythmic symptoms diagnostic of an inner-ear (CVS dysfunction).

And three of the four short cases from Chap. 13 also improved in ways that clearly included phobias and anxieties as well:

- In addition to *John X's* improvements in reading, writing, concentration, distractibility, balance, and more, he's *no longer afraid of heights and carnival rides; he's not as overloaded and panicky in crowded/noisy places; and his performance anxiety and panic are gone.*
- On non-stimulant inner-ear meds, *Andrew* now feels that he has a brain. Concentration, hyperactivity, impulsivity, anger, hypersensitivity, *nightmares*, and sleepwalking are gone. And he's now able to fall asleep *and is no longer afraid of the dark or being alone, going to school, or getting on the school bus. He can now go up and down elevators and escalators without panic. Also, he's no longer fearful of sounding stupid as before. And he's more assertive and so speaks up.*
- After *Sheila* responded favorably to anti-motion sickness medication, her *phobic/anxiety and agoraphobic symptoms dramatically improved. She's no longer fearful of leaving her house alone. Her panic is gone when having to cross a street unassisted, and she no longer fears losing balance and fainting with cars coming and going.*

Step II: Scanning the Scientific Literature for Phobia Links to the Inner Ear

Once a linkage between cerebellar-vestibular system (CVS) dysfunction and phobias seemed possible—even certain—I realized that there had to have been hidden clues and overlooked historical evidence supporting this amazing and exciting connection. So, I reviewed these respective topics in the scientific literature with a new, unbiased, and thus re-focused mind. And I'm sure you'll be as interested in what I found, as I was.

Despite my knowing that recently discovered insights often have independent historical roots, I was still surprised to learn that several clinicians dating back to the late 1890s reported correlations between phobias—including agoraphobia—and the inner ear. However, what did not surprise me was that the vast majority of traditionalist researchers and clinicians completely ignored or denied these amazing historical insights—as I initially had. Similarly, they had also overlooked my past data indicating the inner-ear/cerebellar's hidden role in phobias, as well as the coexistence of dyslexia, ADD/ADHD, and phobia symptoms in patient after patient. Again, until my research findings convinced me otherwise, I too was a typical tunnel-thinking traditionalist. As a result, I now consider myself an atypical traditionalist.

No psychoanalyst, psychiatrist, psychologist, or neurophysiologist was ever able to reasonably explain why certain individuals fear heights and bridges, whereas others fear moving vehicles, like elevators, escalators, elevators, cars, trains, planes, buses, and more; or why combinations of these phobias frequently present themselves in patients. It just never occurred to these professionals that CVS-determined imbalance and misperception may trigger height phobias, especially when looking down, or that the rest of the above phobias are obviously motion related and that multiple CVS mechanisms co-occur in both dyslexic and phobic individuals.

Also, agoraphobics, if you listen to them, will tell you that they experience imbalance and directional/orientational impairments, even dizziness—which explains their symptoms' quality and combination for the first time ever. Recall Maria's remarkable description of agoraphobia in the opening pages. Or that both sensory and motor (or motion) shielding environments providing insufficient stimulation may trigger claustrophobic anxiety of enclosed spaces like tunnels, rooms without windows, elevators, and even of feeling motion-trapped—waiting on lines and in traffic, unable to move, or wearing tight clothes. And I explained the universal phobias (snakes, rodents, roaches, etc.) as a failure of the CVS to continue suppressing/inhibiting archaic warning signals and as phobic responses that may have had an adaptive value in our evolutionary past—but which are currently just maladaptive anxiety intrusions into consciousness—previously buried within our subconscious.

There were, however, exceptional psychiatrists who did provide brilliant insights. For example, Otto Fenichel, one of Freud's most gifted and loyal disciples, clearly recognized a relationship between motion phobias, anxiety, dizziness, and the inner-ear. But he was so fixated on the sexual origins of neurotic anxiety symptoms that he overlooked the *primary determining role* of the inner-ear. Instead, he complicated his observations by adding in an unnecessary Freudian theoretical factor he couldn't shake loose from. Thus, Fenichel mistakenly postulated that *primary* early sexual conflicts *secondarily* accrued to the inner-ear, thereby overstimulating it.

However, in formulating this theory, Fenichel correctly highlighted another of Freud's concepts—the brilliant notion of somatic compliance. This suggests that emotional conflicts accrue to physical/somatic weak spots, e.g., the inner-ear. This insight is best illustrated by Bonnie, whom I briefly mentioned in Chap. 7. She was a patient of mine with hysteria who desired to regain her deceased mother and so heard her voice until she was successfully treated with both psychotherapy and inner-ear-enhancing meds. As you might also recall, Kathy and a few other dyslexics—with inner-ear/CVS dysfunction—reported hearing their thoughts as well as the words they read.

Had Fenichel maintained the simplicity of Occam's razor in order to explain his clinically observed correlation between phobias/anxiety and the inner ear, he would have long ago been credited with a major discovery. But similar to other researchers, he couldn't shake off his previously ingrained theoretical foundations, even when they didn't fit.

Way back in the 1930s, Paul Schilder, a truly brilliant and remarkably productive neuropsychiatric researcher and theorist I previously mentioned, highlighted a vestibular role in both neuroses and psychoses. In fact, he even emphasized that the inner ear processes gravity signals—a hypothesis I independently arrived at to explain a few of Kathy's symptoms. Although his highly original insights were ingenious, they were never properly followed up. And by now you probably have an inkling as to why, since the repetition of these scientific CVS-related oversights appears to exclude just chance errors.

Despite all of these uncanny past insights, as well as those in my own publications, no psychological professional seemed able to objectively recognize and analyze the possible *somatic* origins and specific mechanisms responsible for phobias—and so, to truly find the best treatment methods possible. Instead, some remained narrowly focused on *counting* and/or *naming* the phobias—giving them Latin and Greek names, like catapedaphobia (fear of jumping from high and low places), didaskaleinophobia (fear of going to school), and illyngophobia (fear of vertigo). Does this labeling tendency for phobias not sound similar to the synonym-coining compulsion for dyslexia I noted in Chap. 1? Might there be a common motivation—naming rather than understanding?

Fortunately, psychopharmacology and neuroimaging studies have made significant advances since I initially published my findings on phobias and related anxiety disorders many years ago. So, there is now greater recognition that there is a neurotransmitter-based—somatic—causation for phobias as well as an anxiety-releasing brain center(s) within the CNS.

However, these advances alone cannot explain the quality of even one phobia—whereas my inner-ear/CVS theory clarifies most of them in referred patients. And only kryptonite can explain why no other researcher came close to hypothesizing that impaired functions and disorders which overlap with one another so frequently, and are thus considered comorbid, may likely have a common underlying origin. And also, why all these simple and obvious inner-ear—and especially cerebellar—links were overlooked or denied, despite their staring at and calling out to us.

Although a few other investigators have also postulated a vestibular origin of phobias based on special inner-ear testing (refer to Chap. 19), no one else had previously recognized the crucial role of the cerebellum in both triggering and regulating anxiety signals; nor has anyone else been able to explain the quality, combination, and causation of these phobias. And despite my past publications, no other clinician has arrived at, or advanced, the CVS insights needed to best understand and treat these varied anxiety disorders. My well-published secret—that dyslexia, ADHD, phobias, and related anxiety disorders overlap in approximately 70–90 percent of people seeking help for these conditions because they are CVS-caused—may have to await rediscovery until after this book is published and read. Importantly, milder, non-referred cases have much less overlap.

Step III: Analyzing New Cases for Phobia Links

Now let's look at additionally obtained content derived from *new patients, some referred primarily because of phobias*. This clinical data will prove vital in further clarifying and validating the amazing scientific connection between the inner-ear/cerebellum and phobias, dyslexia, and ADD/ADHD.

Two New Cases of Phobias and Their Mechanisms: Joanna and Her Mother Nancy

The presenting symptoms of a dyslexic child named Joanna and her loving but phobic mother Nancy appear completely different on the surface. However, a careful analysis of their clinical details will help illustrate how previously hidden causal mechanisms can be recognized and understood *once you know what to look for*—via what I call *the hindsight phenomenon*. In Nancy, the hidden inner-ear/cerebellar dysfunction underlying her phobias and anxiety disorder was discovered only *after knowing to test for it* using specific CVS-detecting diagnostic methods.

Joanna Herron is 8 ½ years old. She is a beautiful young dyslexic girl—with coexisting phobias and panic—who responded well to inner-ear enhancers.

Joanna's Mother Nancy Writes About Her

I, her mother, am a "retired" special ed teacher. So, given my experience with learning disabled kids, I recognized Joanie's learning problems early in kindergarten and before.

Before Treatment: *She worked hard at learning, then as now; reading slowly—painfully so—always needing to check, double check, losing her place,* etc.

Her language development as a preschooler was creative and telegraphic. She packed as much meaning as possible into very few words. Her language was extremely abbreviated but very entertaining. For example, she said, "Doing? Doing?" to ask, "What are you doing?" into her third or fourth year.

She makes up words even now. And she will often say the exact opposite of what she means, for example, "No one over 16..." when she means no one under 16.[1]

---

[1]Traditionalists regarded the speech-related symptoms of Joanna and others as "proof" that dyslexia was a language disorder of thinking-brain origin—despite the fact that a majority of dyslexics, including those in this book, have superior verbal functioning. And those dyslexics with speech and language symptoms have only CVS dysfunctioning. Importantly, most so-called Freudian slips—including speech slips— are really CVS determined.

As you will read later on, the speech symptoms displayed by dyslexics are inner-ear/cerebellar-determined and are as qualitatively different from language or aphasic disorders as are the reading symptoms in dyslexia vs. alexia. Most importantly, the speech symptoms of Joanna and other dyslexics improve on inner-ear-enhancing medications, whereas aphasic or thinking-brain symptoms do not—unless there are coexisting but overshadowed CVS difficulties present as well.

She completely avoids all team sports and eye-hand coordination sports. She is a strong swimmer, but many of her strokes are a "creative" mix of what she has been taught and what she manages to put together when she can't coordinate the stroke as it's taught.

Joanna, when younger, would often seem unduly fearful and would panic in situations that did not warrant it. As a kindergartner, Joanna was invited to a roller skating birthday party. I spent half an hour with her choosing skates and trying them on. She was miserable and frightened until we took them off. We never related her fears and anxieties to dyslexia until we began reading your research.

Joanna's memory, both auditory and visual, is weak. When she is at home with her siblings, she will often cry out in frustration, "You made me forget!" With family hubbub in the background, she loses her train of thought easily. Her teachers report similar distractibility at school.

Joanna wants to do well in school. She works very slowly, partly because she is constantly double-checking, erasing, and losing her place. She spends much energy just trying to stay focused. As a first grader, her attempts to read were so fruitless she'd study the details of each picture endlessly.

I asked her once, "Joanna, what is reading like for you?" She sighed and said, "When I'm trying to read, I can see the letters. When I'm not trying to read, they're just black lines." That response gave me insight into what incredibly concentrated effort it takes for Joanna to make any sense of the written word.

She wants very much to be truly competent in school. But she is presently way over her head. She lashes out at siblings, all of whom are excellent readers. And we fear her anger and frustration will also be turned inward if her feelings of incompetence continue to increase.

Joanie's interaction with friends is becoming difficult. She says, "I'm dumb." Then she tries to entertain her friends by being silly. Her feelings of insecurity are starting to push kids away. This is a very sad thing to watch.

We are anxiously looking forward to our trip to your clinic. I have more hope than most who may come to you, for a very simple reason. On our insistence, our family physician read your research and placed Joanie on a trial of medication. Sure enough, her teacher reported that for the first time she could read her own writing, and she would try reading without blowing-up. She was less frustrated, less anxious and panicky.

After Treatment: *A year ago, after only two months following her first appointment with you, we were thrilled because Joanna had risen from a pre-primer to a low second grade instructional reading level. The progress continues! And yet, if we miss a day or even an afternoon dose of her medications, her father and I will both see the distractibility and stumbling over familiar words return. Her anxiety level rises too. Miraculous!*

Joanna's fourth-grade teacher says she is now academically "cooking up a storm" in class. She was recently tested and qualified for Talented and Gifted. Amazingly, she is currently reading Charlotte's Web. And I recently suggested Ribsy (of Henry Huggins fame) because she is such an animal lover. Chapter books!

When I look ahead, I shudder—so much more homework. But then I sit back and look at where Joanna was two years ago. A big strong second grader struggling to make "the" say "the" each time she saw it. Who frequently cried out, anxious and frustrated, "Why do I have to try! Why can't I just do it!" An angry, hurting young girl. Her progress has not been overnight but rather steady. And Hallelujah, it continues! And it affects all areas of her life: academics, speech, memory, attention, coordination, mood/anxiety and behavior, and, best of all, self-esteem.

Indeed, were dyslexia derived from a language disorder, then gifted speakers and orators like Winston Churchill couldn't be dyslexic. Yet Churchill *was* dyslexic.

Nancy Herron (Age 42)

Nancy is a phobic adult *without any apparent* coexisting dyslexic, ADD/ADHD, or inner-ear balance and coordination symptoms—even after a careful history was taken. She responded favorably to a combination of inner-ear enhancers after being neurophysiologically diagnosed as having a CVS dysfunction. As I've mentioned, pure phobics like Nancy—those without obvious links to other CVS-related disorders—appear clinically atypical when examined by clinicians, *recalling that these referrals are highly selective, usually more severe samples of the total phobic population.* However, prior to my research, all phobics were mistakenly considered "pure" when their impairment was viewed in a tunnel-visioned way. In other words, clinicians never saw the many overlapping CVS-related symptoms in phobics because they failed to look or listen for them, not because they weren't there.

> ***Before Treatment****—As for myself, my problems of inner-ear/cerebellar dysfunction are not academic but rather are in the area of anxiety and phobic symptoms. I look back now on basically my entire adult life and can see how this medical condition, unknown to myself, colored my experience of life: my longstanding self-perception of incompetency, despite my advanced education and successful experience as a teacher of Learning Disabled children; my inordinate sense of anxiety in what others considered to be perfectly normal, hospitable environments, such as classrooms, crowded church gatherings, grocery stores. In attempts to explain my distressed responses to normal life, I would look to my childhood and my rather imperfect parents. Realizing that I had not been terribly mistreated, abused, or neglected led me to conclude that I was just one incredible screw-up. And that I managed to attain "screw-up" status on my own. I was so hard on myself.*
>
> ***After Treatment****—Now two and a half months since seeing you, diagnosed with a CVS dysfunction and on all the medications you advised, I am in awe of the changes I am experiencing. Life and decision-making are no longer dire and difficult. My schoolgirls are delighted to see me when I arrive in their classrooms for my volunteer work. Hey, my sixth grader even jumped out of her seat to give me a big hug when I arrived today!*
>
> *With the first medication (Atenolol, [a beta-blocker used for stage fright and performance anxiety, and even dizziness]), I noticed an immediate sense of "okayness." I noticed it in my ability to look people in the eye, and in a new sense of normalcy—in situations such as watching a daughter's soccer game or talking with a small group of friends in a crowded restaurant. Being in the spotlight, or being worried that the spotlight might come my way, is no longer a big deal.*
>
> *Crowds can still be a problem at times, and fluorescent lights are most certainly "not my friend," but the overall level of my daily anxieties has gone way down, especially after adding the inner-ear meds. Life is not one endless string of trauma after trauma.*
>
> *My longstanding mindset of being deficient, inferior, and unworthy has not evaporated entirely. But I have made great strides towards normalcy or just a calm inner state. I now feel an obligation to share my and Joanna's experience with other educators and parents. I know Joanie and I are just the "tip of the iceberg" here in Oregon. I now recognize so many of Joanna's symptoms in my former students. Knowing what is causing their problems is incredibly empowering.*
>
> *And as for myself, I feel I can roll with the punches now. I am no longer frozen by fear or self-hate. Wow, these medications are allowing me to be real, not fragile and brittle as before. Previously, I felt betrayed by my body. My body was in control—not my mind, not my "self."*
>
> *Being relaxed is, well, awesome! I really am an incredibly blessed individual: four marvelous children and a loving and loony nerd of a husband to call my own. Before, my*

recognition of my many blessings was clouded with self-doubt and foreboding. What a difference normalcy makes.

The only sorry side to this story is the ignorance of the mainstream. Doctors, teachers, other parents... have never heard of your work. This is a crime. Your work should be as commonly known and accepted as the use of insulin to treat diabetes, and antibiotics for bacterial infections. So many people suffer needlessly. Much education is much needed. When (not if) I return to teaching LD kids, I will share my knowledge and experience with any and all who will listen.

I feel like my life is just beginning now at age 42. There is an amazing calm in this realization. Again, thanks to you from my daughter Joanna and myself.

The Benefits of Meaningful Insights and Helpful Therapies

Nancy Herron's insightful words offer two very important interrelated points that may have escaped your attention: (1) the tendency of CVS-dysfunctioning phobics to blame themselves for their treatment failures and (2) the significant therapeutic benefits derived by phobics when they really understand the triggering mechanisms underlying their anxiety disorders, such as those previously discussed.

The repeated failure of many phobics to respond to traditional therapies alone is typically internalized by patients as feelings of hopelessness. And their well-intended, but sometimes "theoretically narrow-focused," therapists seldom share the blame for these therapeutic failures—further reinforcing the patient's conviction of being too far gone or just too crazy for help. How do I know this? Because I once believed that phobias were neurotic manifestations and so unwittingly mistreated them according to the mistaken psychological theories prevalent at the time—as did all my traditionalist colleagues.

I have often observed this very same self-blame and negative self-esteem spiral when dyslexics refuse to seek new help—fearing they are hopeless and therefore attempting to avoid yet another devastating therapeutic disappointment. In fact, many fear their very first consultation, expecting their gut conviction and fear to be verified—that they're just dumb or brain damaged or crazy and beyond any help.

So, I cannot sufficiently emphasize the therapeutic value of insights such as those provided within this book by patients, including my clarifications, in helping the CVS-impaired improve—especially phobics in whom learned anticipation and new triggers often lead to spreading anxiety and even panic. Also, as previously noted, nothing beats the therapeutic synergy created by valid and in-depth insights as well as favorable med and other helpful treatments.

A Genetic Consideration and Explanation for Universal Phobias

Because Nancy and her daughter Joanna both have phobias and CVS dysfunction, it's possible that there may be some genetic links, despite significant differences in their phobic and non-phobic manifestations. Indeed, phobias and anxiety do run in families as do dyslexia, ADD/ADHD, and CVS dysfunctioning.

Believe it or not, I've had phobics in whom the very exact and extremely rare anxiety trigger had to have been genetically transmitted, since no other sensible alternative could be found. Thus, a patient of mine named Angelina was fearful of *green* flying birds, butterflies, insects, and crawling caterpillars. And guess what? When she discussed this fear with her mother, Angelina learned that her mom had these exact green fears—but had never revealed it to anyone, believing others would conclude she was crazy.

Although there are many possible explanations for this "green genetic phobia," there is one that appears most likely to me based on my clinical experience. Similar to my explanation for universal phobias, such as fears of rodents and snakes that pop up in individuals throughout most societies without any obvious causation, I assumed that these green configurations also had a similar specific adaptive quality to our evolutionary ancestors. And so, an equally unique genetic or acquired cerebellar-related inhibitory defect allowed this normally suppressed phylogenetically ancient trigger and mechanism to consciously manifest in "more recent family members."

Interestingly, this very reasoning may easily explain why dyslexia and/or SLD and/or ADD/ADHD is inherited, as well. All we need to assume is that they are genetically determined delayed or impaired developmental CVS states having variable characteristics.

Therapeutic Considerations

By and large, the CVS enhancers were found significantly helpful in treating CVS-determined phobias. In addition, the SSRIs (selective serotonin reuptake inhibitors) and SNRIs (serotonin-norepinephrine reuptake inhibitors), as well as other meds and nutrients, tend to significantly decrease the intensity of the input overload and/or over-reactive anxiety responses emitted from impaired anxiety-releasing center(s) within the brain. Thus, when indicated, combinations of these meds often provide the best and most rapid therapeutic responses possible (refer to Chap. 21). In addition, nonmedical add-ons, including psychotherapy, CBT (cognitive behavioral therapy), and desensitization, can also be highly effective. This is especially so when the primary CVS-determined phobias become secondarily contaminated with, and reinforced by, emotional factors—including the anticipated dread of anxiety/panic—and so are fueled by multiple overlapping sources.

Concluding Thoughts

In many ways, discovering the inner-ear or CVS causal connections to phobias/anxiety disorder and dyslexia as well as ADD/ADHD represented a completely unexpected pinnacle in my clinically based and continually evolving research career. Clearly, none of the vital insights needed to make these amazing phobic connections were based on prior theoretical formulations or traditionalist teaching. And so, none of them were predictable. None!

Rather, the opposite was true. Each and every important insight forced its way into my awareness—having to penetrate layers and layers of my previously biased "resistance filters" that were leading me to see and hear only those things my traditionalist teachers and training considered significant. And what these filters allowed me to see represented only a tiny and often distorted fragment of the four-dimensional clinically revealed connections portrayed throughout this book.

Embarrassingly, all the truly vital insights into the above phobia links were initially sidestepped or denied by all of us. This is especially so since once CVS-determined phobias are triggered, patients learn to secondarily anticipate and fear these and even look-alike "triggers." And so, these learned triggers can then mentally trigger the phobias—thus leading many professionals to confuse the obvious secondary conditioned or learned psychological result with the real but hidden primary somatic cause.

Now that the phobia connections to dyslexia, ADD/ADHD, and the CVS have been significantly clarified, really summarized, it's time to backtrack a little and add fascinating depth to the evolving portrait of dyslexia and its encompassing CVS syndrome. Accordingly, Chaps. 16 and 17 will now provide incredible insights into the 4-D reading process in dyslexia as well as the super-ten basic CVS mechanisms capable of explaining all, or most all, of dyslexia and related ADD/ADHD signs and symptoms. And these very same super-ten mechanisms can similarly explain the CVS phobias.

Chapter 16
The Reading Process in Dyslexia

In many ways, the discovery and clarification of all the basic underlying inner-ear/cerebellar-related determining mechanisms responsible for first the reading symptoms and then the non-reading symptoms characterizing the dyslexia or CVS syndrome was yet another of the many challenging and stimulating aspects of my evolving research efforts. Needless to say, these efforts did not proceed smoothly or in straight lines. Once again, backtracking and zigzagging were commonplace. And only after many years of listening and questioning, observing and treating thousands of dyslexics did I eventually see that the reading disorder in dyslexia was similar, by analogy, to a 4-D hologram in which the more you looked, the more complex the reading portrait became. And this "hologram" continually changed over time in patients—due to a host of dynamically interacting compensatory vs. destabilizing variables. Eventually I was even forced to recognize that the multidimensional reading hologram was but one of 18 comprising the dyslexia syndrome.

However, just before providing you with the details that emerged from this fascinating research journey, I thought it important to reemphasize the traditionalist two-dimensional view of dyslexia so that it might serve as an immediate point of contrast. As I've repeatedly stressed, the traditionalist misunderstanding of dyslexia was and is quite simple: Dyslexia is a severe and "pure" reading comprehension disorder of alexic-like cerebral processing origin with a poor prognosis.

An Unexpected Discovery

So, how did I put together the holographic dyslexia picture or cosmos? you might be wondering. In retrospect, it was really simple. All it took was enormous patience and determination as well as the ability to follow Thomas Huxley's brilliant suggestion: "Sit down before fact as a little child, be prepared to give up every preconceived notion, follow humbly wherever and to whatever abyss nature leads, or you shall learn nothing."

H. N. Levinson, *Feeling Smarter and Smarter*,
https://doi.org/10.1007/978-3-030-16208-5_16

In other words, all of my efforts would have come to naught—as did those of the traditionalists—had I not abandoned all the preconceived notions about *dyslexia = alexia* and had I not followed the balance/coordination/rhythm neurological inner-ear/cerebellar signs "humbly wherever and to whatever abyss nature leads." And as you know by now, listening to dyslexics and their favorable responses to a CVS enhancing treatment was the key to this discovery.

By collecting all the signs and symptoms characterizing thousands upon thousands of dyslexics, and then grouping their CVS-triggered favorable med responses under related symptom categories (e.g., reading, writing, spelling, math, etc.), I was able to outline the best 4-D sketch of the entire dyslexia syndrome, as detailed within the Self-Diagnostic Test.

And once all of the possible symptoms, to date, for each category (e.g., reading) were identified, I then attempted to explain the causal mechanisms responsible for each and every symptom—via a process I called neuroanalysis (akin to psychoanalysis)—keeping in mind that these dysfunctioning mechanisms would most likely be compatible with known and/or newly discovered inner-ear/cerebellar functioning.

Not infrequently, patients like Kathy revealed the causes of their dyslexia-related symptoms spontaneously and naturally, as if these symptoms should have been known all along by everyone, especially professionals. And so, I merely listed these symptoms and their casual mechanisms. Then I asked other patients if they too were similarly affected, eventually gaining the collective insights provided by thousands of patients.

After years of painstaking effort, I eventually began to see the common inner-ear/cerebellar-related mechanisms that could explain not only the reading category of symptoms but all 18 symptom categories—all 18 holograms. And to this day, I am still filling in new details.

Additionally, I will be discussing the super ten basic mechanisms that I discovered to be responsible for all of the symptoms characterizing the dyslexia/CVS syndrome in the very next chapter. But here I will focus only on the reading symptoms and mechanisms, since they were the ones that I, and all others, initially identified with dyslexia.

Finding the True Reading Hologram: Three Clinically Based Tools

My understanding of the reading "hologram" in dyslexia came about through three essential clinical steps, identical to those I've taken before and reviewed in Chap. 5: *Step 1*, questioning dyslexics about their reading problems and listening to their answers; *Step 2*, observing dyslexics in the process of reading, especially aloud, and analyzing their difficulties for underlying causes; and *Step 3*, identifying the previously hidden dyslexic reading symptoms and mechanisms by virtue of their favorable responses to inner-ear/CVS-enhancing meds.

Although these steps were initially used with children, I later applied them to dyslexic Kathy-like adults—as soon as they began seeking my help—and so obtained significantly greater amounts of information and insights.

Step I: Questions and Answers

As a psychiatrist for the New York City Board of Education, I was, as you know, asked to examine and help severely impaired reading-disabled or dyslexic children. The majority of kids I questioned found it difficult to answer the general questions I initially asked them, including: Why do you have trouble reading? Can you explain your difficulties? I would then follow up by asking lots of other questions, depending on circumstances.

The reason my questions were initially general was simple. At the very beginning of my research, I didn't know anything specific to ask. And according to psychoanalytic principles, I was trained to give patients as much leeway as possible to answer freely—without biasing them ahead of time with specifics.

But I learned very quickly that this open-ended "free-association" technique didn't initially work too well with dyslexic kids. Most of them didn't know what was really wrong with them, since many hadn't yet developed the perspective needed to distinguish normal from abnormal. Some refuted even having a reading disorder at all—psychologically preferring denial to admitting underlying feelings of stupidity.

And so, I was forced to seek new insights via Step II.

Step II: Observation and Analysis of Reading Errors

As a psychiatrist I had no sophisticated neurophysiological tools with which to examine the dyslexic kids at the time—even were I permitted to do so within the school system. Which I was not! So, I did the next best thing. I simply had the children attempt to read both silently and out loud so I could observe and record their errors. I hoped that by analyzing their errors and difficulties, I could determine the specific mechanisms underlying their problems. This method of investigation was very similar to listening to the symptoms reported by my psychiatric patients and then attempting to figure out what caused them.

This simple technique proved substantially more helpful at first than only the Q&A method. For example, it soon became clear that these dyslexic kids, when reading, often reversed letters such as *b* and *d* and words such as *was* and *saw*. So, it became apparent to me that they must have a *directional or orientational visual dysfunction*. The traditionalists had also noted this symptom and mechanism as well. But they failed to recognize its inner-ear/cerebellar causation. Kryptonite?

Very frequently—over 90 percent of the time—dyslexics were observed to lose their place while reading, and so they skipped over letters and words or inserted letters and words from the periphery or out of sequence. To compensate for losing their place, many would deliberately use a finger or marker or slow down their reading speed so that they might consciously guide their eyes during the reading process. So it became clear that these kids had a primary *visual fixation and a sequential tracking problem*. For this reason, they found it easier to read big and dark print, exceptions aside.

This eye tracking difficulty evidenced by dyslexics was also observed by MacDonald Critchley, as pointed out earlier. But since he believed in the alexic/dyslexic reading model, he mistakenly *assumed—really concluded*—that the tracking errors of dyslexics were merely secondary random searching movements characterizing patients who are literally blind or were "word-blind" due to an alexia-like inability to understand the meaning of the words they clearly saw. Thus, to minimize the confusion, their eyes reflexly began searching for a recognizable marker. As you may recall, Critchley failed to test out this assumption—really conviction. His failure to do so was, no doubt, bias-determined.

In trying to teach these children letters and words they didn't already know, it became obvious that repetition was vital to their learning. They had a difficult time learning to visually recognize the letters and words to begin with. And they had an easy time rapidly forgetting what they had previously learned—until overlearning, if and when it occurred, set in for keeps. So, they also had a *visual memory instability for letters and words.*

I often noticed that when reading, dyslexics had *difficulty concentrating and would become easily distracted.* But, interestingly, they would often concentrate for longer periods and with less distraction when there were only a few words on the page. So, their recognition and concentration capacities were frequently found determined by, and/or in proportion to, the word density on the page. This suggested that they might become *visually overloaded* far more easily than normal readers—probably because they had difficulty filtering out and/or maintaining separation of adjacent/background visual "noise." They also performed better in one-to-one situations where external distractions were minimized or better filtered, and focused concentration was maximized.

Upon further analyzing their reading errors, I realized that these children often read only the first letter or two of a four-plus-lettered word and then either skipped or guessed at the rest of them. However, when I pointed my finger at each letter in sequence, this skipping tendency lessened or disappeared. And when specifically asked why my finger made reading easier, a few would comment: "Because I can only see one or two letters of a word at a time—not the whole word." Thus, in addition to their fixation and tracking problems, it appeared they also had *tunnel vision* when reading. This insight explained why these dyslexics found it easier to read small words. By contrast, those with sequential tracking problems frequently skipped past two-or three-lettered short words—without even seeing them. Thus, they found it easier to read big words—because this gave them a larger overall target to fixate on and then retarget so as to eventually recognize and/or guess at.

Not infrequently, kids would experience delayed recognition or understanding of words and sentences they had just read—indicating the presence of *delayed visual processing*. This often led to secondary comprehension and/or misinterpretation errors when tested. And for a very, very few, this delayed recognition was severe enough and persistent enough to resemble a primary visual reading comprehension difficulty of an alexic-like nature.

Interestingly, some kids would occasionally read better when tracing the letters with their fingers. It thus appeared as if a compensatory tactile channel was helpful for recognition purposes when visual and/or phonetic channels were blocked.

I also observed kids moving their lips or vocalizing when reading. Again, when asked why, they would only say it was easier. Was it easier because the movement of the lips/voicing motor movements compensated for visual/phonetic recognition difficulties as did the word tracing finger movements? And some even *heard the words* they read, as previously noted in Chap. 11. Similarly, some read better aloud. However, most did not since they experienced difficulty reading and talking at the same time.

Others were observed to tilt either their heads or the page when reading. And when asked about this, some replied, "I see the print on an angle. And so, I tilt my head or the book so everything is lined up correctly." Might a *gyroscopic disorder* be present?

Many a kid with normal vision would read with their eyes very near to the page as if they were severely nearsighted. And when asked why, they didn't know except that it was easier to read this way. Only later on did I realize why. It was easier for their eyes to fixate on a close target than a distant one and so minimize their word blurring and/or movement. This appeared to be a compensatory symptom, just like deliberately slowing down the reading speed or using a finger to minimize losing one's place. So there were both dysfunctioning and compensatory reading symptoms at play here.

Occasionally, kids were seen shielding their eyes while reading, often blinking and squinting. Only belatedly did I realize that they were *light sensitive*—especially after some told me they also hated fluorescent lights. And parents periodically mentioned that their kids preferred reading in the dark or wearing a baseball cap to avoid glare and direct light. Thus, they appeared to have *difficulty filtering* out light, just as many had problems in adaptively filtering background sound distractions and/or processing too many visual forms on a page—a mechanism I called *overloading* or *flooding*.

Needless to say, I also observed a series of *phonetic recognition and memory difficulties*. Many reading-disabled children seemed not to clearly hear and/or remember specific sounds or blends. Some were *unable to integrate and hear sound sequences*, similar to the way that other kids were unable to see and integrate visual letter sequences. And still other kids experienced *difficulties in simultaneously connecting or integrating the letters and words on the page with their corresponding sound or phonetic counterparts*.

In summary, the observation of dyslexic kids as they read aloud, and the analysis of their reading errors, suggested the presence of numerous dysfunctioning as well as compensatory mechanisms, many of them often operating simultaneously. Although the additional insights derived from listening to dyslexic *adults* reading aloud added to my slowly evolving understanding, the real insight accelerator materialized only after I began successfully treating both children and adults with medications.

The dysfunctioning reading mechanisms observed, pre-medication, included:

- Visual perceptual and/or memory instability
- Visual fixation and sequential tracking difficulties
- Visual orientation and directional difficulties
- Tunnel vision
- Visual overloading and/or light sensitivity
- Visually related concentration/distractibility difficulties
- Gyroscopic difficulties
- Delayed visual processing
- Delayed phonetic and/or auditory speech/sound processing and/or related memory difficulties
- Auditory sequencing and/or integration problems
- Simultaneous visual-phonetic integration impairments
- Impaired comprehension—secondary to all the other dysfunctioning mechanisms, especially delayed visual and, no doubt, phonetic/phonological processing

The compensatory reading mechanisms observed, pre-medication, were:

- Slow reading speed
- Finger-pointing or use of a marker
- Head and body tilting
- Near-point fixation or shifting near/far fixations
- Mouthing or voicing, or "hearing the words" during reading
- Reading aloud is better for some, worse for others
- Repetition for memory reinforcement
- Reading in darker surroundings and/or wearing a hat—which some kids refused to remove in classrooms, despite the inevitable consequences

Step III: Insights Gained Through Favorable Responses to Medication

My understanding of the initially hidden symptoms and mechanisms characterizing the dyslexic reading disorder was dramatically enhanced once children and adults responded favorably to medication. As noted many times earlier, the disappearance of a symptom led to the clear recognition that something had changed—improved. And this change was often easy for both children and adults to describe once I at last knew what specific questions to ask, as well as how to listen and observe more effectively.

Not only were all of my prior dyslexia-related insights independently verified through favorable medication responses, but also a whole slew of previously unrecognized reading (and non-reading) symptoms suddenly revealed themselves via their disappearance. These symptoms included word blurring, double vision, word movement, reversal of light/dark background/foreground word patterns, poor visual and auditory form perception or recognition, and shifting and scrambling of letter and word sequences. Still other patients reported the disappearance of curved lines moving across the page or words now glued down rather than in flight while they were reading; and others reported the disappearance of auditory or phonetic distortions. All in all, it became apparent that there existed a *fine-tuning dysfunction* in dyslexia analogous to the one that scrambles the picture and sound in a faulty TV set—rendering these coexisting signals disjointed in both space and time.

On and on went these startling and unanticipated patient responses and observations. For example, many a dyslexic suddenly reported, "My eyes are no longer glued to each letter or word as I read. And I no longer have to blink or close my eyes for them to let go and move on to the next letter and word." Suddenly it became apparent that for normal sequential reading to occur, the eyes had to stop fixating on one letter or word in order to start targeting another. And so, we had a *stop-and-start mechanism* that was found to be impaired in dyslexics—creating a symptom medically described as *ocular perseveration.* Interestingly, this symptom was referred to by one patient as *reading stuttering*. And this insight eventually led me to better understand an important mechanism responsible for *verbal* stuttering—and perhaps obsessive thinking and compulsive behavior (*thought and motor stuttering*). Even persisting phobias!

Additionally, I suddenly understood why some dyslexics needed to repeatedly blink in order to read better. Blinking enabled the eye to unlock. I also understood the atypical observation that for some dyslexics it was actually *difficult* to read enlarged words and even to use their finger to compensate: Their eyes would fix so strongly onto an oversized word and/or a guiding marker that they couldn't let go enough to continue reading. Also, by simultaneously enlarging the distances between words and sentences via magnification, these patients' eyes would get lost moving from word to word. Hence, both the typical and atypical observations were readily explainable and compatible once their differing triggering and compensatory mechanisms were clearly understood. Perhaps you may now better understand why explaining the exceptions more clearly highlights the rule—or gestalt.

Many successfully treated dyslexics reported the disappearance of headaches, dizziness, nausea, or motion-sickness symptoms while reading, suggesting the preexistence of *motion-sickness and/or psychosomatic mechanisms*. And a few patients were forced to *rapidly scan* words, sentences, and even paragraphs to avoid the visual overloading and related motion sickness responses that resulted from slower and more prolonged reading. Jenny further clarifies these mechanisms in Chap. 20.

So, I was excited to add the following dysfunctioning vs. compensatory reading mechanisms to my evolving insights.

Dysfunctioning reading mechanisms revealed after medication treatment:

- Impaired fine-tuning and perception of reading—and all other signals
- Difficulty stopping and starting ocular fixation and tracking functions—resulting in ocular perseveration
- Impaired filtering of light and sound overloads during reading
- Abnormal triggering of motion sickness/psychosomatic mechanisms during reading

Compensatory reading mechanisms revealed after medication treatment:

- Blinking to refocus
- Use of large print
- Avoidance of finger pointing to minimize fixation on finger vs. reading content
- Mentally hearing the words looked at—phonetic "imaging" (refer to Chap. 11)
- Deliberate and enhanced interest and concentration, to compensate for rapid secondary concentration burnout—or pseudo-ADD
- Rapid scanning and processing of words, sentences, and paragraphs—often just their periphery—to avoid visual overloading and motion sickness responses triggered by viewing one word at a time. (The latter is highlighted by Kathy in Chap. 6 and Jenny in Chap. 20.)

Eventually, an updated list of reading symptoms and dysfunctioning vs. compensatory mechanisms was compiled. These insights significantly increased my understanding of what was really wrong with the reading process of dyslexics. Clearly, this new and dynamic multidimensional CVS perspective on the dyslexic reading disorder was altogether different in both depth and scope than the traditionalist and neotraditionalist *dyslexia* = *alexia* concepts allowed for.

As you can now easily see, and as I've previously mentioned, the thinking brain often plays a crucial *compensatory* role in dyslexia—a likely genetically determined descrambling one, rather than the primary dysfunctioning impairment assumed by prior theorists. Perhaps now you can also better understand how it's possible for the thinking brain, and perhaps also the higher cerebellum, to compensate for impaired reading scores and mechanisms despite the continued presence of an inner-ear/cerebellar determined impairment and resulting dysfunctional mechanisms and symptoms.

The Differing Reading Experiences of Dyslexics

Although the vast majority of dyslexics share recognizable similarities with one another insofar as their reading performance goes, there are also obvious and even dramatic differences between them. The similarities result from common determining mechanisms shared by the majority. The differences are due to patterns of dysfunctioning vs. compensatory mechanisms that are unique to each individual. Needless to say, this belated understanding clearly highlights our oversimplistic and mistaken tendency to define this complex reading disorder by a single variable, e.g., a visual fixation and tracking dysfunction or a severe alexia-like reading-score deficiency or a phonological impairment....

Armed with an understanding of the above reading symptoms and mechanisms characterizing dyslexics, it is now possible for parents and professionals to truly empathize with the incredibly difficult struggle dyslexics face when trying to overcome their disorder as well as compensate for their devastated self-esteem.

Just imagine trying to read when you're simultaneously experiencing:

- *Memory instability* for letters, words, and sentences... both seen and/or heard
- *Letters, words, and sentences skipped over* and mixed in with others from the surrounding page, resulting in confusion and guessing of content
- *Blurring, scrambling, doubling up, and movement* of words and sentences on a page, as well as similar disturbances of phonetic counterparts, resulting in rapid fatigue and burnout
- *Confusion or disorientation* with regard to letters and words, e.g., mixing up *b* and *d*, *was* and *saw*, etc.
- *Misperception* of similar appearing and sounding letters and words, akin to Kathy's magnificently described reading and hearing errors
- *Light sensitivity and visual overloading*
- *Difficulty concentrating and easy distractibility or impaired filtering*
- *Delayed processing* of words so that recognition/comprehension occurs seconds or minutes later, when attempting to deal with new content
- *Gyroscopic slanting* of words and sentences in one direction or in jumbled up/down patterns
- *Tunnel vision* of the whole word, resulting in seeing only one letter at a time and then having to consciously string together all the letters so that a total word view and meaning can be formulated
- *Oscillation and reversals* of the white background with the dark print, which creates a flicker-like effect
- *"Gluing" of the eyes to letters and words* and then having to blink in order to let go of one configuration and move on to the next one
- *Compensatory* near-far focusing, head and body tilting, blinking, light shielding, enhanced concentration, using a finger or marker, slowing down reading speed, self-isolation to minimize distractions, and/or even the paradoxical use of music to absorb or filter out background noise of fluctuating intensity, etc.

In retrospect Were all these dysfunctioning and compensatory mechanisms and symptoms—or even just a few of them—going on simultaneously while you were reading, would you not then more easily become overwhelmed? Thus, the complex primary dyslexia-caused impairment would further intensify. And what if you then become anxious and even depressed by the inevitable frustration that arises—would this not also further impair your eventual recall and understanding of the read content? *In many ways, I found it much easier to understand the failure of dyslexics than to fully comprehend their uncanny ability to compensate and succeed, often without professional help.*

By comparison, the traditionalists, completely unaware of the above-described reading hologram, merely measured the *outcome* of all this complex dysfunctioning vs. compensation. And they oversimplistically and mistakenly concluded what was initially believed to be true: that the cerebral alexia theory of dyslexia was correct. And only because of their *denial* of 99.9 percent of the reading symptoms and mechanisms affecting dyslexics were they able to preserve their mistaken century-plus-old belief in the *dyslexia* = *alexia* connection.

In fact, were it not for their recognition of reading reversals, the traditionalists would have been 100 percent wrong, although they failed to either explain the occurrence of reversals or recognize/acknowledge the reversals' inner-ear-determined directional/orientation mechanisms. Nor did they question and/or explain why no alexic manifested reversals or any other typical dyslexic symptoms and mechanisms. Is it any wonder that dyslexics remained puzzled, frustrated, and devastated by their disorder until this inner-ear/cerebellar research and treatment enabled them to feel smarter and smarter?

Finally, the remaining 17 non-reading symptom categories in dyslexia were then similarly elucidated and clarified in a manner identical to the way I came to understand the reading hologram. Eventually, the entire hidden holographic portrait called the *dyslexia/CVS syndrome* was unmasked. Just as the reading mechanisms were clarified, so were all the non-reading determinants. And as you will see in the next chapter, I was led to discover ten simplified but generalized super-mechanisms that could easily explain all reading and non-reading dyslexic symptoms comprising the eighteen major symptom categories. And thus, they easily explained all of Kathy's symptoms.

The Normal Reading Hologram: Another Zag

Before we end this chapter, it is imperative that I reemphasize a prior insight that may have been overlooked. The above CVS-dysfunctioning vs. compensatory reading mechanisms likely highlight and mirror the very same complex mechanisms characterizing the normal reading process. Why is this important? Because we often oversimplistically assume that there is only one decoding reading mechanism for both dyslexics and normal readers—likely based on the alexia-related reading model which suggests that we either comprehend written signals or not. Or the phonological model. Or even my initial ocular fixation and tracking concept.

And by clearly recognizing this reading hologram, gifted teachers will be better able to specifically target, remediate, and so better compensate for specific dysfunctioning dyslexic reading mechanisms while also more efficiently enhancing the mechanisms used by non-dyslexic normal readers.

Chapter 17
The "Super-Ten" Basic Mechanisms Explaining the Dyslexia Syndrome

In this chapter, I intend to present a truly unique insight: *the"super-ten" general mechanisms responsible for causing and so explaining all—hundreds—of the reading and non-reading symptoms comprising the entire dyslexia syndrome.* However, before describing these mechanisms in detail, I thought it important—as a symbolic and clinical reminder—to present three more verbatim accounts of favorable medication responses typical of the thousands from which most of my insights were derived and continue to accrue.

Three Clinical Vignettes—Favorable Medical Responses

1. ***Johnny's*** *writing is straighter, better formed, smoother, and more rapidly performed. His spelling is almost normal—he's no longer reversing or inserting letters nor leaving them out. It's as if he can see the letters within his mind and not rely on only phonetic cues. He now claims, "I have a brain."*
2. ***Anne*** *is no longer fearful of going to school. She's even better with heights. And I'm not sure this is related to the medications, but she no longer has nightmares as before and can now sleep alone and in the dark. And another thing, she can now dance better. It's as if her sense of timing and rhythm is suddenly present, and she's no longer tripping over her feet and turning in the wrong direction.*

   *Her speech, too, is better. She can articulate her words more clearly, and her stuttering suddenly disappeared. Anne puts it simply: "My eyes no longer stutter when I read, and my mouth moves smoother too." Are these really related?**

   Suddenly she is riding her bike and participating in group sports. Before, she just avoided these events, tending to stay alone.

   Now she's never alone. There are friends over the house all the time, and she just talks and talks with them. Before, she was a loner and a listener. Speaking of listening, she now responds rapidly to what is told her—without saying "What?" and without us having to repeat things three or four times before she seems to

H. N. Levinson, *Feeling Smarter and Smarter*,
https://doi.org/10.1007/978-3-030-16208-5_17

grasp them. And her verbal responses are faster too, which is probably why she now enjoys socializing. (Imagine the benefit to autistics when these CVS improvements occur!)

Anne was always fearful of going shopping with us in busy, crowded places and stores. She was always afraid of getting lost—and often she did. It's as if she became easily disoriented and would forget or confuse the entrance with the exit. This fear is also gone. Suddenly she knows right and left. And east/west and north/south now seem as simple to her as the multiplication tables.

Speaking of these tables, she finally learned and retained them. This was not possible before, despite all our efforts. And her mood is terrific. She sings and dances all the time, just like we always hoped but never thought possible before. Her life just seems easier—normal.

3. *My son **Jamie** is now getting all A's and B's in school. That makes us happier than he is. But what made the biggest difference to him was his suddenly improved sports ability. He can now catch and throw a ball. And his batting is so much better—except when he forgets to take the medications, especially on weekends. He now reminds us to give it to him before he goes to little league.*

How These Super-Ten Mechanisms Were Found

Again, each improvement reported by a CVS-dysfunctioning individual on inner-ear/CVS-enhancing medications highlighted the presence of a previously existing inner-ear/CVS-related and caused symptom. And by carefully analyzing their neurological determinants, I found that they could be classified within *18 major dysfunctional categories—interrelated via a common underlying inner-ear/CVS dysfunction.*

Eventually, the symptoms within each of the 17 non-reading categories were analyzed for underlying determinants, as was the Reading category in the preceding chapter. And after all of the recognized determining mechanisms were condensed into their most general expressions, I was eventually left with ten primary or "super" ones. Important to mention: many symptoms can be explained by more than one determinant—suggesting that either the mechanisms are too generally defined and/or more likely, that *the symptoms have overlapping CVS determinants.*

Also, all the characteristics previously deemed typical for dyslexics, and those with related CVS disorders, were found to vary in degree from one extreme to another—from gifted to severe. No single quality or quantity, symptom, or mechanism came close to capturing the essence of, and so properly defining, this overall impairment. Thus, for example, the dyslexia in each dyslexic was obviously different—since there appeared to be infinite possible combinations of CVS-dysfunctioning vs. compensatory mechanisms which manifested uniquely in each individual with the dyslexia or CVS syndrome—thus far best illustrated by Kathy, whom we've used as a key frame of reference.

Yet, defying the apparent odds, a clearly recognizable 4-D portrait of dyslexia as well as the CVS universe around which it orbits was eventually unmasked—illustrated by the functions and symptoms characterizing the Self-Diagnostic Test. And this complex overall super-portrait proved capable of unifying and encompassing all of this syndrome's typical, atypical, and seemingly paradoxical features while leading to the amazing super-ten explanatory mechanisms as well as a fully encompassing and explanatory CVS theory of the dyslexia/CVS syndrome. However, unlike the Mona Lisa, this portrait as well as its CVS theory will never be complete—forever remaining a dynamic work in progress.

The Super-Ten Mechanisms

The following super-ten inner-ear/CVS-determined mechanisms explain, in remarkable detail, all the many and diverse dyslexia-related symptoms and functions comprising the 4-D holographic dyslexia or CVS syndromes.

1. *The CVS acts like a missile's guidance system—"navigating" our eyes, hands, feet, and various mental and physical functions in space and time.* Thus, a disorder with this system may deflect our eyes while they're attempting to fixate and sequentially track letters, words, and sentences during reading—a process that is normally reflexive and automatic. As a result, the dyslexic's reading process is characterized by fixation and tracking difficulties, requiring compensatory slow reading, finger pointing, using cards as markers, etc., and even moving a thumb vertically down the margin to guide the eyes from line-to-line without distracting them from the main word text.

What's more, the resulting visual-motor scrambling will trigger the insertion and omission of words, as well as the illusion of new words formed from word-parts separated by unseen distances. Words will frequently seem to blur or move around on the page, requiring compensatory blinking, squinting, and concentration in order to re-stabilize the drifting input.

Inasmuch as the tracking in dyslexics is frequently coarse and jerky, the reading process becomes tiring and unpleasant. Often, these discoordinated or clumsy eye movements retarget or become stuck on words, resulting in ocular perseveration or "reading stuttering."

If our hands, feet, speech, and even our thinking mechanisms are not accurately guided in space and time, a wide range of discoordinated, clumsy acts, or "Freudian slips" ("dyslexic slips") will occur. If the hand holding a pen is misguided in space and time, our writing will look discombobulated or dysgraphic. And typically the writing will drift off the horizontal if unlined paper is used and if compensatory concentration and effort are not exerted to extraordinary and thus tiring degrees.

The writing samples presented earlier in the book clearly highlight the graphomotor, spelling, and grammatical errors characterizing the CVS dysfunctioning of dyslexics. And these errors in writing coordination obviously mirror those in reading coordination.

Importantly, if our thoughts and speech are misguided in space and time, then we can readily understand the CVS-determined speech/language impairments—mistakenly attributed to cerebral or thinking brain mechanisms.

2. *The CVS acts like the vertical and horizontal holds on a television set—although a four-dimensional one. It fine-tunes in 3-D space—plus in time—all (voluntary and involuntary) motor responses leaving the brain and all sensory responses coming into the brain.* If voluntary motor responses leaving the brain are improperly fine-tuned, one's motor functions become discoordinated and imbalanced. This may result in delays or difficulties in fine, gross, and rhythmic motor activities. Specifically, the following symptoms may occur: delays or problems with crawling, sitting, walking, tying shoelaces, buttoning, zippering, holding and using writing implements and scissors, and playing various sports. Also, speech delays and/or symptoms such as stuttering, stammering, articulation errors, and "Freudian"/dyslexic slips of the tongue, mind, and hand are not infrequent. And when involuntary motor responses leaving the brain are improperly fine-tuned, toilet-training delays may arise as well as such symptoms as bed-wetting and soiling.

If the sensory input to the brain is improperly fine-tuned, this input will drift or scramble. The thinking brain, however bright, will have difficulty perceiving, interpreting, remembering, and concentrating on drifting, scrambled inputs. If the drift is 180°, typical $b = d$ reversals may occur. And as you've read, CVS dysfunctioning dyslexics often see, write, read, and navigate at tilted angles or even backward. Also, Kathy-like misperceptions are typical.

Even a genius watching and listening to a "drifting TV channel" will have great difficulty remembering and concentrating on the slanted or scrambled picture and soundtrack. Variations in the amount of drift will account for variations in the degree of clarity. Some segments of the TV program may be seen and heard clearly, while others will be only partially seen and heard. And some will be completely blurred, resulting in compensatory guessing and even illusions. Additionally, when the visual and/or auditory or other vital components are out of sync in time, further symptoms invariably arise.

If asked about the content of a scrambled TV show, a viewer will not be able to answer too many questions. Similarly, if unaware that their "secondary comprehension" difficulties are due to a drifting "TV image/sound," dyslexics will instinctively feel stupid, regardless of their IQ. In fact, the smarter a dyslexic is, the more frustrated he will become, and the dumber he will feel.

For this reason, compliments don't work too well with dyslexics, although explanations for their failure can be helpful! These kids *know* they are not able to grasp, remember, and reproduce information as well as their classmates or as well as their instincts convey they should. So, they often feel compliments to be insincere, otherwise they wouldn't be needed.

Although reassurance does not reverse feeling stupid, making some feel worse, it is crucial nonetheless since encouragement keeps many striving until compensation occurs. If it occurs. By contrast, criticism and misunderstanding are felt very keenly and reinforce dyslexics' gut feelings of stupidity, resulting in an even deeper sense of inadequacy.

In the absence of this vitally needed understanding, it is very easy for teachers and even parents to mistakenly believe these children are stupid, indifferent, lazy, and defiant. Especially if the parent or teacher is processing the same content as the child, but, by analogy, receiving it on a clear "TV channel." Moreover, the child watching the drifting TV channel will inevitably lose his concentration and become distracted and restless. He'll want to get away from this frustrating input as soon as possible and switch the TV channel.

This experience is very similar to how one reacts to motion sickness or any overload and related dysfunction. Instinctively one wants to eliminate the distressing input, either by fight or flight. If a child can't play hooky or "change his channel" in school by means of distracting mechanisms, he will fight. If his anger is acted out, he will be viewed as a behavior problem with disruptive tendencies. Children, in an effort to escape a frustrating and humiliating situation, may sometimes unconsciously behave in a manner that provokes authorities to suspend or expel them from school. Thus, they may also become bullies, truants, or dropouts.

If children's anger and fight are inwardly directed, they will become depressed—feel guilty—and give up. At times, guilt from feeling stupid and inadequate will trigger mechanisms that invite punishment and being bullied, and thereby alleviate guilt—a most unfortunate cycle. If, on the other hand, children are impelled by triggered anxiety to avoid the frustrating drifting channel altogether, they're labeled "school phobic."

In order to understand all the variations and complexities of the dyslexic disorder, one has to carry the TV analogy a few steps further. Picture the brain as a giant TV set with millions of channels. Imagine each separate event as being independently processed on its own wavelength. Thus, one channel may drift, while another remains fine-tuned. One channel may drift only mildly, while another is completely blurred out. One channel may drift vertically, while another drifts horizontally. One channel may drift from right to left, while another drifts from left to right. On and on the possibilities go, accounting for the diverse combinations of symptoms seen from dyslexic patient to patient—also accounting for their reading from right to left in Hebrew fashion and even bottom-up.

And similar variations occur with motor functions, perhaps better explaining how and why even gifted athletes with the CVS syndrome may often manifest function-specific imbalance and dyscoordination.

Furthermore, the fine-tuners themselves may vary in function from moment to moment, depending on known and unknown variables and circumstances. Spontaneous fluctuations in the fine-tuning mechanisms may result in corresponding variations in symptoms, usually beyond the individual's control. Allergies of various kinds may trigger signal drifting, which can account for regression in spring and fall or when gluten, sugars, and dyes are present in the diet. Similarly, altitude and barometric changes, as well as endocrine variations and even the full moon and gravitation, may trigger fluctuations.

By far, the most frequent destabilizing factor is fatigue. Once concentration burns out, pseudo-ADD sets in—even PTSD. And then most mental and motor systems regress—even shut down. Additionally, in a vicious cycle, ensuing anxiety and depression further diminish functioning and thereby intensify frustration and failure. Thus, sleep and frequent rest periods are essential to recharge the dyslexic's "batteries." Also very helpful are concentration enhancers such as interesting topics, teachers, and even stimulant medications.

3. *The CVS serves as a three-dimensional compass system. It reflexively tells us spatial relationships such as right and left, up and down, and front and back.* If this 3-D compass system isn't working efficiently, then one must consciously devise compensatory methods such as wearing a ring or a watch on one hand or recalling which hand has a scar or was broken or was used to pledge allegiance. Related difficulties in sensing, knowing, and even understanding east and west, and north and south, may also occur—often triggering anxieties about getting lost.

The compass system directs all body functions: sensory, motor, speech, thought, and even biophysical patterns. Moreover, one sequence may be misdirected, while another remains unaffected or compensated for, *and yet another operating at a gifted level.* And recall the role directional and orientational uncertainty plays in triggering agoraphobic and related anxieties—which can secondarily further destabilize this impairment.

4. *The CVS acts as a timing mechanism, setting rhythms to motor and even sensory, cognitive, and language tasks.* A disturbance within this system may result in difficulty sensing time and learning to tell time. Dyslexics may not know *before* from *after* and can't sense whether a minute, an hour, or several hours have gone by. As a result, they may become "compulsively" late or early—the latter to compensate. Speech timing may be off, resulting in slow or rapid talking and even dysrhythmic speech or stuttering. Even rapid or slow thinking can be similarly explained. And for some, the rates of thinking and speaking may be out of sync. The CVS system, primarily the cerebellum, must also serve to inhibit or modulate the speed of the various sensory input signals. Accordingly, dyslexics may experience visual, auditory, tactile, and related signals as being faster, and thus they may blur out these sensory sequences at lower thresholds than do normal subjects. In fact, many dyslexics with phobias of driving experience cars, their own included, as racing far faster than they really are—and so panic, fearing they are losing control. The opposite—slowed perception—can occur, as well, leading to other symptoms. (These speed-related symptoms will be more thoroughly described in Chap. 20 in relation to my diagnostic 3-D Optical and Auditory Scanners.)
5. *The CVS serves as a dynamic filter, substantially blocking out non-adaptive and potentially contaminating/distracting sensory-motor and mental "background noise."* Impairments or "holes" within this CVS filtering mechanisms can account for the sensory-specific and other distractibility symptoms of dyslexics,

including those with ADD, as well as the internal or subconscious "leaking" of archaic and suppressed maladaptive thoughts and impulses. This "leakage" can result in such diverse manifestations as daydreaming; impulsive stealing; hitting others; universal phobias of snakes, rodents, and more; and obsessions and compulsions. Similarly, background motor movement must be inhibited or filtered out in the interest of smooth, rhythmic, and goal-directed "foreground" action; otherwise, clumsiness and dyscoordination result.

6. *Integration of sensory-motor functioning is inner-ear/CVS related.* Dyslexics sometimes experience a breakdown in integrated or composite movement patterns, as well as in sequenced sensory-input experiences—called *decomposition* of sequences or patterns. Thus, "klutzy" individuals must slow down movement speeds and attempt a conscious, deliberate, and cerebrally directed *recomposition* of these individual steps so as to complete an intended action. Similarly, dyslexics characteristically experience tunnel-vision during reading—often seeing only one or two letters of a word sequence at a time. They are then forced to look at, and sound out, each letter of a total word sequence, one at a time. Finally, they must attempt a conscious reintegration/recomposition of the total sequence so as to complete the reading task. And often central and peripheral visual mechanisms are compromised—decomposed—forcing dyslexics to use one or another rather than both visual mechanisms simultaneously. And at times peripheral vision is exaggerated via compensation or impaired filtering—intensifying background distractibility.

Sound sequences are also decomposed for many dyslexics, explaining some auditory input processing lags and distortions as well as a need for extra time and repetition before speech can be "sequentially heard," compensated for, and understood. In fact, this mechanism frequently explains the misperceptions experienced by dyslexics, which lead to disparities between what they are told and what they hear and recall.

Interestingly, some dyslexics cannot look at and listen to people talking at the same time—since they are distracted by facial expressions. Thus, these dyslexics are often mistakenly considered autistic-like. And the opposite appearing mechanism—over-focusing on facial movements may be vital for some so as to compensate for their ADD-distractibility. Others cannot compensate for their impaired auditory processing unless, like the hearing impaired, they look directly at the speaking person for communication clues. This latter mechanism is sometimes responsible for telephone phobias—since needed facial and body communication clues are then absent.

Crowd phobias often have similarly impaired sound and visual overloading and/or distracting/disorienting triggers—perhaps also related to a disintegration of a separation mechanism maintaining gestalt or stimulus integrity. Too often, this overloading impairs word crowds on a page or conversations in a room with background noise. Thus, some dyslexics like Kathy cannot normally see letter, word, and sentence separations, while others cannot properly hear distinct sound gestalts.

Additionally, disintegration of composite sensory and/or motor sequences, as well as filtering, may also affect the simultaneous processing of multi-sensory visual, acoustic, position-sensing, motion-related, and motor-related—as well as the sticking and separation—mechanisms involved in reading. These impairments then result in the various "types" of reading difficulties characterizing dyslexics, as well as their special compensatory styles. As a result, many a single-variable professional unaware of the complex CVS reading hologram presented in Chap. 16 has named/described rather than understood these diverse fragments. Thus, you may have heard of linear dyslexia where dyslexics skip lines, and paragraph dyslexia—where their vertical skipping is just greater. And you certainly have heard of phonological dyslexia, not to mention the list of synonyms described in the first few chapters. Have we not all unwittingly used these dyslexia-related disintegration mechanisms in our attempt to unmask this complex CVS syndrome?

7. *The CVS is connected to various mood, anxiety, activity, and autonomic nervous system centers of the brain and thereby modulates these and various other functions*. Accordingly, a failure in these diverse functions may result in secondarily related and interconnected anxiety, mood, and self- and body-image disturbances, as well as impulse and activity disorders—symptoms often characterizing ADD/ADHD and phobias. Additionally, a failure to modulate the autonomic nervous system may result in a series of so-called psychosomatic symptoms: difficulties with swallowing, breathing, heart rate, temperature, sweating, motion sickness, urinary and gastrointestinal functions, and even eating. And as we've read, a failure to properly send and regulate anxiety triggering signals and responses can result in phobias/anxiety disorders. Similar difficulties may also trigger mood fluctuations, including depression, thus explaining the reported improvements of these symptoms on CVS enhancers.
8. *The CVS serves as a gyroscope for the brain*. This mechanism maintains stable visual alignment and perception relative to the positions of the head, neck, and body. Dysfunctioning in this mechanism readily explains such dyslexic symptoms as seeing print that appears to be on an angle and the compensatory need for head, neck, and body tilting in order to effect a neurophysiological realignment. Similar repositioning is experienced during writing—for analogous reasons—and also during sports and other motor activities.
9. *The CVS processes muscle tone and gravity signals*. Impairments in muscle tone not infrequently lead, or contribute, to "double-jointedness," slouching, and/or head and shoulder tilting, possibly even facilitating scoliosis and flat feet (*pes planus*) in those physiologically predisposed. Indeed, tonal imbalance may intensify strabismus (failure of the eyes to work together in synch) and trigger "jelly legs." Improper processing of gravity may contribute to the sensations of falling or being pulled to one side and even to irresistible feelings and fears of being pulled to the ground when looking down from heights. It may also contribute to a person's moving up when they intend to move down, as exemplified by Kathy—who also had severe directional difficulties.

10. *The CVS is assumed to facilitate the processing of starting and stopping numerous motor, sensory, and even mental functions.* Thus, it is not unusual for inner-ear/CVS dysfunctioning dyslexics to have difficulty stopping a motor sequence once started—which can lead to the repetition or perseveration characterizing their reading, speaking (i.e., stuttering), and writing errors as well as the mental and behavior symptoms characteristic of OCD and persisting anxiety triggers—phobias. As often noted, inner-ear/CVS-enhancing medications, and even corrective conditioning, often help improve this impairment.

For proper sensory perception, sequencing, and flow, there may also be a very rapid stop-and-start regulating function as well—a symptom when prolonged I refer to as "sensory stuttering." Sensory perception might therefore be impaired if this mechanism malfunctioned, thus missing or distorting or sticking within intervals along the stream. Interestingly, good music and rhythm may facilitate smooth sensory and motor flow—thus also explaining why memory is enhanced and why stutterers may sing well. By contrast, dysrhythmic "music" and/or distracting sound sequences may trigger symptomatic intensification in dyslexics while creating dyslexic-like symptoms in non-dyslexics.

Summary

In many ways, I believe the above-described insights—although highly condensed and perhaps overloading—represent another major high point in the understanding of dyslexics and their complex disorder. Now every parent, loved one, and caring professional can truly understand just about every known facet of this heretofore puzzling impairment. And every dyslexic can understand himself/herself with the depth, scope, and conviction needed for insight to become therapeutic. Armed with these powerful insights, it is now possible for every dyslexic to replace their self-blame with confidence and begin to feel as smart as they really are!

And equally important, for the very first time, healers can direct their diverse treatment techniques at the *super-ten specific mechanisms* responsible for the many and diverse symptoms characterizing the dyslexia or CVS syndromes—and so exponentially enhance therapeutic outcomes.

Chapter 18
Many Helpful Therapies

Many therapies have been reported helpful for those with the dyslexia/CVS syndrome. However, because of my comprehensive CVS theory, it is now possible to holistically and uniquely encompass and properly explain them all and so facilitate their acceptance and use.

Simply put, the following helpful therapies are those that tend to reduce symptoms by (1) improving CVS functioning and signaling, (2) enhancing cerebral and higher-cerebellar descrambling and other compensatory mechanisms, and/or (3) minimizing/avoiding destabilizing factors.

A Heads-Up and Explanation

So, before we start, I have an important heads-up for you: Some of these effective CVS improving methods were initially refuted defensively and were condescendingly called "magic cures" by those mistakenly believing faulty cerebral dyslexia vs. CVS-related theories. Others were incompletely and even incorrectly explained/theorized and so were negated rather than better clarified. And I've even included a therapy that most had rejected and/or found highly controversial and "politically incorrect" so as to stimulate your thinking.

Just remember: All of these methods have one thing in common—patients have been helped by these therapies to varying degrees. None are harmful. And as you will read, there is much to be gained by reviewing and so better understanding them all.

H. N. Levinson, *Feeling Smarter and Smarter*,
https://doi.org/10.1007/978-3-030-16208-5_18

Medical/Neurophysiological Treatments

Medical Treatment

The first and only *medical* treatment for dyslexia and its syndrome resulted from my discovery that this disorder was of a primary inner-ear/CVS origin. Since the anti-motion sickness meds were known to improve the balance/coordination/rhythm, vertigo, motion sickness, and concentration symptoms characterizing inner-ear/CVS dysfunction, it seemed reasonable to assume that these same medications might also improve CVS-related reading and possibly the other non-reading symptoms characterizing the dyslexia syndrome. Fortunately for countless millions, this assumption was clinically demonstrated to be valid!

Advantages As the case presentations in this book and in my many other clinical studies demonstrate, the inner-ear/CVS-enhancing medications, including stimulants and nutrients, now offer 75–85 percent of treated dyslexics hope and help—rapidly and sometimes dramatically.

Since this unique treatment is capable of rapidly improving the total syndrome rather than only its reading or academic or ADHD or speech/language or phobic symptoms, it likely should be used first to facilitate educational methods. This is especially so in more severe cases. Best of all, any minimal side-effect risks can be rapidly reduced to almost zero, and even prevented, by test-dosing.

Importantly, this CVS-enhancing method rapidly decreases signal scrambling, thus enabling *all other therapies—all involving signals*—to be more effective. Consequently, most other methods might then be viewed as add-ons to maximize the depth, scope, and rapidity of the medically triggered generalized improvements in fortunate responders.

The risk of using only non-med add-ons as stand-alone therapies The add-on therapies, to be later reviewed, are generally innocuous and so are often used alone by many who fear meds or know very little about them. However, one must consider the risks of using *only* methods that, when compared to meds, take longer to work, target fewer symptoms, and are characterized by lower potency and improvement rates in failing, desperate, and dumb-feeling dyslexics. This is especially true for those who have given up—surrendered—after previously failing or minimally benefitting from educational and other therapeutic modalities. In these cases, meds should be considered a vital add-on.

Playing the odds Importantly, these absolutely safe options are rarely understood in this realistic comparative perspective. And their abovementioned negative consequences or "side-effects" are seldom, if ever, compared to those of medical treatments. Reasoning like a "medical oddsmaker," I maintain that to win you must have the odds in your favor. That said, not all of these non-med therapies are slow and limited. And some should be tried first—especially the educational methods, often in combination with others.

Just remember, my reasoning is based on having medically treated a significant majority of patients who failed to adequately respond to prior therapies, especially the vital educational ones. So, my comments are biased by my rather limited or secondhand experience with how well these other methods work in those who have no need of my help.

In the final analysis The best chance of winning—maximally and rapidly improving—with the least overall risk is to truly understand all of the therapeutic options as well as their attendant positives and negatives. Only then should you decide what is really best for you, your child, and/or your patient and what to try first and next.

I have commented throughout this book, especially in footnotes, why I believe that inner-ear meds are potent CVS enhancers and that placebos are atypical when the results are clinically analyzed, and also why needed formal validating double-blind controlled studies, designed according to my clinically determined specifications, must be performed by independent, unbiased (non-"triple-blind") investigators. Hopefully, this book's content will override any prior resistance to perform them.

Allergic/Neurotoxic Avoidance

Dr. Ben Feingold, a noted allergist, many years ago recognized that sugars, dyes, and various other allergenic substances may intensify and even trigger such ADD/ADHD-related symptoms as hyperactivity, impulsivity, impaired concentration, and distractibility. And I have noted how adding/changing color to meds often inactivates them for some patients and especially how kids may fly off the handle or really become revved up after consuming sugar and/or specific dyes. Accordingly, the avoidance of these and other so-called "neurotoxic" substances, now including gluten and even dairy products, in select individuals is crucial, despite a refuting study or two. Although atypical, this toxic mechanism is 100 percent obvious and potent in those affected. Fortunately, it seems to be "outgrown" with age.

Non-chemical, Non-medical, Neurophysiological-Based Therapies

There are a number of non-chemical, non-medical, neurophysiological-based therapies that have been helpful in improving the varied symptoms characterizing the dyslexia syndrome. I've referred to them as add-ons or stand-alones. Some are more helpful than others and faster to show results. All play a vital therapeutic role, whether used alone or in combination or first, second, or third. Clearly, pedagogic methods, especially those guided by neurophysiological and psychological insights, should be used first and continued for those children with academic symptoms, no matter what other therapies are implemented, my own included.

Although the varied psychological therapies are important to minimize the emotional fallout resulting from frustration and failure as well as to modify behavior, I've decided to skip them within this presentation. However, I believe the psychotherapeutic value of this book's insights, especially when reinforced by the favorable overall symptomatic responses of those with the dyslexia syndrome to CVS-enhancing treatments, provides the best catalysts for rapidly correcting impaired self-esteem and self-blame while often triggering an immediate sense of emotional well-being. This insight will once again be demonstrated when you listen to Jenny in Chap. 20.

Fast ForWord (FFW)

FFW is a cognitive training modality designed to improve language and reading skills using software products evolved from the research of a number of highly respected neuroscientists, including Michael Merzenich and Paula Tallal. This method is based on data supporting a previously discussed neotraditionalist dyslexic theory proposed in the late 1990s. It claimed that many children who have language and reading difficulties, assumed to be of a primary cerebral origin, have problems with rapidly processing sounds. Thus, their FFW cognitive training method is stated to improve defective sound processing, which then generalizes to enhance phoneme awareness, language, and reading.

Although this method has been stated to help large numbers of children worldwide, some researchers have raised questions about the extent of a rapid auditory processing deficit in children with language and reading disabilities. And a few question Tallal's claim that: "Ninety percent of the kids who complete the program made 1.5–2 years of progress in reading skills."[1] Still others challenge the assertion that her program even helps kids' language deficits at all, claiming that improvements were coincidental to her method.

I have had no direct experience with using this method and so cannot properly judge the scientific data and claims, pro and con. However, as mentioned earlier within this book, I developed and patented a 3-D Auditory Scanner in the 1970s that measured the auditory processing speed of word and sentence signals heard. Thus, I have personally verified that these rapid and other auditory signals may be distorted or improperly processed in some dyslexics. I also found that my ability to accurately obtain the desired measurements were significantly more complicated than I had initially thought, and the conditioned gains were less than expected. However, my method was completely different and significantly less robust and accurate than that appearing to characterize FFW, requiring further study.

Importantly, there are many overlapping dysfunctioning vs. compensatory sound and non-sound processing determinants in dyslexics, as reviewed and clarified in

[1] Begley, S. "Rewiring your gray matter." *Newsweek*, January, 2000, pp. 63–65.

Chap. 16. Thus, improving only one important reading mechanism of many may not lead to significant overall reading gains in some, despite FFW's efficacy.

Also, the reading and language impairments these distinguished scientists considered to be of a cerebral linguistic origin were, in fact, determined by my research to be CVS-caused. As you might recall, the speech and language symptoms rapidly improved in many of my CVS dysfunctioning dyslexic patients when treated with CVS enhancers, including Michael Schultz, who opened this book and was again described in Chap. 14.

Considering this FFW method's inherent complexity and probable misassumptions, is it any wonder that some researchers attempting to further validate Tallal and colleagues' results justifiably obtained conflicting or refuting data? Thus, the true efficacy of this valuable therapeutic tool may have been somewhat statistically diluted by mistaken assumptions and convictions.

Despite the refuting claims, it seems very likely that this method does enhance both CVS and related cerebral functioning. And so, it leads to improved reading as many favorable validating studies attest to. You may also now wonder: What mechanisms are likely motivating these frequent and often intense conflicts over scientific acceptance and rejection while simultaneously ignoring invaluable and obvious insights?

The Tomatis Listening Method

Because impaired sound processing and its improvement are important in dyslexia, I decided to review another sound theory and therapy, one less known and significantly more controversial than most. This method is based on an auditory listening dysfunction considered by Tomatis to be initially triggered by a middle-ear impairment.

While attempting to help opera singers and others improve their vocal performance, this well-known French otolaryngologist many years ago developed a device called an Electronic Ear. It enhances the uppermost missing sound frequencies as well as improves sound stimulation in patients. Thus, Tomatis was able to help Maria Callas, Sting, and other vocalists.

Unbelievable claims As an ear specialist whose father was a famous opera singer, Tomatis proposed that sound therapy—especially listening to classical music—helped patients with dyslexia, ADHD, impaired auditory processing, poor motor skills, depression, ASD (autism), and schizophrenia.

Unfortunately, most experts were turned off by both Tomatis' claims and method, as was I initially. Thus, upon first "hearing," one aspect of his theory really seemed preposterous: that by repeatedly listening to their mother's voice, those afflicted by ASD and schizophrenic disorders would be helped. How, you might wonder? Tomatis believed their core impairments were caused by faulty fetal-maternal sound communication in the womb. And he also theorized how and why listening to music also helped the other varied disorders noted in the above paragraph.

All of his theories involved the middle ear. And some, like the womb theory, were difficult to initially listen to—no pun intended. But Tomatis may have independently captured an important insight about the negative effects of auditory misperception and flow—albeit his theory, like all others, was based on, and highly biased by, his own unique background.

Clarification So, readers must be wondering, why did I risk presenting his highly controversial content here? Because I believe there's something of value to be learned—and taught—by doing so. In my opinion, Tomatis' musical listening therapy may have helped some patients he was treating for the above disorders by adding compensatory timing and rhythm capabilities to their defective CVS-determined scrambled sound transmissions.

In other words, I reasoned that compensatory timing and rhythm may decrease sound/listening scrambling or "auditory stuttering" in a similar way to the well-known cessation of speech stuttering when singing and/or using a metronome. And we all know that when memory chains are rhymed, they are significantly easier to recall! Might improved auditory timing and rhythm using sound therapy improve other dyslexia-related functions too via a spreading improvement mechanism previously described by Tallal? I now believe so—especially after really listening to my patients and then to Tallal and Tomatis!

However, much in the same way that Fenichel added unneeded Freudian concepts to his correct phobia/inner-ear observations, Tomatis mistakenly complicated the reason why some of his ASD and schizophrenic patients, likely suffering from a hidden co-existing and relatively minor CVS impairment, improved with his sound correcting therapy. It's highly improbable—likely impossible—that he normalized previously impaired fetal-maternal communications or even that this dysfunction really existed or that it caused ASD or schizophrenia.

But as an otolaryngologist, this was the best theory Tomatis could arrive at to explain the improvements he apparently observed. As is often the case, the observations may have been correct even if the explanatory theories were not. Thus, some independent studies validating Tomatis' therapeutic listening method were mistakenly discounted by most other professionals—unsurprisingly.[2]

By contrast, Tallal and colleagues working within the thinking brain considered a similar appearing auditory dysfunction to result from a cerebral linguistic defect that responded to cognitive phonologically based sound therapy. I, on the other hand, viewed this impaired sound component as only one of many CVS dysfunctioning mechanisms contributing to the reading, speech, and non-cerebral language impairments in dyslexia.

[2]Although the fetus may hear maternal and non-maternal sounds and even have some discriminatory capability, Tomatis's theory is more simply and accurately explained by the fact that the CVS enhancers improve all of the above impairments without the use of any sound or maternal voice therapies. And my CVS theory explains all the varied disorders and therapies best, whereas Tomatis's theory is highly limited and improbable, at best.

As you are by now well aware of, I determined that CVS dysfunction causes learning problems, ADHD, impaired auditory processing, and poor motor skills, as well as secondarily complicating ASD and schizophrenia. And as you will read more about ASD and even schizophrenia in Chap. 22, the coincidence of these overlapping insights in both my and Tomatis' research is truly remarkable, despite our differing clinical and research backgrounds, and disparate interpretations.

Although the Tomatis method initially "sounded" way too strange for me to take seriously, I did see and treat some patients from Canada, where this method held credence, during the late 1970s and early1980s who benefitted from his therapy. And only much later on did I read about these concepts in more detail and reviewed some of the independent validating studies. Yes, I know—placebos? But this is a term too often unwittingly misused by those resisting alternative explanations.

Overcoming first impressions Certainly, there were refuting studies as well. But I expected those. And yes, I was initially guilty of reflexively and intensely dismissing this theory and its therapeutic results just as the traditionalists dismissed mine, and most of the others now reviewed. Frustratingly, we are all beset by bias mechanisms. But in the end, I very belatedly overcame mine concerning Tomatis and others. And so, I was left wondering about the uncanny link between my theories and those of Tallal and Tomatis.

And as you read more about all of these varied helpful therapies and their therapists, might you wonder as did I: Were we not all—like puppets—scientifically dancing to nature's hidden CVS-related tunes, although we heard them very differently?

Neurofeedback: A Simple Explanation

When scanned by EEGs, many patients with ADHD display unique qualities in their brain wave frequencies that distinguish them from those of non-ADHD patients. And these differing wave frequencies are often linked to concentration, distractibility, and even hyperactivity symptoms.

Since behavior and brain function influence each other, neurofeedback was hypothesized to possibly correct this brain wave difference by training ADHD patients, via interactive computer programs, to use their brains differently during concentration tasks. By thus normalizing the patients' brains' electrical wave frequencies, it seemed likely to eliminate the resulting ADHD symptoms. Sounded very logical—but…?

Over the years, I've had ADHD and dyslexic patients report benefits from neurofeedback. It certainly made sense to me and was somewhat consistent with my CVS theory—but only after some thought. Clearly, most experts believe that ADD and ADHD, and specific brain wave frequencies characterizing those with these impairments, are of a primary cerebral origin—*and they may well be correct.*

However, being somewhat adversarial while also attempting to maintain a simple unified primary CVS theory of the total dyslexia syndrome, I wondered if these brain wave frequencies measured atop the cerebral cortex might not be secondarily influenced or even triggered by a *primary dysregulation within the higher interacting cerebellum.* Perhaps neuroimaging studies may help resolve this vital consideration by examining both cerebral and higher-cerebellar activations when patients are self-regulating their brain wave frequencies during silent concentration exercises?

Once again, I have had no direct training and experience with neurofeedback. So it is difficult to properly analyze conflicting data supporting and refuting this method's efficacy. However, since I've had ADHD patients benefit from neurofeedback, including Joey in Chap. 14, I'll support it unless proven incorrect. As there are no side-effects, except for its high cost and slow therapeutic onset, what do patients with these symptoms have to lose, especially those failing to respond to medically based stimulant and non-stimulant therapies as well as the add-ons or stand-alones?

Overall, there is one thing I'm certain of: No matter what the theory or therapy, and however well designed validating studies appear to be, there will always be refuting/skeptical critics, as well as an important need for them. And the reason is simple: Nature is just too complicated for anyone to completely or perfectly capture any complex disorder or system, hence the value of insightful free and open discussions such as these, as opposed to defensive/closed group-think ones.

Occupational and Sensory-Motor Integration Therapies, Reflex and Optometric Treatments

Sensory-motor-integration and occupational, vestibular, reflex, ocular, as well as other therapists have reported academic as well as coordination improvements when dyslexics perform various motion-related and/or eye-training exercises. Although their benefits were initially refuted by traditionalist experts because these therapies cannot reverse primary cerebral deficits, and so were condescendingly/defensively called "magic cures," I reasoned differently—alternatively. If indeed these and related therapies do improve dyslexia-related and CVS functioning but cannot reverse primary cerebral impairments, then should not dyslexia be considered of primary CVS rather than cerebral origin!

More specifically, I postulated that the inner-ear or CVS modulates all body and most eye movements as well as motion and sensory-related activities. Since repetition often leads to improvement in the specific functions repeated, it seemed reasonable to assume that the specific underlying CVS-related mechanisms modulating them were enhanced.

However, one must still account for the reported academic, concentration, and related higher improvements which occur when only sensory and/or motor exercises are performed. In other words, why will a child given eye exercises and asked to participate in various balance/coordination and reflex tasks often read, write, speak, and concentrate better? The likely answer resides in the following paragraphs.

Transfer of Function: Specific vs. Generalized Improvement

Perhaps the following reasoning will help explain how and why all of the CVS-related exercises help improve the varied symptoms characterizing those with the dyslexia/CVS syndrome, using eye exercises here just to illustrate the point. For example, if we assume:

- That repetitive *E*ye tracking (and similarly all of the other mentioned conditioned motor-, sensory-, and reflex-enhancing techniques) improves underlying *CVS circuit/mechanism E*—which then leads to enhanced fine-tuning of the signals sent to *Processor E* within the higher cerebellum and thinking brain.
- That this conditioned *circuit/mechanism E* improvement is also transferred to neighboring and interconnected *CVS circuits/mechanisms R*, *W*, *M*, *C*, *T*, etc.—which then also fine-tune the signals sent to *Processors R*, *W*, *M*, *C*, and *T*.
- Then it's likely that the specific *R*eading, *W*riting, *M*ath, *C*oncentration, and *T*ennis *Processors* within the cerebral cortex and higher cerebellum will more easily descramble, or otherwise compensate for, the clearer signals received—thus resulting in the above corresponding improvements. (It's also possible for one circuit/mechanism to radiate signals to multiple brain processors, etc.)

Limitations of Functional Transfers

Although positive transfer of function is important for therapeutic purposes, it might be helpful to illustrate just how restrictive functional transfers may be, thus accounting for the limitations characterizing the above therapies.

When astronauts being readied for space were spun in various directions, an interesting observation was noted. Rotating someone repeatedly in a counterclockwise direction often led to an improved tolerance for only counterclockwise rotations. Contrary to initial expectations, this exercise did not necessarily lead to an improved tolerance for clockwise and other directional rotations. These results clearly indicated how the body uniquely adapts to specific stimuli and conditions while resisting more generalized or transferred responses. Although this limitation on spreading effects may be adaptive in preventing generalized "flooding," it can be frustrating to healers for the therapeutic purposes we are considering.

Athletics improve concentration and cognition Fortunately, transfer of functional improvements to neighboring circuits does occur, at least in certain contexts. In my clinical practice I've repeatedly noted the existence of an initially puzzling phenomenon: Dyslexic/ADHD athletes often do their best academically when in sports training or competition, despite the limited study time they have. However, upon termination of their sports activities, due to either a changing season or an injury or even as punishment for prior academic failures, a significant number of athletes report and manifest a corresponding decrease in their concentration, memory, and overall academic functioning.

At first glance, one might interpret this correlation as an excuse conjured up by athletes to justify continuing their sports and training time. However, this was not the case in my experience. Most often, it was their parents who reported this fascinating but puzzling correlation.

My educated guess is that sports activities resulted in a transfer of function to neighboring and/or underlying inner-ear/cerebellar-related circuits, which in turn resulted in better fine-tuned signals reaching higher brain processors. And because of decreased signal scrambling, there resulted greater descrambling capability as well as concentration and academic improvements.

Unfortunately, the cessation of sports-triggered CVS stimulation/enhancement led to a regression in this conditioned functional transfer. And so, the ensuing signal fine-tuning and resulting cognitive improvement was then eliminated.

In other words, CVS-enhancing exercise therapies act similarly to the CVS-enhancing meds. And so when clearer or less scrambled signals are sent to higher CNS processors, they are more easily descrambled and interpreted. And when the meds or exercises stop, so does the improvement—unless neuroplastic and/or neurochemical changes occur. Accordingly, the reported generalized cognitive and concentration improvements triggered by the varied exercise therapies can more readily be explained.

"Practice Makes Perfect… Sound Body, Sound Mind"

The unexpected clinical observation that physical exercises for dyslexics may result in increased mental capacity is in accord with the adages "Practice makes perfect" and "Sound body, sound mind." And it is in perfect harmony with the sensory-motor and reflex inhibition/enhancing therapies developed by Jean Ayres and both Peter and Sally Goddard Blythe, respectfully. In fact, Peter Blythe, using reflex therapy, independently concluded in the 1970s that there was a vestibular basis for the very same disorders as I did. (Refer to Appendix 8 for a description of Reflex Therapy by Sally Goddard Blythe and my commentary as to how these concepts and my own mutually validate each other.)

Moreover, these insights may help explain why there are so many seemingly "crazy joggers" running miles and miles in the early morning prior to work—perhaps to jump-start and fine-tune their mental day. Obviously, it makes them feel better. So, it may be more than just endorphins kicking in!

In the final analysis, these CVS-improving, fine-tuning, and varied other therapeutic exercises tended to further substantiate the CVS origin of dyslexia while further—"magically"—refuting the primary cerebral theories of dyslexia. Interestingly, most all of these therapists focused on the inner-ear and vestibular system, yet none had initially factored in the crucial role of the cerebellum or "little brain."

Yoga, Meditation, and the Inner-Ear/CVS Connection

The growing popularity of yoga and meditation—along with their beneficial therapeutic results—has, until recently, defied a proper neurophysiological explanation. After meeting with Ila and Garrett Sarley as well as Stephen Cope at The Kripalu Center for Yoga & Health many years ago, and belatedly reading their illuminating works, I wondered: Might the improved movements, timing, rhythm, concentration, and cognition developed through yoga and meditation be CVS modulated, at least in part?

Might many of the benefits of yoga and meditation—decreased anxiety and stress, feelings of well-being and contentedness, a sense of being in greater touch with one's body, mind, and surroundings—be related to enhanced CVS-stabilizing and fine-tuning mechanisms as well as other CNS structures?" Then cut the next sentence, "Why did I think so?" and then use the final sentence as is. The reason for cutting "Why did I think so?" is because it sounds like you're asking a question, which the reader assumes is going to be answered by the next sentence's "Because". But the next sentence is not set up to provide an answer to that question. Instead, it goes off on its own direction.

Due to ever-present bias/resistance, most medical traditionalists, myself included, did not initially take yoga, meditation, and their long noted and reported positive effects seriously. However, MRI studies have definitely shown significant and somewhat rapid increases in both gray and white brain matter corresponding with improved memory, learning, as well as concentration, behavioral, and emotional benefits. So, the reported mental benefits were based on CNS improvements—and not placebos. But the studies thus far have not shown greater cerebellar changes than those observed in other important CNS structures.

Tinted, Glare-Free, and Magnification Lenses and Special Typeset

The use of tinted lenses has been recognized to help minimize or compensate for some of the symptoms characterizing the reading disorder in dyslexia. Since some inner-ear/cerebellar dysfunctioning subjects may be light-sensitive or photophobic due to impaired light-wave filtering, often frequency-specific, it seems reasonable that specifically tinted and/or glare-free lenses may be helpful for these affected dyslexics by minimizing their visual signal-scrambling and/or overloading.

As might be expected, there are conflicting reports as to this therapy's efficacy—possibly related to an existing failure in properly explaining the neurophysiological reasons for this method's benefits and relationship to the CVS.

There are also data suggesting that bottom-heavy typeset may minimize word movement (oscillopsia) and reversals for some dyslexics. And there are dyslexics who can read one typeset significantly better than others, suggesting just how specific and complex these visual processing mechanisms may be. In fact, Kathy, in Chap. 7, clearly and convincingly described the visual processing complexity involved when reading. And her descriptions were significantly more insightful than those in most other studies—combined.

To explain the possible benefits of bottom-heavy typeset in anchoring print to the page, you might have to consider a somewhat comical sounding insight taken from the non-reading realm: A patient of mine who was afraid of heights solved some of his residual balance and related phobic symptoms by using heavy shoes. *Feeling better anchored*, he became more balanced, and so his fear of falling from heights disappeared. Perhaps *seeing* bottom-heavy typeset serves a compensatory function similar to the way that visually fixating and concentrating on a target in otherwise open, endless space enhances both overall inner-ear and CVS functioning, including its specific orientation mechanism—and so decreases motion sickness and agoraphobic anxiety.

One thing is certain: none of the abovementioned visual reading aides would have helped an alexic reading comprehension disorder, or even a phonologically based impairment, except for the following possibility.

A transfer of CVS dysfunction I've observed dyslexics whose writing and other *non-reading functions* sometimes improved when wearing tinted lenses. Since this phenomenon begged for an explanation, I eventually found one, instead of just denying this puzzling fact or calling it a placebo so as to easily dismiss it.

Just as I previously reasoned that there is often a transfer of favorable CVS function when using helpful therapies, *there may also be a transfer or spreading of CVS dysfunction and signal scrambling* when light and glare sensitivities are in active play—destabilizing other interrelated non-visual functions. So, correcting for light and glare reverses this existing *negative* CVS and related spreading effect.

In other words, by eliminating the currently existing light-triggered negative spreading and signal scrambling effect, and thus eliminating/minimizing the generalized cognitive-related symptoms it previously caused, there may result corresponding non-visual reading (phonetic, etc.) and non-reading (writing, math, etc.) improvements.

Interestingly, I surprisingly found tint/glare-related reading or clarity improvement to often be print-size specific—beneficial for only one of several word sizes. This suggested that tints were not needed for well-compensated fixated and processed print sizes. And a previously helpful tint—that patients reported made the size appear bigger— was frequently noted to be unhelpful once a favorable med response took hold. This suggested that the meds "cured" the problem that the tint had previously helped.

I doubt that these and many other little known clinical insights were factored into enhancing this method's efficacy as well as the design of validating studies and the interpretation of the resulting data.

Educational Therapies: Special and Otherwise

Educational therapy is as complex as it is crucial. And since each child or adult with the dyslexia syndrome is uniquely defined by their normal vs. abnormal pattern of sensory, motor, memory, concentration/distractibility, and related cognitive and even anxiety functions, it is imperative that educators attempt to better understand their students' assets and deficiencies as well as the responsible mechanisms.

Needless to say, this rather daunting task is easier described than performed. It requires that educators be armed with a vast array of educational techniques combined with gifted intuition and empathy as well as the crucial neurophysiological insights provided by books such as this one. In the final analysis, teachers are expected to perform "Herculean wonders" on large groups of desperate children and adults, often without the help and guidance of clinically experienced professionals. The fact that they often succeed is nothing short of miraculous.

My general advice to teachers is to find and utilize clear and open (non-scrambled) sensory, motor, and related channels in LD students while also attempting to improve their minimally impaired functions/mechanisms via repetition and other compensatory conditioning and reinforcing techniques. Thus, there is great value in attempting a multi-sensory/motor and cognitive approach initially—until more specific insights are obtained during the teaching/learning process. Although devised by Orton (and Gillingham), based on his (mistaken/incomplete) cerebral dominance theory of dyslexia, this method is completely consistent with the many dysfunctioning mechanisms characterizing the CVS-determined reading disorder in dyslexia. Once again, the method was right even if Orton's theory was not.

Difficulty in phonological processing and awareness has more recently been recognized by traditionalists as a defining determinant of the reading disorder characterizing dyslexics. While important, this mechanism is but one of the many contributing to the dyslexic reading impairment. And to ignore all the other causal determinants, including the incredible compensatory or descrambling capabilities of the higher cerebellum and cerebral cortex, is to engage in tunnel-thinking and denial—or 2-D reasoning.

Nevertheless, enhanced phonological training and phonetically based teaching methods should be emphasized within a multi-sensory approach. Indeed, most gifted teachers have long used phonemic awareness training in priming children for later phonetics and reading.

Hopefully, my research has now made it possible for educators to newly develop and/or apply the best possible pedagogic techniques to help dyslexics better compensate for their impaired academic-related reading and non-reading symptoms and mechanisms. Thus, favorable outcomes will inevitably occur more rapidly and easily.

New Therapeutic Insights: New Research For Professionals

Interestingly, my attempt to explain the many helpful methods using CVS theory led me to greater insights into the CVS theory itself—all of which now require new research efforts. Thus, I was forced to ask, and then answer, the following questions.

Question: *Why do some therapies work better and faster than others?*

Answer: Because some therapies must likely target more CVS circuits/mechanisms than others, as well as better enhance those that are more able to fine-tune signals. And some conditioning/compensatory methods are more efficient and so faster to take hold than others.

Question: *What determines the amazing differences between individuals?*

Answer: There are likely innate differences among individuals in (1) the ability of their CVS circuits/mechanisms to be conditioned and transfer conditioned responses, as well as to determine CVS fine-tuning, (2) their resistance to transfer, which may help them adaptively avoid generalizing (flooding), (3) their higher CNS descrambling capabilities.

Question: *Might these differences also apply to medical and chemical therapeutic efficacies?*

Answer: Very likely, since each individual responds uniquely to specific meds, doses, and a host of other variables, as elucidated in Chap. 21. Since meds can rapidly and simultaneously target a great many CVS circuits/mechanisms and so also quickly facilitate signal fine-tuning, it's easier to now explain their favorable overall response patterns and speed.

Question: *Might similar differences apply to the compensatory therapies as well—including the varied educational methods?*

Answer: Very much so, since there are innate differences in compensatory descrambling and cerebral conditioning/learning capabilities among those with (and also without) the dyslexia syndrome. And so, different educational methods will no doubt function akin to different CVS med and non-med therapies.

Summary A varied assortment of medical and non-medical therapies have been presented and discussed. Hopefully, this clinically based presentation of helpful methods and related insights will advance every dedicated professional's ultimate aim: to better understand and identify the best possible multidisciplinary approach so as to maximize the benefit that can be provided to all those who suffer with the dyslexia/CVS syndrome, young and old.

I have little doubt that the probable synergy (1 + 1 = 3) some of these methods, when properly understood, combined, and selectively implemented by dedicated healers and educators, will lead to more effective outcomes. Perhaps it may also enhance normal CVS and related cognitive/educational-targeted functions?

Chapter 19
Four Steps to a Certain Diagnosis

My unique way of medically diagnosing the dyslexia or CVS syndrome developed in conjunction with my continuously evolving understanding of this complex four-dimensional disorder. As you'll recall, I ultimately recognized that the many possible symptomatic outcomes in dyslexics, as well as their respective intensities, were due to four major variables:

1. The primary CVS dysfunctioning (and compensatory) site(s) within the overall anatomical structure of the CVS, and the degree of signal scrambling
2. The diverse cerebral-cognitive (reading, writing, spelling, etc.) and related CNS brain sites receiving scrambled signals of varying intensities and the degree to which these structures are endowed to adequately process/descramble the "dizzy" signals
3. The overall compensatory ability of the CNS (central nervous system) to neutralize symptom formation by utilizing other physiological and/or psychological mechanisms
4. The presence and nature of decompensating physiological (toxic, infectious, metabolic, traumatic, etc.) mechanisms as well as negatively impacting psychological/educational and environmental factors

Considering the above insights in determining symptom formation, it became vital to arrive at a diagnostic format capable of measuring *only core CVS and related CNS dysfunctioning* variables 1 and 2, above. And to do so, I had to eliminate or minimize the important overlapping masking effects of secondary compensatory vectors and even tertiary decompensatory triggers—variables 3 and 4—which tend to distort the key primary CVS causal symptomatic determinants.

To simplify things, I've broken this CVS diagnosis down into four steps so that parents, adult dyslexics, and especially professionals can clearly understand what is involved in a proper medically determined diagnostic process.[1] By contrast, all

[1]Although dyslexia may start out as a pure inner-ear or CVS (Type III) disorder, patients are often emotionally traumatized by poor schooling and by feeling dumb, ugly, etc.—Type I events. In

H. N. Levinson, *Feeling Smarter and Smarter*,
https://doi.org/10.1007/978-3-030-16208-5_19

other dyslexia-based diagnostic methods rely entirely on reading and related psycho-educational test scores.

However, because many different medical disorders can result from CVS dysfunction, and because even lookalikes exist, only an experienced physician can make a reliable diagnosis.

Four Steps to a Certain CVS Diagnosis

Step I: "History is 90+ Percent of Diagnosis"

By listening to my many patients, you will inevitably find, as I eventually did, that the only way to obtain a true and meaningful sketch of the symptoms and mechanisms defining the entire dyslexia CVS syndrome is to ask questions. Not just any questions, but diagnostically important ones—such as those characterizing the Eighteen Major Symptom Categories of the Self-Diagnostic Test in Chap. 7.

Obtaining a 4-D Portrait By obtaining a history and sketch of the dyslexia/CVS syndrome found in each patient, as well as a clear picture of how and why these symptoms vary over time and in response to specific triggers (e.g., fatigue, allergic phenomena, ear and sinus infections, etc.), you will accurately arrive at the true portrait of this disorder as well as its determining mechanisms. This is not only the best way of obtaining such a sketch, it's the only way. Neither psychological scores, blood tests, CT (computerized tomography), MRI (magnetic resonance imaging), nor any other sophisticated neurophysiological techniques will ever come close to capturing this vital and crucial holistic perspective. *Once the true portrait of all the symptoms and determining mechanisms is qualitatively obtained and defined, then each of the important parameters characterizing a patient may then be quantitatively investigated and measured, depending on specific needs—e.g., comparing pre- and post-treatment results, obtaining more detailed and specific insights,* etc.

Knowing what questions to ask and how to ask them properly will reward clinicians with answers that lead to a reliable diagnosis of the dyslexia syndrome in close to 100 percent of tested individuals. And almost as important, these same answers may help determine which of the dyslexia-related symptoms and mechanisms respond most favorably to specific medications and/or their categories as well as nutrients (refer to Chap. 21 and Appendix [2]).

---

addition, poor parenting and emotional conflicts (Type II mechanisms), when present, further complicate the learning and concentration process, resulting in a symptomatic and diagnostic mixture that requires more than medication and related therapies. Moreover, patients occasionally present with mixed neurological patterns involving both CVS and non-CVS (Type IV) CNS dysfunctioning. As a result, the diagnostic process can be more complicated than presented above. Nevertheless, these exceptions aside, the CVS diagnostic and related therapeutic process remains a crucial cornerstone in medical management. And once the basic CVS (Type III) parameters can be better clarified, the other determinants, if present, also become more recognizable and treatable.

Despite a positive history, no patient with the dyslexia syndrome will manifest all CVS signs and symptoms, most will demonstrate some, and a very few will appear neurophysiologically normal—highly compensated. In fact, there is often a surprising counterintuitive disconnect between the number of symptoms and their intensity per patient and the number and magnitude of the diagnostic neurophysiological signs found.

These surprising clinical observations should once again remind us that there were very few accurately predictable assumptions or straight lines found in this dyslexia research effort. Most all investigatory paths curved—especially since we were invariably "blindly" dealing with multiple overdetermined mechanisms, some dysfunctioning vs. compensatory vs. decompensatory.

As a result, I became more and more convinced of the importance of first obtaining a clinically reliable overall sketch of the dyslexic disorder and its many diverse manifestations. I have done so by listening to dyslexics before quantitatively investigating single theoretically derived variables in the dark, or even worse—unwittingly following mistaken *dyslexia* = *alexia* "triple-blind" convictions.

Step II: Traditional Neurological and Neurophysiological Testing—Something Old

Since the dyslexia syndrome has been shown to be of an inner-ear or CVS origin, the tests that prove most helpful diagnostically are, of course, those measuring inner-ear/CVS functioning and dysfunctioning. After taking a thorough and focused medical and CVS history, the accepted inner-ear/cerebellar diagnostic procedures and tests include neurological examination (including visual acuity and audiological examinations), electronystagmography (ENG), and ataxiometry. When combined, these tests will provide experienced clinicians with a certain diagnosis. For those of you unfamiliar with these tests, let me review them briefly.

Neurological Examination

This methodology consists of a series of clinically based diagnostic parameters commonly administered to assess the integrated function of the cerebellar-vestibular system (CVS) as well as other central nervous system (CNS) functions/structures. Many of the CVS signs tested for are typical of those indicative of dizziness, imbalance, or drunken driving and so may be familiar. To minimize compensatory factors which mask important diagnostic CVS indicators, I've learned to test patients, whenever possible, while they are distracted and/or with eyes closed, since enhanced concentration and visual fixation mask CVS signs and symptoms, exceptions aside.

A Few Typical CVS Neurological Signs

1. *Ocular fixation and tracking dysfunction*, or "clumsy eyes," are most often due to the eyes receiving faulty directional signals from an impaired CVS. Not infrequently, these faulty signals cause repetitive, to-and-fro, horizontal, vertical, and even circular eye movements called *nystagmus*. Sometimes this nystagmus is obvious clinically. You can actually see these rhythmically beating eye movements just by observation. Most often, however, nystagmus is suppressed or appears to disappear when individuals fixate and concentrate on objects around them. To maximize the detection of these *hidden or subclinical*[2] abnormal eye movements, individuals must be tested with their eyes closed and during non-focused states—using electronic eye movement detection equipment and the ENG technique (see below).
2. *Strabismus*—refers to a malalignment of the eyes and is caused by a primary weakness of eye muscles. However, this malalignment may be *secondarily* intensified in dyslexics by a hidden CVS dysfunction that further impairs eye muscle tone—and so intensifies dyscoordinated fixation and tracking.
3. *Romberg instability*—refers to body swaying due to impaired balance of CVS origin while standing with eyes open and then closed—and then while standing on one foot.
4. *Dysdiadochokinesis* is a CVS-determined disturbance resulting in rhythmic difficulty rotating outstretched arms in opposing directions, especially when the rotations are accelerated. Clinically, these movements appear "herky-jerky" and "out-of-sync."
5. *Finger-to-finger-sequencing* is a CVS "target-finding" function. CVS-dysfunctioning patients will often skip or misdirect the thumb while attempting to move it sequentially from finger to finger, although dyslexic musicians and others may perform superbly—yet show other CVS signs of dysfunction.
6. *Finger-to-nose testing*—involves another CVS-targeting or direction-finding function. Thus, dyslexics often "overshoot" or "undershoot" their nose when their forefingers attempt to reflexively hit it from outstretched arms. Occasionally, their arms may even reverse directions entirely, heading away from the nose when they should be heading toward it. Accelerating the speed often reduces or eliminates compensatory masking—rendering this impairment more obvious clinically.
7. *Tandem walking and instability*—describes a CVS-determined inability to walk in a heel-to-toe, straight-line fashion while looking ahead. The feet are often observed to miss their intended heel-to-toe targets; balance is also occasionally lost, a CVS-determined symptom called *ataxia*.
8. *Impaired muscle tone*—suggests the presence of CVS dysfunctioning when primary muscle function is found intact. Low muscle tone often results in overly loose joints, double-jointedness, flat feet, and even "jelly legs."

[2] These signs are more evident when the task is rendered more difficult (by speed and/or complexity) and compensation is minimized by distractibility, etc.

9. *Fine-motor intention tremor* of the hands due to a CVS dysfunction is frequently mistaken for a primary anxiety response, although there are other causes of tremors.
10. *Dyspraxia or dyscoordinated movements*—reflect CVS temporal and/or spatial motor dysfunctioning. This impairment may affect, in varying degrees, any combination of fine, gross, and rhythmic motor activities involving any and all body parts (hands, feet, upper and/or lower trunk) as well as speech (e.g., slurring, stuttering, etc.). Although this impairment may lead to generalized klutziness and accident proneness, it may also exist in athletes and so may be function-specific.

Traditional Neurophysiological "Inner-Ear" Testing

In order to provide you with the essence of this important but rather complex evaluation, I will merely summarize the basics of two neurophysiological tests traditionally used to diagnose and validate the presence of inner-ear or CVS dysfunctioning. The intricate details of these methodologies will be discussed in Appendices [4–7].

- *Electronystagmography (ENG)* is a standardized neurophysiological test in which inner-ear-determined reflex eye movements are electronically measured under various triggering conditions. These conditions include having the patient (1) observe and track moving targets; (2) reposition their head, neck, and body; (3) respond to middle ear stimulation with warm and cool water—called caloric testing; and (4) rotate in a spinning chair or moving table. The quality and degree of the triggered eye movements, electronically measured, suggest the presence or absence of CVS dysfunctioning. Because of the complexity of the CVS as well as its ability to compensate for, and thus mask its own dysfunctioning, testing is advised for as many diagnostic parameters as possible. (Refer to Appendix [5] for greater detail.)
- *Ataxiometry* is a standardized diagnostic methodology that assesses overall balance functioning as well as its dependence on vision and proprioception—the internal sensing of all body parts in relation to one another and to space. This test provides computer-generated scores that serve as an objective measure of balance dysfunction as well as of medication-triggered and other compensatory improvements. It also helps determine whether seemingly inner-ear-caused symptoms (e.g., imbalance, dizziness, motion sickness, etc.) may actually result from non-CVS disorders (e.g., extreme stress and anxiety, dysfunction of cerebral and related CNS structures). Importantly, this method also provides exercises that may improve imbalance.

Step III: 3-D Optical and Auditory Scanning—Something New

3-D Optical Scanning

This is a new means of measuring and detecting CVS-impaired ocular fixation and tracking. As you read earlier, this method was originally designed by me to rapidly measure and verify the CVS-determined ocular fixation and tracking defect I first assumed was responsible for reading scrambling and related symptoms in dyslexics (refer to Fig. 19.1).

The 3-D Optical Scanner—which measures the speed at which visual "blurring" of accelerating words and objects occurs—is now, after repeated upgrading, substantially more reliable for rapidly diagnosing inner-ear/CVS dysfunction. As a result, it can also screen for those young children likely to develop the reading and/or non-reading symptoms characterizing the dyslexia/CVS syndrome. And the analysis of all the typical—and atypical—data it generates has led to invaluable insights into the complex dysfunctioning and compensatory mechanisms that frequently confound test results as well as researchers, often leading to mistaken conclusions.

But for now, we'll stick to the basics of how the scanner works: Because dyslexics frequently have a CVS-determined ocular fixation and tracking dysfunction, their clumsy eyes cannot follow and clearly see accelerating visual sequences as can the eyes of CVS-normal non-dyslexics. So when the eyes reach their maximum tracking capacities, they suddenly stop moving and the moving sequences (e.g., letters, words, pictures of elephants, etc.) suddenly blur out at target speeds significantly below those of non-dyslexics—or even dyslexics who do not have ocular fixation and tracking problems.

In addition to measuring tracking capacity, this test can also detect and measure the narrowing of the fixation and tracking span (tunnel vision) that characterizes some dyslexics (whereas others may have superior peripheral vision), as well as the presence of inner-ear-determined visual and motion illusions (e.g., seeing stationary elephants move and/or feeling oneself in motion while at rest). Overall, the more abnormal parameters found, the more likely is the presence of a CVS dysfunction—since unknown compensatory mechanisms often played havoc with clinicians and researchers like me who initially expected to find simple straight lines rather than complex twisters.

As a result of this insight: *The 3-D Optical Scanner was also found capable of measuring compensatory fixation and tracking mechanisms.* Additionally, this blurring-speed exercise may be utilized, via conditioning techniques, to somewhat improve the very function and dysfunction it aims to measure.

3-D Auditory Scanning

Just as I designed the 3-D Optical Scanner to measure the eye-tracking and related visual processing speed in CVS-dysfunctioning dyslexics, I also invented the 3-D Auditory Scanner to measure the auditory processing speed of rapidly heard words and phrases—clinically noted to often be impaired in those with CVS dysfunctioning. Simply put, this device speeds up words, phrases, and sentences listened to without distortion, in both the absence and presence of background interference—"noise." Typically, those individuals exhibiting slow or poor auditory processing or related central auditory processing disorder (CAPD) during conversations will likely have decreased auditory processing speeds, many fascinating exceptions aside. And the exceptions, upon investigation, revealed significant insights about compensatory functioning as well as possible errors made in interpreting these and related auditory processing scores.[3] Interestingly, repetition of this and other auditory processing parameters may result in some compensatory improvements. (For further insights into my 3-D Scanners, refer to Appendices [6 and 7].).

Step IV: Neuropsychological Testing

Analyzing Performance: Qualitatively

Although I employ or advise a wide range of standardized neuropsychological and neurological assessment tests when indicated, I have also found that *observing the quality of impaired performance* in dyslexics tends to be significantly revealing, diagnostically.[4] Thus, when I need to confirm the responses to the historical questionnaire (Step I), I frequently ask patients to read, write, draw (Bender Gestalt visual designs and Goodenough figures), spell, calculate, perform memory tasks, etc. Then I record and analyze the type of errors they make. A qualitative analysis of the errors and difficulties observed most often confirm the data previously obtained from Step I, History. (Again, see Fig. 19.1.), although exceptions are the rule.

---

[3] The exceptions I have encountered, upon investigation, revealed significant insights about compensatory functioning as well as about possible errors made in interpreting these and related auditory processing scores. For example, those with mild degrees of the so-called CAPD can compensate when tested, using substantial degrees of concentration, especially over short periods, and thereby obtain "normal" or "false-negative" scores. And by contrast, when impairments in concentration ability affect normal speech-processing mechanisms, "false-positive" auditory delays may occur. Indeed, the response delay in some dyslexics can reflect difficulties in properly recalling and/or sequencing the words normally heard and/or mentally thought of, as well as motor or expressive delays.

Although many other variations were discovered during my testing of thousands of dyslexics, the above examples will hopefully prove sufficient to highlight the need to consider quantitative test scores within the overall context of clinical experience and "knowing your patient." In other words, the most reliable data and insights are obtained when both qualitative *and* quantitative analyses are performed by open-minded clinicians who recognize that "unexpected exceptions often highlight the overall hidden rule." Thus, this method requires further study.

[4] Although not emphasized here, it is crucial to note that standardized quantitative assessment tests and scores are absolutely vital in measuring before-and-after treatment results and in establishing baselines for the varied functions found impaired in dyslexics.

During my diagnostic examinations (Steps I–IV), I also carefully observe family interactions while engaging the patients in as much "chit-chat" as possible—attempting to informally evaluate their mental and cognitive status. And when noting unexpected results and/or "symptoms" during these interactions, I ask the test subject and/or family members as many questions as possible in order to fully understand both expected and unexpected responses. Once again, I find this technique—especially when guided by the obtained history—highly useful in estimating IQ and a host of other social and communication skills vital to diagnostic assessment of their total syndrome, including the coexistence of ASD.

Before continuing further, let me provide you with a few examples that illustrate the qualitative value and meaning of the diagnostic procedures often referred to as "neuropsychological tests" (Figs. 19.1, 19.2, 19.3, 19.4, 19.5, and 19.6).

Reading Errors

Interestingly, I discovered that it was possible for the higher cerebellum and cerebral cortex—via compensatory descrambling mechanisms illustrated in Chap. 9—to enable some patients to recognize the sentence by viewing its peripheral/scrambled parts. Amazing!

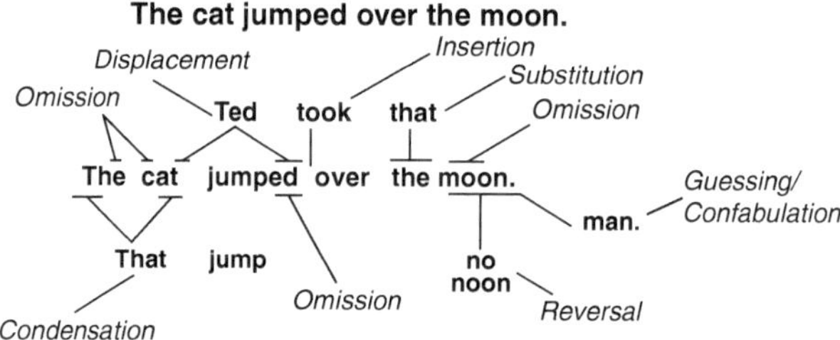

Fig. 19.1 The "typical" dyslexic errors and mechanisms triggered when a reading-disabled patient with the dyslexia syndrome attempts to read a sentence, "*The cat jumped over the moon.*" By means of an error analysis and diagram, the mechanisms underlying the dyslexic reading performance are reconstructed. Typical errors include omissions, insertions, displacements, condensations, rotations/reversals/scrambling, substitutions, and guessing/confabulation. (Refer to the similarity of these dyslexic error mechanisms to Freudian dream mechanisms, discussed in footnote 4, Chap. 9.)

Writing Errors

When copying the text using printing rather than script, the task was more rapidly completed. However, capitalization was both omitted and improperly added. Letters were omitted, reversed, and poorly constructed and spaced.

Fig. 19.2 An 8-year-old dyslexic was instructed to copy "*It was pet day at the fair. The children were waiting for the parade of animals to begin. They had trained their pets to do many tricks.*" Copying and translating the printed form to script were very difficult. It took 10 minutes to complete two sentences. Grammatical detail was lost and letters and words were omitted, reversed, and poorly formed and spaced

Copying—Script (10 min.)

Copying—Printing (more rapid)

Spelling Errors

Fig. 19.3 Graphomotor-related spelling errors of a bright 10-year-old dyslexic girl. A neurodynamic analysis of the spelling errors suggests a dysfunction in the visual-motor memory of letter sequences, along with the compensatory use of phonetic recall. Letters and letter pairs are perseverated and at times inappropriately fused or condensed. Moreover, the spelling disorder is complicated by graphomotor incoordination, drifting, and the omission of grammatical details. *Interestingly enough, this girl's oral spelling was found to be superior to her graphomotor spelling, suggesting that the motor channel selected to test spelling may significantly alter the performance*

Mathematical Errors

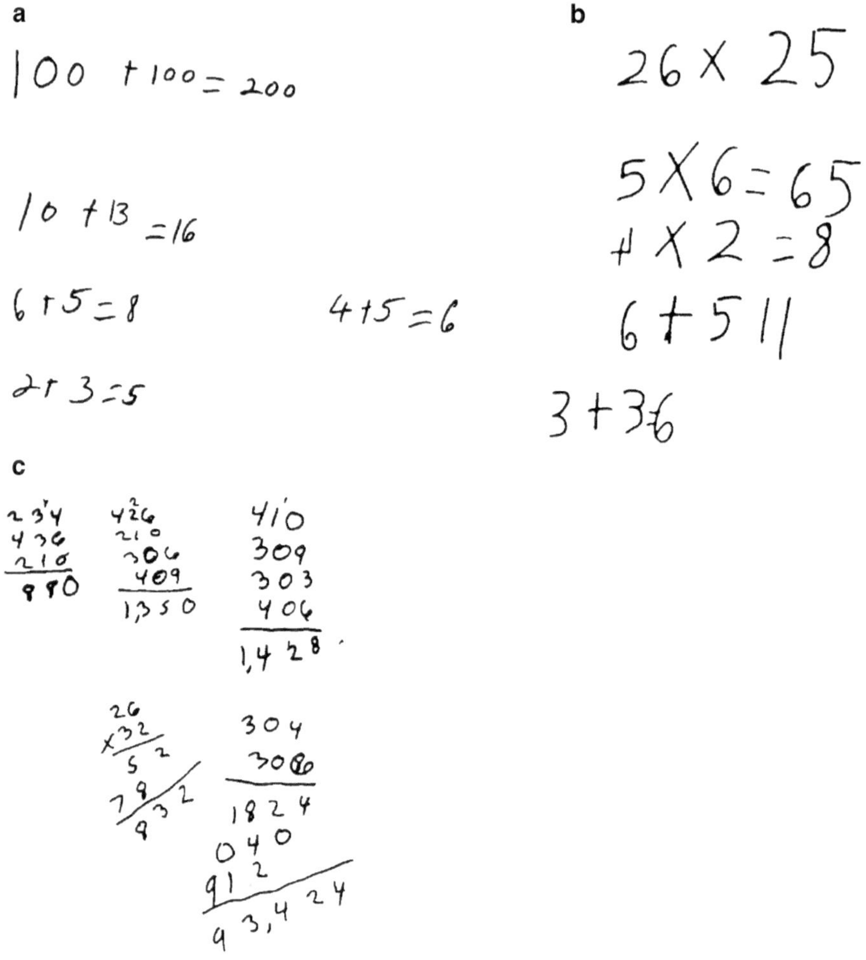

Fig. 19.4 The mathematical errors in dyslexia may be of several distinct, overlapping types: (**a**) "Simple" addition calculations such as 100 + 100 and 2 + 3 are remembered, whereas more difficult calculations are forgotten and the answers guessed at or confabulated. The above 9-year-old recalled the answer but forgot to put in the equal sign when adding 6 + 5, and belatedly added it to the eq. 3 + 3 = 6. (**b**) A similar memory instability for multiplication. When asked to write and multiply 2 × 6 and 2 × 5, this patient mentally condensed the numbers, writing 26 × 25. When asked to write and calculate 5 × 6, he guessed at an answer, and the guess was merely a combination of the two numbers written. In the 4 × 2 = 8 equation, he reversed the 4. (**c**) The limited multiplication ability of a 9-year-old dyslexic. The numbers are occasionally poorly formed and the column alignment drifts to the right. Needless to say, graphomotor and spatial incoordination may result in careless errors, despite superior conceptual and memory ability

Normal Bender-Gestalt Designs

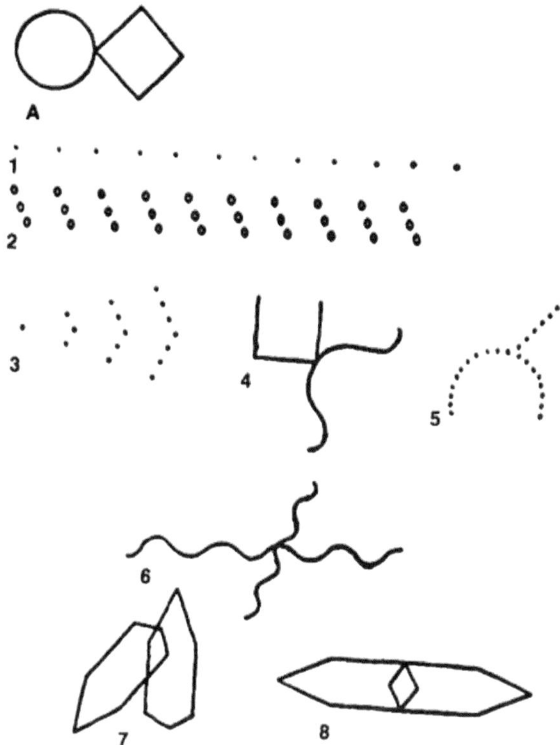

Fig. 19.5 The Bender-Gestalt stimulus cards. Individuals are requested to draw nine Bender-Gestalt stimuli; the graphomotor drawing performance should closely approximate the provided Bender-Gestalt stimulus figures (as above)

Abnormal Bender-Gestalt Designs and Goodenough Figure Drawing

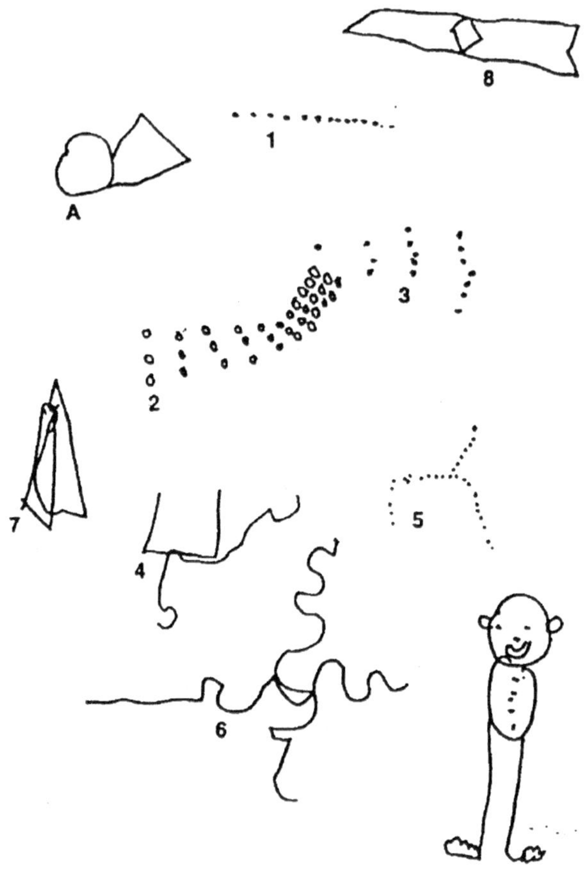

Fig. 19.6 Bender Gestalt and Goodenough figure drawings of a 10½-year-old dyslexic boy. Cards A, 4, and 8 were found to trigger angle formation errors. Orientational and directional disturbances were provoked by card 2. Card 6 triggered zigzagging. The human figure that dyslexics are requested to draw is simplified, detail is minimized, and the arms and hands are omitted due to impaired fine-motor coordination

Summary

I've just presented a four-step diagnostic process capable of successfully revealing the CVS-determined impairments underlying the dyslexia syndrome in over 96 percent of cases examined.[5]

[5] Despite the fact that all four diagnostic steps were initially required for a certain diagnosis, I eventually recognized that shortcuts were possible—thus substantially shortening the diagnostic time and effort, while preserving accuracy. Clearly, all the diagnostic results provided unique insights—especially those obtained from my 3-D scanners. But over time and with experience, I separated those results that were vital from those that merely added "whipped cream" to the diagnostic pudding.

By simply turning the page and reading about Jenny in Chap. 20, you will readily appreciate the value of a certain CVS diagnosis—and how it led to a fascinating life-changing improvement in a gifted mother of three that otherwise might never have occurred. And in Chap. 21 you will learn about the vital therapeutic insights required to obtain the amazing benefits available from a "life-saving" medical treatment and nutritional add-ons. (For additional observations on the diagnostic process, see Appendices [4–7].)

Chapter 20
"I Didn't Want Medical Treatment, But...": Depression vs. "Dyslexia Without 'Dyslexia'"

We live in a culture currently dominated by health and nutrition concerns. There's a preference for organic foods—everything natural; a mistrust of anything "unnatural," including vaccinations, antibiotics, medications of all sorts; and a preference for a range of non-medical "medicines," such as nutrients and vitamins. In addition, there's a desire for "alternative treatments," such as health spas, yoga, acupuncture, and body detoxifications.

As a clinician, I now occasionally examine severely impaired dyslexic/ADHD/phobic children who are brought in by parents seeking *only* diagnosis and non-medical treatment. I also see adults with varied disorders—who adamantly refuse meds. Accordingly, I spend an inordinate amount of time attempting to allay their anxieties and moderate their belief systems. Sometimes I succeed, humoring them with a challenging but sobering comment: "Don't worry, the meds may not work. So then you all will be very happy and relieved not to take them." Those who laugh will usually cooperate, albeit reluctantly.

As chance would have it, just when I was "certain" this book's content was complete, in walked Jenny. I didn't realize until much later that this gifted and accomplished young stay-at-home mom of three was highly medication-averse.

Since her clinical content was packed with fascinating insights, including the important fact that she was *seemingly depressed* and "dyslexic without 'dyslexia'," I couldn't resist presenting Jenny right here and now. She also stands as a rather typical example of how a patient's "anti-medication" belief can be quickly reversed upon recognizing her treatment's remarkable benefits and especially how a seemingly depressed, anxious, and "crappy"—feeling mom can be rapidly transformed into the healthy, loving, and caring one that she always instinctively was.

H. N. Levinson, *Feeling Smarter and Smarter*,
https://doi.org/10.1007/978-3-030-16208-5_20

A Very Brief Case Introduction

Jenny is a 31-year-old mother of three who sought my help because of stress-related depressive and anxiety symptoms, which she believed—based on reading about my research—were possibly due to a CVS dysfunction. Although superbly articulate, intellectually gifted, and an avid reader, Jenny can't spell or write well and is poor in math. Following this very brief introduction, I'll let Jenny speak for herself—and then reserve my detailed commentary for later.

Had Jenny not read of my research and instead sought treatment elsewhere for her most distressing symptoms, the following bulleted content would most likely have been told to her psychiatrist and/or psychotherapist(s):

- Easily irritated by her kids and husband—feeling like a "crappy" mom and wife
- Fatigued all the time
- Poor sleeping habit
- Prefers to be alone—frustrated by others and often fearful of social communications
- Severely abused physically and emotionally in childhood—sustaining several concussions inflicted by her stepfather; her real father abandoned the family shortly after her birth
- Significant medical neglect and poor care
- Endured very poor socioeconomic and educational circumstances, was eventually placed in a girls' home—which she ran away from as a teen, raising herself
- Attended mediocre schools—when attending school at all
- An avid reader, very intuitive

Without any further information about Jenny's clinical evaluation obtained from my four-step diagnostic process, is there any doubt what most psychiatrists/therapists would conclude—or how they would treat her?

Jenny's Self-Report

Now I will finally present Jenny's typed self-report—edited so as to illustrate how she would have verbally expressed it—given her outstanding language skills. However, by doing so, I have eliminated her minor dysgraphic sequencing, spelling, and grammatical errors—which she made despite her compensatory use of word-processing and spellcheck. In fact, Jenny wrote her report in spite of inner duress and defensive resistance—in hopes of helping others as she was just helped.

> *My spelling is so bad that I have to use substitute words regularly because I don't even know where to begin to try to spell some words. Auto-correct would not even recognize my efforts. This has already happened, in fact, while writing these notes. I wanted to use one word, but realized I had no idea how to make that word manifest on paper, so I substituted a different word which did not perfectly capture what I wanted to say.*
>
> *I really like to be alone. People stress me out. Only after taking Dr. Levinson's motion-sickness medication did I understand why. I used to think I was just a crappy mom—that I*

did not have the maternal instincts and patience my friends have. That I was flawed in that aspect.

Then I started taking this medication and suddenly I had the patience of a saint when with my family. My irritability became a non-issue. Now my kids and husband can be jumping around, all talking to me at once, and I am cool as a cucumber. This is in sharp contrast to the way I felt before taking motion-sickness medication.

After a while, I stopped taking the meds for several days due to weight gain. I was talking to a woman I'd been working with for a couple of weeks when I suddenly realized that conversing with her was irritating me and I needed to move away from her. I recognized that she moved a lot when she talked. Her face was moving in many directions as she expressed herself verbally. I only noticed this now that I was off the medication. And suddenly it was too much for me to be around her. Standing with her face-to-face and watching her move around that way made me feel disoriented and put me into overwhelm/irritability mode. I needed to turn around and shut her out.

The first time I met Dr. Levinson was an interesting story. I am one who does not like to take medication and who very rarely makes an exception to this rule. So, I walked in his office thinking I would get tested for dyslexia. And if in fact I was diagnosed dyslexic, I would not take the medication. But I would at least walk away with a greater sense of understanding and self-compassion.

In speaking with Dr. Levinson about my test results, he discreetly asked me, mid-conversation, if I would mind just taking a quarter of this little pill. "Its just an antihistamine," he said. Knee-deep in conversation, I replied, "Sure, I'll try it. No problem." I took the quarter of a pill.

We continued in the conversation, which I found fascinating, and somewhere along the way he asked me to try another quarter of this pill. Sure, no problem, I took another quarter of the pill.

The conversation continued and he stopped me to ask me how I was feeling. When I paused to assess myself I was surprised to report, "Wow, I feel way more relaxed!" I did not realize the base level of stress that I carry when having one-on-one conversations with people. Previously, his subtle body movements when he spoke would have stressed me out, but this was happening somewhat unconsciously. Typically, I try to find one part of a person's face to focus on—one eye usually—and I just concentrate on that one eye when we speak, and negate all else. Though this technique "worked" for me for years, I was unaware of the base level of stress/disorientation having a conversation with another human being created in me. After taking the medication during my conversation with Dr. Levinson, suddenly his movements stopped bothering me. I no longer noticed or tracked them as I had before. This enabled me to just relax and enjoy the conversation and his company. What a gift!

After that experience, I knew I would try this medication. And after I did, there was no way I was going to stop taking it until my condition resolved itself. As mentioned earlier, I did stop taking it for several days after noticing some weight gain, but I quickly started to experience burn-out and irritability with others again. I concluded that my quality of life was way better when taking the medication than when not taking it and being disoriented all the time with people. The possibility of weight gain was a price I was willing to pay.

History and Background

I'm a 31-year-old stay-at-home mom with two small boys (three and five years of age) and a two-year-old girl. No family medical history is available since I was raised in a girls' home.

I've had chronic ear infections since childhood. Because the doctor did not want to put tubes in my ears, I would get ear infections left and right and was on antibiotics often. And my eardrum would rupture once or twice a year in the wintertime from the pressure, and clear/yellow fluid would ooze out. This happened well into adulthood—the last time was about three years ago. As a result, my right eardrum has lots of scar tissue.

I come from a highly abusive family. My stepfather used to hit me in the head repeatedly—one time I was diagnosed with a concussion and contusions. That was one of the only times I saw a doctor, yet my stepfather hit me often.

I remember being traumatized in school. Perhaps because of the severe abuse, I do not have a lot of memories about school or my childhood, but I remember struggling with math. I was great at English and creative writing, despite my spelling. Spelling contests were never an option for me. There were even times I was on the honor roll.

Generally speaking, I have anxiety speaking in public and to groups of people. Even if it's just one or two people, I can have overwhelming anxiety. I am managing this now, but that is definitely an issue.

I read a ton. I love to read! Reading was never an issue for me but it's questionable if perhaps I have memorized the words. I cannot sound out words well. My handwriting is horrible, and I remember it used to slant up to the right really badly. (Thank you, lined paper and computers!) I use an index card when reading to help me keep place on the lines.

I read fairly quickly, and I speak rapidly as well. And I can often intuit the answer or the outcome of a situation or conversation very quickly—after listening to only a few words. My right brain is very much awake. So I am highly intuitive.

Questions, Answers, Considerations—and Review

Where else, besides this book, would you have learned how CVS-determined motion sickness and related mechanisms might trigger so many emotional and stress-related symptoms? And even a highly unique dysfunctional reading mechanism? Do not such clinically derived insights justify both the usefulness and validity of Step 1: History, and also the three other diagnostic steps? Especially since a proper diagnosis led to a medical treatment which simply, rapidly, and dramatically dissolved Jenny's emotional distress, frustrations, and related fatigue—including anxiety and apparent depressive symptoms.

Dyslexia is not language based Considering that Jenny is linguistically gifted, as was Kathy, and that self-acknowledged dyslexics such as Winston Churchill are world-renowned *orators, it should be crystal clear to all that dyslexia is not a language-based disorder of primary cerebral origin—despite mistaken theories claiming so. It's the reverse: Dyslexia, or rather its CVS causation, may negatively impact language and speech in some—as many of my patients have revealed!*

Phonological processing is CVS-based Jenny was also helpful in dispelling yet another mistaken dyslexia conviction: that cerebrally impaired phonological and phonetic processing causes the dyslexic reading impairment—and so is often assumed to be incompatible with avid or normal dyslexic readers. Little do traditionalists know that phonological deficits, such as those characterizing Michael, Jenny, Kathy, Joey, John Whitney, and my other dyslexic patients, are of CVS vs. cerebral origin and so often respond very favorably to CVS enhancers.

Genetic vs. acquired dyslexia As you may recall, Jenny's father had spelling problems—suggesting her own difficulties may be of genetic origin. However, it is also possible that concussions, multiple ear infections, and ruptured ear drums may have caused, or intensified, Jenny's assumed genetically predisposed CVS dysfunction and resulting dyslexia syndrome.

An atypical reading mechanism Importantly, Jenny's gifted reading capability due to rapid visual scanning and processing as well as to intuitive grasping of subliminally absorbed reading content had already been added, in part, to my list of dysfunctioning vs. compensatory reading mechanisms in Chap. 16. However, upon later questioning, Jenny added significantly more understanding as to how her speed-reading with full comprehension, requiring minimal concentration and tracking, is possible.

How Jenny reads As repeatedly emphasized, my clinical method of finding answers to previously misunderstood dyslexic symptoms is to simply ask and listen to my patients for additional explanations. Accordingly, Jenny's follow-up email further elaborated upon her rather unusual—dyslexic—reading style, which resembled Kathy's scanning of sentence tops to enable decoding (refer to Chap. 6), while also somewhat illustrating Jenny's misspelling and dysgraphic tendency:

> *"In speaking with Dr. Levinson he asked me to focus on how I read. I have noted the following:*
>
> *1) Confirmed that I do a version of speed reading but its more of a intuitive paragraph surfing. I at best visually look at every third to fourth word and I am not fully focusing on the third of fourth word even then. Its what I would best describe as visually surfing the paragraph. Visually surfing the sentences.*
>
> *The eye tracks the top of the sentence. There is not an intention to look at the word itself fully. Or even strait [stare] on. I literally skim the top of the sentence looking at the the top part of the third of fourth word and there is a quick grasping of the context of the sentence/ paragraph.*
>
> *I skip almost entirely the small words (to, the, it's, and – and so on.)*
>
> *I do use a note card of something to hold my place – track which sentence I am on if the font is smaller. I prefer paper print outs as reading things in Word on email or reading emails – its harder for me to keep track on which sentence I am on.*
>
> *I can slow down and read the words slowly but ironically, it makes me feel kind of cross eyed/disoriented/motion sick/visually stressed. I have yet to take the motion sickness medication right now, I will do so now. But its an interesting discovery. I imagine if I take the medication it wont bother me to read slowly and focus on the words one by one. I still will likely speed/intuit read as that is my default way of reading apparently. But if I chose to focus on words and slow down, I imaging with the motion sickness medication it would not bother me so much. It is clearly a tracking issue.*
>
> *Without motion sickness medication, it generally speaking stresses me out to have a conversation with someone that moves when they speak (head, hands, body.) Its kind of like that with reading I see. It stresses me out to see all of the letters around each other in a paragraph. So I apparently trained myself to surf the context of the whole paragraph.*
>
> *2) it also arose again that I have a difficult time making certain sounds of letters. I found myself spelling out my name again, and my email on the phone and I have a very difficult time pronouncing the Z sound. It slurs and sounds like a C sound when I make it.*
>
> *Thank you*—Jenny"

Some Additional Insights

A dyslexic without "dyslexia" Quite obviously, Jenny's clarification of her dysfunctional vs. compensatory reading process assuredly qualifies her as a reading-impaired dyslexic, despite enhanced reading comprehension. Thus, Jenny should be diagnostically considered a *dyslexic without "dyslexia"—one without an obvious reading comprehension/decoding disorder.*

In many ways, both Jenny's and Kathy's compensatory reading styles were remarkably similar, by analogy, to somehow grasping a book's entire content by just skimming its book cover. This mechanism once again highlights the remarkable capability of the thinking brain and/or the higher cerebellum in gifted dyslexics.

Real vs. placebo favorable med response No doubt, some may believe that Jenny's favorable therapeutic responses were due to a placebo effect—perhaps because her improvements dramatically challenge all known traditionalist dyslexia concepts. However, were this placebo assumption or conviction correct, one would have to explain how wishful thinking could be so selective and effective—considering Jenny was against meds and improved before even realizing she'd taken two test doses. And that she lost her improvements upon stopping meds—only to regain them upon restarting them.

In addition, how might a placebo-assumption explain her weight gain? Surely this atypical side effect is not a placebo—since she stopped the med initially to get rid of this *undesirable negative.* And she never even knew weight gain was a potential side effect until I later informed her of the possibility. Had Jenny wished her improvements into existence, why couldn't she similarly wish away her weight gain? For that matter, why didn't her wish that nutrients and natural therapies help—without a need for meds at all—lead to a placebo improvement? Although placebos do play a role in all therapies and must be accounted for, they are often used by some to negate results that differ with their expectations and theories.

Enhanced emotional immunity By the way, can anyone explain how Jenny survived her devastating emotional, socioeconomic, and physically abusive background—alone, without therapy or even assistance, while also devastated by her severe CVS symptoms?

Well, I can. Having examined a few other similarly traumatized cases, including Holocaust and war survivors, I reasoned that some individuals are endowed with "enhanced emotional immunity and survival instincts" as others are blessed with "enhanced physiological immunity." Some have both, while others have neither. And most fall in-between with varying degrees of both.[1]

[1] So, why is this important here? Because we as professionals often overlook crucial insights such as these and many others, when too rapidly assigning unproven emotional (and also incorrect neurological) causes to Jenny-like mental symptoms without carefully examining the soma. In fact, all of this book's insights resulted from the unmasking and correction of these and related misassumptions.

By sharp contrast, it's possible that Jenny's dysfunctional parents illustrate the deadly pitfalls that occur when dyslexic children become adults without treatment—and perhaps without emotional immunity.

Obsessed I was also able to determine, by simply asking her, why and how Jenny became "obsessed" with healthy foods and fearful of meds: She wanted to make sure her kids would be healthy—presumably by caring for her kids as she herself wasn't. So, Jenny became, or always was, the loving mom she never had.

How Jenny Might Have Been Diagnosed by Other Professionals Without This Book's Many and Vital Insights

Emotional "red herrings" Without knowing Jenny's true dyslexia or CVS hologram, most psychotherapists/psychiatrists would have mistakenly pursued only the *obvious psychological clues—"red herrings"*—and so assumed primary emotional causes for Jenny's symptoms, ignoring all the others that seemed to them unrelated or irrelevant. And who could blame them—given Jenny's severely traumatic emotional background and her speaking-related and social anxiety/phobias. And even her autistic-like need to fixate on one eye or body part to avoid looking at those she conversed with.

No doubt, the psychiatric treatment of choice for her anxiety and her seemingly depressed and partially burned-out, irritable and fatigued state would be a trial of SSRIs or SNRIs. But given her dislike—or fear—of meds, she would likely have refused. Clearly, a psychotherapeutic trial(s) would have taken many years, given her complex and severely traumatic past. And given the hidden CVS origin and mechanisms underlying her emotional symptoms, significant positive results from only psychological treatment(s) would have been highly unlikely.

An ENT "red herring" Perhaps Jenny might have been sent to an ear, nose, and throat specialist for her repeated ear infections and severe motion sickness. What is the probability that this expert would have connected her seemingly unrelated emotional problems with ear symptoms—especially had Jenny not told them? Would such a physician have obtained a thorough history that revealed *all* her symptoms—especially those defining her dyslexia or CVS syndrome? Doubtful. He/She would have justifiably focused primarily on whether or not Jenny should now have her tonsils and adenoids removed, along with the possible insertion of draining tubes, and also on whether this surgery might eliminate her motion sickness as well as repeated ear infections.

A likely tutorial misdiagnosis Now let's assume Jenny then went to a tutor to improve her spelling, math, and writing. No matter how pedagogically gifted, would this teacher have considered Jenny to be dyslexic—given her superior reading comprehension? Do many teachers or experts properly understand my tongue-in-cheek paradox: *dyslexics without "dyslexia."* Clearly not! Indeed, given Jenny's traumatizing history, it is likely that the cause of her "relatively mild" or masked academic (writing, spelling, and math) symptoms might also have been attributed to her impoverished emotional, social, and educational background.

Considering that Jenny reads well, would these tutors have even thought to search for underlying reading dysfunctioning or her coexisting *compensatory sentence-scanning mechanisms, needed by her to avoid the motion sickness triggered by rapidly inputting too much visual detail were she to read word after word as most of us do?* Very unlikely! No other tutor or expert has done so.

Psychological testing confusion Had psychological testing been advised and performed, what might the results have been? And how beneficial? From my experience, in a case like Jenny's, the tests would have probably generated multiple diagnoses—likely including depressive and anxiety characteristics—and at least 20–30 pages of data that would have overloaded any busy healer or tutor. And in the end, most recipients of such data would have abstracted *only* what they initially believed to be important in the first place—and ignored all else. Sort of what we all do. So, this massive data input would probably have only enlarged Jenny's "quantitative haystack" without qualitatively revealing the vital hidden causative "CVS needle."

No doubt, some readers will challenge this cold-sounding assertion. However, I can sadly justify it with only one word: kryptonite! And then crown my assertion with a rhetorical question of my own: Why hadn't all the traditionalists combined solved the dyslexia-syndrome riddle—found the "CVS needle"—despite all the evidence-producing dyslexics repeatedly telling them—and now readers—the answers? Denial, obviously!

A likely neurological oversight Suppose Jenny's "imaginary tutor," having learned about her history of abuse-inflicted concussions, had sent her to a neurologist for evaluation. How likely is it that her significantly masked dysgraphic-like writing, as well as her spelling and math problems, would have been diagnosed as CVS-determined rather than due to Jenny's concussion and/or emotional causes, if indeed these masked symptoms were properly diagnosed at all? Were I to guess: possible, but unlikely.

Vitally needed CVS insights And if CVS signs were perchance found, they would probably be used to explain only Jenny's inner-ear determined motion sickness and justifiably reasoned that they were due to her many ear infections. Without the benefit of this book's or Jenny's anecdotally obtained insights, it appears unlikely that the neurologist would have felt a need to take a comprehensive history similar to the one recommended in the preceding chapter. Instead, Jenny might have been subjected to an MRI or CT scan—which would have come out normal, except for possible evidence of her past abuse-inflicted concussions. And none of the CVS-specific diagnostic tests would likely have been advised or performed.

As you can see, CVS-suffering *atypical* patients like Jenny, and many *typical* others, are seldom properly diagnosed and treated.

Conclusions

Perhaps you can now better understand why I chose to inject Jenny's case in-between the crucial diagnostic and medication chapters. Her presentation validates my clinical experience which suggests there is a preventable wide-spread misunderstanding of *all* dyslexics and their CVS impairment—as well as how to best diagnose and treat the vast typical majority, especially dyslexics without "dyslexia."

Importantly, I also hoped to demonstrate here, via Jenny, that many emotional disorders—especially depression, anxiety states, PTSD, and others—may be primarily predisposed, and/or secondarily intensified, by CVS dysfunctioning. And so, these impairments may be helped by CVS enhancers and insight. But *help* is based on the premise that clinicians will consider CVS impairments and their many and varied symptoms as part of their differential diagnosis—despite the presence of other more obvious, but non-causative, Jenny-like "emotional red herring" clues that often appear on "center clinical stage."

Another Zag

Born depressed Finally, I'll leave readers to consider another fascinating Jenny-like insightful clinical experience. I've successfully treated two CVS dysfunctioning young adults with CVS-enhancers who were *born depressed*—after they had previously failed all traditionally accepted treatments for their depressions. Although recognizing and describing children *born anxious*, I have yet to read about their depressed counterparts—*born depressed*. Like many of my other clinical insights, their existence seemed obvious, but only in retrospect. Thus, I urge you all to consider my belatedly conceived clinical CVS motto: "When in doubt, test them out."

Chapter 21
Real Smart Drugs and Treatment

Feeling Smarter and Smarter has thus far highlighted the dramatic improvements possible when dyslexics are properly understood, diagnosed, and medically treated. These improvements, typical of many thousands, have been presented to you through the personal accounts volunteered by my many patients and/or their loved ones.

Now all you need—especially if you are a clinician—is information on the vital therapeutic insights and real smart drugs that are capable of helping millions of other bright but dumb-feeling individuals with the CVS-syndrome (refer to Appendix 2). So, here goes.

Getting Started

The aim of medical treatment is simple: to maximize improvement in as many dyslexia/CVS-related symptoms and mechanisms in each patient as possible. The task, however, is quite complex and dependent on a wide range of crucial variables. Of these variables, the following four are most important:

1. The clinical experience of the treating physician
2. The four-step, diagnostically determined dysfunctional pattern of CVS signs, symptoms, and mechanisms characterizing those seeking treatment
3. The number of effective drugs and chemical substances available for helping both dysfunctioning and compensatory mechanisms
4. The unique chemical or metabolic reactivity of individuals with the dyslexia or CVS syndrome to the specific drugs and doses required

H. N. Levinson, *Feeling Smarter and Smarter*,
https://doi.org/10.1007/978-3-030-16208-5_21

Maximizing Chances for a Successful Med Treatment

Clinical experience is crucial Only God knows beforehand, or with certainty, which of the effective drugs and doses are best for any individual's chemical system—or how to completely prevent negative effects. However, well-experienced physicians following my diagnostic/therapeutic guidelines can provide substantial, rapid, and even dramatic medical benefits to 75–85 percent of treated dyslexics—both young and old. And by test-dosing patients, these benefits carry only a very slight risk of minimal side effects, which can be immediately reversed.

At this point you may be wondering: What do these introductory remarks mean for me, my spouse, my child, or my patients? They mean simply that physicians are only "God's oddsmakers"—not Gods themselves. Despite this limitation, however, physicians can maximize the chances for a successful outcome if they truly understand their patients and are committed to fully implementing their own scientifically based art—armed, of course, with my 50-plus years of clinical insights.

Med benefits far outweigh avoidable risks What I tell patients and loved ones, especially those who are fearful of medications, is this: Remember that there are also great risks—for children and adults—when *avoiding or delaying medical treatment* and/or relying exclusively on minimally helpful, non-medical options. *Clearly, there are significantly greater risks to choosing non-helpful "pipe dream therapies."*

However, when meds are started early in very small doses and side effects are either absent or immediately eliminated, the very short-term risks of using a prescription or helpful chemical are minimal. And as you've repeatedly read, medically triggered responses are often rapid, dramatic (in about one third of the favorably responding cases), effortless, and known to improve a wide range of symptoms beyond just reading, writing, or spelling. Effective medical treatment can also render all add-on therapies substantially more beneficial. However, only effective meds can result in dyslexics *rapidly Feeling Smarter and Smarter.*

All can be helped Let me reassure you that *every* dyslexic can be helped—especially if we consider the benefits of the non-medical add-ons discussed in Chap. 18. But the really great news is that 75–85 percent of dyslexics favorably *respond to medical treatment alone, including the use of nutrients: one third dramatically, one third moderately, and one third mildly*. Prior to my research, zero percent were medically helped.

Considering the fact that there has not been one new drug marketed in the world for CVS dysfunction or dyslexia in way more than 50 years, the dramatic increase in my improvement rate resulted entirely from a better understanding of existing chemical substances, their combined use, and their respective optimal doses. As new and more targeted drugs become available in the future, I have little doubt that 100 percent of medically treated dyslexics will eventually benefit.

Adults benefit as do children Although dyslexic children are usually the focal point of early diagnosis and help, adults with the dyslexia syndrome are too often therapeutically bypassed—probably because they're considered less amenable to remediation or are mistakenly believed to have outgrown their childhood disorder. Or maybe because adults are believed to be just disinterested in time-consuming and costly add-on therapies.

But unfortunately, adults who remain medically untreated (or *mis*treated) and left to deal with their daily humiliations alone are at a severe risk of suffering a host of acute and chronic conditions, including pathological lifestyles; failed marriages; severe mood, anxiety, and behavior disorders; addictions; unemployment; and more.

Sadly, escalating failures in untreated adults metastasize far more widely and deeply than those affecting children and often lead to vicious cycles, including rapid burnout and PTSD. But fortunately, dyslexic/ADHD adults respond as favorably to my medical treatment as do children—despite the chronicity of their core CVS-based symptoms. And clearly, their risks from non-treatment are far higher than any minor transient side effect they might incur by using medically supervised inner-ear/CVS enhancers, stimulants included.

Medication fears are symptomatic The misguided, almost cult-like, tendency to focus only on the perceived *danger* of medical treatment is similar, by analogy, to obsessing over fears of flying from New York to California—without comparing flying risks to the dangers of walking, driving, or biking there or without considering the downsides of not going to California at all, if crucial to get there.

Thus, in my professional opinion, fears of medical treatment for those with dyslexia/ADHD, phobias, etc. should most likely be considered more like an anxiety symptom than a valid and rational choice—and so must be dealt with accordingly.

Two Basic Groups of Medications

Medical treatment for the dyslexia syndrome is entirely dependent on understanding the *primary* origins of symptom formation and *secondary* compensation. As a result, two general groups of medications or chemical substances have been found helpful:

- *Group I* – medications/nutrients that primarily improve inner-ear or CVS functioning and thus minimize or eliminate the scrambled signals sent to initially normal central nervous system (CNS) processors and/or to those possibly even predisposed to developing impairments
- *Group II* – medications/nutrients that can enhance signal transmission, processing, and regulation throughout the CNS and secondarily improve compensation in normal—and even abnormal—brain centers and functions

Thus, by both decreasing CVS-caused signal scrambling *and* enhancing the ability of the CNS processors to descramble "dizzy" signals, these Group I and II chemicals, when properly combined, can impart substantial potency to a successful medical treatment plan.[1]

Clinically Based Therapeutic Insights

Before discussing the specific chemical groups and subgroups, let me tell you what this "clinical oddsmaker" has learned about medically treating dyslexics and their many and diverse symptoms:

- Statistically, one drug or substance alone will not typically provide maximum improvement, some exceptions aside.
- Each and every medication tends to target unique symptoms and segments of the dyslexia/CVS syndrome—even if it's in the same drug family as other medications. And each medication has a specific chance of working.
- A clinically guided combination of medications and related chemical substances from *both* Group I and Group II will deliver optimal results in most cases. By analogy, one star athlete alone, however gifted, cannot win a baseball game—without a team. Similarly, physicians often need a "team" of chemical substances (not to forget an important range of non-med, nonchemical add-ons) to provide maximum benefits for a majority of their patients suffering from the dyslexia/CVS syndrome.
- Remember, we're not just interested in improving reading but also writing, spelling, math, etc. and all eighteen major symptom categories! We want to win the entire game if possible, not just hit a single, a double, or even a triple.
- Doses must be adjusted to the individual. And the best or optimal dose is often independent of age, weight, etc.—and even of the average doses commonly advised. To find the optimal dose for each patient, we have to *test-dose*—start low and work our way up to a maximum without any side effects. And by no side effects, I mean just that. Tiredness, moodiness, or other negatives should not be accepted by patients or their physicians. If there are no short-term negatives with these medications, there will be none in the long term, atypical exceptions aside. If side effects are unnecessarily endured, then patients, parents, and/or their physicians, rather than the drug, must bear some responsibility. By analogy, if a child is told to cross a busy intersection without caution or proper supervision, are we to blame the intersection or auto for any ensuing accident?
- If no side effects of any kind are accepted by the patient, parent, and/or physician, then there's nothing to lose and everything to gain by initiating med treatment. Also, by relying on a combination of chemical substances—all contributing to an overall chance of improvement—the optimal dose of each substance is

[1]Some chemical substances may have overlapping Group I and Group II functioning.

sometimes lower than were only one drug used alone, many exceptions aside. *Best of all, most successfully treated patients with the dyslexia/CVS syndrome will not have to remain on medications indefinitely.*

There are also many other fascinating and vital essentials to consider:

- *Chemically triggered brain learning*—After 2–4 years on some CVS-enhancing medications, 80 percent of improved dyslexics will do as well off medications—or on decreased doses—as they previously did when on them. This type of medicine-catalyzed compensation also occurs for many other disorders, including epilepsy, asthma, hypertension, specific allergies, and more. The brain and body appear to learn and so compensate in a manner similar to the way the medications helped. Surprisingly, therapeutic doses must often be *lowered* over time. Thus, optimal doses given to young children often remain constant—or may require reduction—even after the child doubles in age and weight. Importantly, when meds and/or doses are less needed, side effects may suddenly appear—warning clinicians that patients have "outgrown" their prior requirements. These unexpected observations led me to wonder: Might these CVS enhancers, as well as other meds, trigger neuroplasticity or a chemical equivalent thereof? Since lasting improvements can atypically occur in some patients after only a month or two, further research may enable us to identify and utilize this amazing compensatory mechanism for all.
- *Drug tolerance and immunity*—By contrast, drug tolerance and immunity may also occur. If tolerance is significant, especially with stimulants, the specific med must be discontinued and a new stimulant tried. When immunity occurs, it tends to be complete and irreversible; therefore, dose increases are often ineffective, fortunate exceptions aside.
- *Drug pseudo-immunity*—Atypically, it is also possible for a med to stop working in a way that *resembles* true drug immunity. However, by switching brands, the drug's efficacy and potency often immediately return. This suggests that the inert mix that is part of a branded drug's specific formula is what sometimes triggers this rejection or prevents absorption. Why is this important? Because there are only a very limited number of potent inner-ear enhancers available for each person. So, you don't want to waste a potential winner. And guess how I discovered this insight about switching brands or manufacturers? You're right—patients or their observant parents told me.

Occasionally, a co-occurring illness will temporarily neutralize a drug's efficacy. And over time, improvements reoccur. (Refer to Abe in Chap. 22.)

- *Drug sensitivity responses*—Not infrequently, patients may suddenly develop overdose-like responses to previously well-tolerated and favorable therapeutic dosages. Although substantially lowering the dose is sometimes helpful, the med frequently needs to be discontinued and replaced.

Real Smart Medications and Nutrients: General Groups

In Chap. 18, I described the way my medical therapy works in general terms; now it's time to present the various groups and subgroups of helpful medications. But first a word of caution: Although I firmly believe that patients should be as informed as possible about all aspects of their disorder, including medical treatment, only physicians have the training and background to properly advise and prescribe medications as well as frequently monitor their effects. All too often, readers are led to believe that over-the-counter drugs are safer to use than those requiring prescriptions. In my opinion, this belief is often unjustified. In fact, I'd go so far as to state that few, if any, drugs should be sold over the counter. And no med—however safe it appears to the layman—should be taken without a doctor knowing about it.

Group I: The Inner-Ear or CVS-Enhancing Medications

When I initially began medically treating dyslexia over 50 years ago, my understanding of this disorder and its helpful medications was indeed limited. At that time, the idea of combining several medications to create greater CVS impact while minimizing side effects was unheard of—as was the use of nutrients and just about every chemical intervention presented here. Yet I was still able to obtain a 30 percent maximum improvement rate, which even today must be considered infinitely better than the zero percent that was medically attainable prior to my research.

However, over many years, I realized that a wide range of different medication subgroups may have CVS-enhancing potency and that each drug in a given category or family was as distinct in its effects as is each child in a family of genetic siblings. By virtue of these and other insights, the percentage of successfully treated dyslexics radically improved t*o approximately 75–85 percent.* And the percentage of *dramatic* responses also increased.[2]

The following subgroups of medications and nutrients were found capable of fine-tuning and improving the CVS-determined signal-scrambling dyslexic impairment.

---

[2] Clearly, placebos invariably play a role in med and other therapies. And as you will have by now seen, any role they play must involve the CVS as must non-placebo responses—since they superficially trigger similar outcomes. And the overall favorable response factor in placebo effects appears to vary significantly with the meds and their chemical/therapeutic categories. Although I have come to clinically recognize this role to be minimal in cases not anticipating favorable responses, only future double-blind studies using a method I have devised will clarify this issue.

Anti-vertigo Antihistamines

Initially, I thought only anti-motion sickness or anti-dizziness antihistamines were helpful in improving CVS functioning. I also mistakenly believed that one anti-motion sickness antihistamine was as effective as another. Thus, if one didn't work, neither would the others. Not so! And I seriously misunderstood the important role of optimal therapeutic doses—not realizing that for some patients, very small or higher-than-average doses are most effective.

How did I arrive at these and other medication-related insights? The simple answer: pure clinical trial and error! For example, patients who feared meds were started on very, very low doses—and in some patients those low doses worked better than the average dose I initially recommended (recall Joey's response to only one eighth of a tablet, in Chap. 14).

Sometimes, despite my carefully explaining the proper dose and writing this information down, "dyslexic errors" occurred. So instead of taking one to two tablets twice a day, patients mistakenly took four pills each time. And that turned out to be the best side-effect-free therapeutic dose for them. Again, had I not been carefully listening to, observing, and monitoring patients, these crucial understandings would never have occurred to me. Nor have they to many others.[3]

Regular Antihistamines

Other chance observations, as well as an insatiable desire to more successfully treat dyslexics, led to yet another unique insight: I belatedly recognized that most antihistamines marketed by drug companies for colds and allergies also had inner-ear or CVS potency. How did I find this out? Patients and/or parents realized that dyslexic symptoms improved only when sick—leaving them puzzled until they read about my research. When sick, they were on typical antihistamines!

So, an additional subgroup of antihistamines was offered to dyslexics who failed to respond to the known anti-vertigo drugs. As a result, the overall improvement rate increased once again—although these typical antihistamines were statistically less effective than anti-vertigo drugs, some exceptions aside. But there were lots of antihistamines to try, as opposed to just a few anti-vertigo meds.

And since each of the effective meds appeared to target some dyslexia-related symptoms more than others, it seemed reasonable to attempt combinations when indicated. And combining worked! So, I was able to improve even more symptoms, on average, per patient. Unexpectedly, in some of my patients, the anti-vertigo meds

---

[3] No doubt, readers will now better understand my prior footnotes in both this and Chap. 5, critiquing a triple-blind study using only one dose of one drug for all dyslexic subjects and attempting to draw reliable conclusions based only on reading score performance after three months of meclizine treatment. Although the researcher, Fagan, was told all about the above drawbacks and advised as to the study's best design, he chose to proceed as he initially thought best. As a psychoanalyst, I can only wonder why he came to seek my advice. And why he chose to ignore it.

even proved to be highly effective in treating allergies. And allergic improvements decreased their dyslexic symptoms. So much for the unchallenged, narrow-minded, and rigid rules and assumptions we all tend to follow as gospel! Thus, I have concluded that without significant clinical effort and involvement—constantly observing, monitoring, and helping patients—"rapid" medical treatment advances such as those seen in this book seldom materialize, unless one is lucky. Thus, I've used, rather than relied on, both involvement and luck.

Importantly, patients are often able to provide vital therapeutic insights to clinicians willing to immediately test out their reported responses. By contrast, absolutely needed formal double-blind controlled validating medication studies—factoring out placebo and other variables—take many years to complete and publish and much longer to implement. So, I reasoned that both these methods might be mutually beneficial when properly combined.

In order to avoid indefinitely withholding valuable treatment and related beneficial insights from suffering patients until meds are "objectively" proven effective in formal or more objective double blind studies, I suggest a sensible scientific compromise: Test and implement known and seemingly helpful available meds clinically as soon as possible when needed, while waiting for formal double-blind validation. In this way, the clinical insights obtained beforehand, if heeded, will also lead to significantly more reliable and effective research designs. Accordingly, I have proposed one such simple and rapid double-blind research method to independently validate my therapeutic data.[4]

As previously stated, I found that a majority of dyslexics had symptoms characterizing ADD/ADHD—even more than 50 years ago, before these terms were so well defined. Thus, I treated some of these dyslexics with stimulants, long before most clinicians had gained the experience to comfortably use them. Not only did the stimulants improve the primary ADD/ADHD part of the dyslexia syndrome, they also secondarily helped with the resulting fatigue and burnout—pseudo-ADD—experienced by many dyslexics trying to compensate for their many primary symptoms and never-ending errors. And surprisingly, the stimulants were sometimes more effective than the inner-ear antihistamines.

Since the reading-related symptoms typically called "dyslexia" overlapped with ADD/ADHD 70–90 percent of the time in referred patients, I initially decided to combine anti-vertigo and stimulant meds for this "comorbid" category of patients—after testing each med, one at a time. As expected, greater benefits were obtained by combining meds, while sometimes minimizing doses and side effects. Importantly, *all* of the symptoms comprising the total dyslexia syndrome were potentially better improved in this way, as opposed to just a few.

---

[4] Percept Mot Skills, 73, 723–38. Levinson, H. N. (1991). pg 736. This study design was offered Fagan, although he declined—no doubt favoring one he initially thought best, despite a complete absence of understanding dyslexia or of the complex intricacies involved in my medical treatment. These many and diverse unanticipated insights occurred slowly over many decades. Thus, his results were doomed to be misleading at best. And they were.

More recently, several non-stimulant meds, such as clonidine and atomoxetine or Strattera were reported and marketed as helpful in ADD/ADHD. However, in my experience, they are significantly less effective than the more typical concentration enhancers—but absolutely worth trying when the stimulants fail. Instead, I found a few of these non-stimulants to be more helpful as add-ons, especially when attempting to further decrease impulsivity, opposition, and even insomnia.

Antidepressants/Antianxiety Medications

Since many dyslexics were observed to be moody, depressed, and/or anxious—and some of the kids experienced bedwetting—tricyclic antidepressants were initially used to combat these symptoms; that is, before a newer generation of these meds was discovered. Unexpectedly, these tricyclics occasionally improved the ADD and even the phobic segment of the dyslexia syndrome as well. And very rarely, some academic symptoms improved too.

Eventually, I recognized that mood, anxiety, and a variety of psychosomatic symptoms, including fatigue and a tendency to burn out, were part and parcel of the dyslexia syndrome or secondarily related. And eventually I found NASA research that clearly documented that the antidepressants—in addition to the antihistamines and stimulants—had mild anti-motion-sickness efficacy and, thus, might also have some CVS potency. These insights, when therapeutically implemented, not only led to a greater degree of improvement, but they also clearly supported my panoramic concept of the dyslexia/CVS syndrome, as well as triggering new insights into ADD/ADHD and how the stimulant medications may affect the CVS.

I then found that the antidepressant bupropion or Wellbutrin, which tends to also increase concentration, as well as the Prozac-like medications (SSRIs and also SNRIs) which decrease anxiety and stabilize mood, were also sometimes helpful—since those with CVS-determined disorders were even more likely to have the latter symptoms than so-called normal controls.

So, these second-generation meds were then tried when needed. These meds not only improved the primary CVS-determined mood and anxiety/phobic symptoms, but they were also helpful in reducing the secondary mood and anxiety symptoms triggered by frustration, failure, and impaired self-esteem. And very atypically, patients surprisingly reported reading and related academic benefits as well.

Non-antihistaminic Anti-nausea/Anti-vertigo and Anti-epileptic Drugs

In my never-ending search for additional medications helpful in dyslexia, I tested out a few marketed primarily as anti-nausea medications, especially in patients failing to favorably respond to the CVS enhancers. These meds were very infrequently shown to be minimally helpful for dyslexics. And in reviewing the literature on anti-epileptic medications, I found that some of these drugs could be beneficial for dizziness and motion sickness as well—though probably utilizing differing mechanisms.

However, their efficacy remains uncertain to date. *They even failed to trigger placebos!*

Over time, I read of a new med that was specifically shown to improve some of the symptoms of dyslexia. Its name was Piracetam and it belonged to a drug category called Nootropils. Upon carefully reviewing the literature, I found that, in addition to helping with memory, it also was an anti-vertigo or anti-dizziness drug. Was this effect due to chance alone? Or did this medication help dyslexics *because* it improved CVS and related compensatory functioning? Although sold over the counter in Europe and Mexico, this somewhat helpful medication is not available in the USA.

Antianxiety, Anti-panic Medications

Because of the CVS-phobia connection, I recognized that the anti-vertigo medications often reduced anxiety and that some anti-panic medications (e.g., diazepam or Valium) frequently helped vertigo. As a result of these reciprocally reported favorable responses, my "team" of medications for phobics was expanded. At the same time, my CVS-phobia hypothesis appeared more independently substantiated, especially after observing the therapeutic benefits of the SSRIs and SNRIs on anxiety/panic.

However, I frequently use a natural neurotransmitter GABA, a highly calming antianxiety agent, before most other substances. In fact, it proved highly effective in two adult patients who had been phobic since birth but had failed all other med trials before I saw them. So, it's a great add-on to other meds I've used for phobias/anxiety. And a miraculous stand-alone—if and when it works. And so was c-Tyrosine.

Group II: Signal and Processing/Regulator Enhancers

Herbs and Natural Substances

Over a period of years, I came to recognize that a variety of vitamins, minerals, and related health products I tested out had somewhat helped my patients. By and large, these nutrients were not nearly as effective as the CVS enhancers—not by a very, very long shot. But remember my motto: Some improvement is better than none! And by adding selected harmless substances to my winning therapeutic "team," I hoped to obtain greater degrees and numbers of improvements per patient, on average. And I did, although a trained nutritionist would no doubt have obtained far, far better results.

Clearly, additional studies and nutritionists are needed to further elaborate upon this highly complex modality in order to obtain the best possible results (refer to Appendix 3).

Clinically Based Med Correlations

Having developed the above insights, I then explored the efficacy of the specific CVS enhancers in improving the various CVS-determined symptoms and mechanisms found to be impaired in dyslexics. And the resulting data enabled me to somewhat better choose which combination of medications would more likely be effective for each patient, notwithstanding a major unknown: each individual's highly idiosyncratic reactivity to specific chemical substances and doses. Although this important unknown will likely be clarified by future studies—genetic and others—I did manage to determine which medications are statistically the most effective as well as their most common side effects and how best to minimize and avoid those negatives.

Summary

By combining medications and nutrients that can minimize CVS-determined scrambling and enhance the compensatory potency of CNS processors and modulators, I have found that the probability of a favorable outcome is significantly increased. However, as noted, each medication within a given category and subcategory is surprisingly different. And each patient typically responds best to only one of three to four inner-ear enhancers.

By and large, the anti-motion sickness antihistamines help the non-ADD/ADHD part of the dyslexic syndrome the most, while the stimulants are more beneficial for the ADHD segment of the impairment. And vitamins, minerals, and nutrients add some potential depth and scope to the overall improvement quality and quantity—with little risk of side effects.

Also, by using a synergistically acting therapeutic "team" of meds and other compounds, the risk of side effects is often reduced, and greater degrees of improvement likely occur.

In retrospect, none of these specifically reported insights and correlations could have been initially predicted by non-clinician theorists in "ivory towers," regardless of their gifted abilities, altruistic attitudes, and/or use of sophisticated instruments. These insights could only be derived *clinically in real time* by directly observing and listening to patients and/or their loved ones—close up—while attempting to figure out and test plausible, scientifically grounded explanations. As a result of my steadily evolving understanding, a majority of dyslexics—children and adults—can now be helped *medically*. And by virtue of their more "normalized" CVS and related functioning, dyslexics are able to respond significantly better and more rapidly to all other non-medical add-on therapies.

As I mentioned earlier in the book, CVS-related dysfunctioning was discovered to *coexist in* a series of distinct major brain disorders, such as autism or ASD, mental retardation, cerebral palsy, bipolar disorder, schizophrenia, etc. Accordingly, the limited but important favorable responses of autistic patients to CVS enhancers will be discussed in the very next chapter, especially as the incidence or recognition of ASD is increasing.

I hope the above insights and med/chemical-triggered improvements will encourage those suffering from the dyslexia/CVS syndrome to now seek helpful treatment while catalyzing pharmacological chemists to design new CVS-signal stabilizers and transmitters as well as CNS descrambling enhancers so that real cures become possible ASAP.

Chapter 22
An Effective Partial Medical Treatment for Autism (ASD) and Autistic Trait Disorder or Pseudo-autism

Three Autistic Children From Three Different Continents, Plus a Fourth Patient with Autistic Trait Disorder

The aim of this chapter is to provide insights into a rapid and effective—but partial—medical treatment for autism or (ASD) and autistic trait disorders (ATD), as well as a rationale for why this treatment works and fails.

Autism affects approximately one in 68 children—often emotionally overwhelming these kids and their loving families by the challenges brought on by impaired social skills, repetitive behaviors, and major speech and nonverbal communication issues. And even worse, this disorder persists throughout adulthood. Thus, any and all safe and especially rapid partial improvements are often considered miraculous by those affected.

A coexisting CVS correlation As previously noted, I unexpectedly discovered many years ago that a CVS dysfunction coexists with the vast majority of autistic patients that I've thus far examined. And since a CVS dysfunction and its resulting syndrome of dyslexia-related symptoms, including ADD/ADHD and phobias/anxiety, responded favorably to CVS enhancers, I decided to treat autistics with these same meds. My reasoning was as follows:

- Autism—or its spectrum—is caused by *major primary brain processing (and/or transmission) impairments of unknown origin(s)*. This disorder was considered medically untreatable *until I long ago began to do so with CVS enhancers, initially on only a research basis.*
- According to my clinical research, those with autism or ASD also have a coexisting signal-scrambling impairment of CVS origin—which sends distorted signals to (1) autistic-causing or triggering brain processors and (2) other non-autistic or

H. N. Levinson, *Feeling Smarter and Smarter*,
https://doi.org/10.1007/978-3-030-16208-5_22

normal brain processors—thus, secondarily resulting in the many and diverse symptoms characterizing the dyslexia/CVS syndrome.

- By decreasing the CVS-determined signal-scrambling to autistic brain processors and related mechanisms as well as to non-autistic—normal—processors, using CVS-enhancers, including stimulants and other meds when needed, it seemed possible to improve overall functioning in those suffering from ASD. However, the core autistic disorder was reasoned to likely persist, albeit perhaps minimally improve.

A successful partial med treatment Fortunately, my reasoning was proven clinically correct. Over the past decades, I have helped mildly, and a few moderately, impaired autistic children and adults using inner-ear/cerebellar-enhancers, although the possible efficacy in severe cases has been difficult to properly evaluate. To demonstrate the rapid and sometimes dramatic improvements possible, I will present autistic children whose loving parents sought my expertise—each having repeatedly failed all other non-behavioral, non-tutorial attempts at help.

Four Favorable Med Responders

All four children—Jordan, Abe, Jack, as well as Barrow—had been diagnosed with ASD since early childhood. Additionally, I diagnosed all four as having a coexisting CVS dysfunction based on my four-step diagnostic process. And as you will read, they favorably responded to my medication regime in different ways and degrees—just as do those with the dyslexia/CVS syndrome. However, Barrow was somewhat atypical—and so was considered by me to possibly have autistic trait disorder or pseudo-autism.

Jordan Johnson: Treating Autism + ADHD + Dyslexia

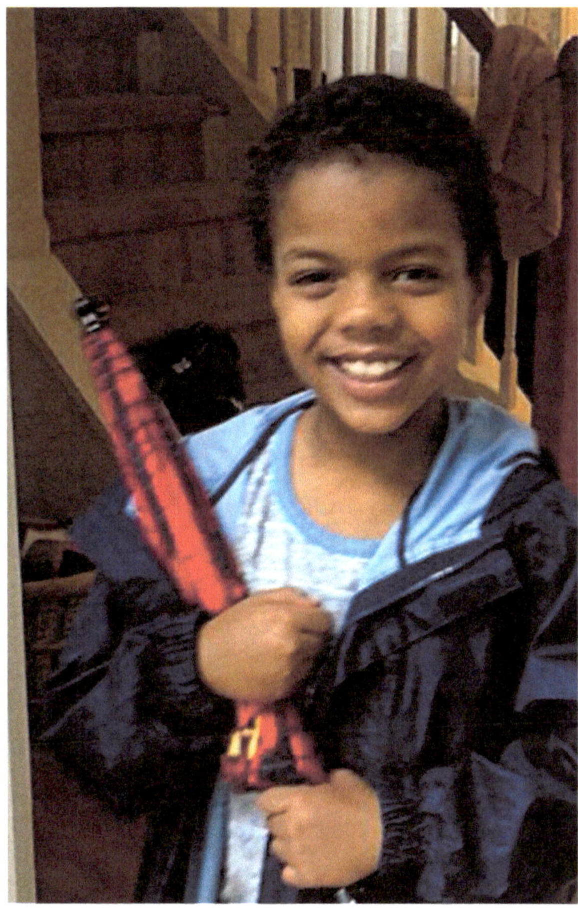

Jordan is 9 years old. He was initially diagnosed with autism when very young, and then later with ADD—prior to seeking my help. During the first six months of my treating him for an underlying cerebellar-vestibular (CVS) dysfunction—coexisting with his primary autistic impairment—Jordan's communication skills, as well as many of his non-autistic symptoms, significantly improved.

His mom describes Jordan's autism as well as his improvements on CVS-enhancing meds as follows:

> *Jordan was diagnosed with autism at age two and a half. At age five he was evaluated at Duke University where his diagnosis was changed to ADD. Before seeing Dr. Levinson, nine-year-old Jordan was "in his own world." He was very hard to motivate. He did things in his own time and was unaware and unaffected by social pressures. It was very hard to follow his train of thought. His statements seemed random, as if he were telling you something from the middle of the story rather than the beginning. It seemed as though he was just a little bit off… as if a switch needed to be flipped.*

But once we started treatment with Dr. Levinson, changes began. The switch was definitely turned on. I started noticing Jordan saying things… as if he was more "in the moment." He said, "Tell me about it." That was a phrase he got from his teacher, and he was using it in context. He actually reminded me that he needed to have his homework done. This meant that he had developed new organizational and planning skills as well as greater memory and interest.

His teacher told me that he seemed more assertive, volunteered to write on the chalkboard, and followed along more during class. He also could relay a story to me of what happened at school, something that he could never do in the past. He bargains more, argues more, and even tries to pull the wool over my eyes. All of those things are typical for his age but something I never saw before.

As we reached our sixth month on Dr. Levinson's program, Jordan's speech and communication improvements continue to surprise me more and more. He asked me what the word "pregnant" meant—he had heard it on TV. We also had a discussion about the razorback boar. He started listening to my conversations and then asking me questions about what was said.

One morning I allowed Jordan to have popcorn for breakfast. And later that day he lied about it to my sister. He told her he had pancakes and eggs. I was so proud and amazed. He showed the understanding that popcorn is not a breakfast food and also had the presence of mind to be embarrassed about it, while attempting to spare me possible criticism.

I now understand a lot more about what he is saying and I can follow his train of thought. As a result of all of his improvements, I am very pleased and very hopeful.

—Lois Johnson

Abe X

Abe was 8 years old when his caring and actively involved parents brought him to me for help. Although his family resides a continent away from most ASD research centers, they repeatedly followed up on every lead—having Abe diagnosed by many autism experts who offered a glimmer of hope, regardless of distance and expense. And they had his private schooling amplified by as many tutors, behaviorists, and trainers as possible. Through her efforts to help Abe—supported by his exceptionally caring father, Abe's mother became a virtual resource for many other autistics in need.

In fact, were it not for his mom's amazing intuition and maternal instincts, Abe would never have significantly benefitted from my medical treatment. And the reason is simple: Autistics are often highly sensitive to metabolic and environmental triggers. However "minor" these triggers might seem to others, they often cause major symptomatic responses. Thus, meds and doses must often be very carefully monitored and repeatedly modified.

Observing, monitoring, and compensating for these fluctuating triggers and the patient's responses are difficult—even for a family living near their doctor and in the same time zone. So, it was truly remarkable to see a mom living a continent and culture away handle this aspect of treatment so well—while speaking another primary language. Somehow—to help her son—she was able to fully comprehend both my Brooklyn accent and the vital questions and instructions conveyed.

Because of the language difference, which influenced this mom's writing, not her excellent spoken English, I will describe most of Abe's rapid and evolving improvements as they were observed and/or communicated to me via frequent telephone consultations and a few visits. And then Abe's mom will summarize her observations in her own words.

My Summary of Abe's Improvements

Abe was correctly diagnosed as autistic shortly after birth. His core ASD symptoms were not unlike those of Jordan's, so I will focus on reporting his improvements while taking CVS-enhancers—as summarized from my notes:

> *Abe's concentration, memory, impulsivity, frustration, and anger management rapidly improved. His screaming in school was greatly reduced. He was quieter, calmer, and exhibited an 80 percent reduction in his anxiety. Abe suddenly spoke more—primarily to himself, initially. Then his speech was directed to his family, and then to others. For the first time he seemed happy.*
>
> *His reading quickly improved but he still manifested difficulty recalling the content within paragraphs read. Abe performed addition problems more quickly. And although he was better able to repeat numbers forward, backwards remained difficult. His spelling rapidly improved—soon he was getting all A's and A⁺'s.*
>
> *Fast forwarding two years: Abe is now considered dramatically better in most respects. His reading has spurted by more than four grades—especially his comprehension. And he* enjoys *reading—particularly when alone. He's asking more and more questions. He's talking more to others and has quite a few friends, although initially enjoying their presence more than conversing with them. He can now go on play dates by himself. Loves swimming and horseback riding—as his below photos reveal—and is extremely good at both. And oh yes; You will see him talking in front of his class—a first. He still regresses in the presence of background noises and when he doesn't get his way—but is so much better.*
>
> *One year later: When on proper doses, Abe's prior outbursts are gone, he's among the top math students in his class, prefers to be with friends—and regresses only with parents. Decreased doses due to med unavailability resulted in diminished functioning—and he reverted back to his norm when optimal doses were once again restored.*

The Meds Used

It's important to mention that Abe was treated only with an anti-motion sickness antihistamine, an anxiety reducing nutrient GABA, and belatedly with small doses of coffee in the morning. Besides caffeine, he could not tolerate any other stimulant meds for his ADD/ADHD symptoms. And importantly, his previous antipsychotic med, Risperdal, prescribed by another MD, was no longer needed to control his outbursts and so was stopped shortly after he began my treatment.

Abe's med doses had to be continually adjusted. For example, his meds appeared to stop working for two months following an appendectomy—whereupon they once again became effective. And his mom had to adjust the doses more than ten times, both up and down, throughout the course of his treatment to date. During periods where the meds were stopped, or not adjusted, his prior symptoms returned.

Abe and his family were fortunate—since there are many similar cases where the meds never again regain their efficacy once lost.

A Vaccination Effect

One more important insight: Following his vaccination at age 5, Abe's autistic symptoms intensified. Since similar intensifications occurred following his other illnesses, it may be reasonable to assume that—many possible exceptions aside—vaccinations may *intensify* autistic symptoms, rather than *cause* them as many parents currently fear. In those rare reported cases *caused* by vaccinations, there may have been a highly atypical chemical encephalopathy—or sterile brain impairment. However, the infection risks of not vaccinating are high, especially since this alleged cause of autism has been debunked.

Abe's Mom's Comments

At the very beginning we knew that something was missing in our life—our son was very different from our other children. It was hard to describe—hard to say for sure—but his difference broke our hearts every second. And so, we passed through a very hard time day by day, year by year.

It was also tough finding a doctor who could help him—us—who we could trust. We spent years going to different countries looking for help, tried lots of medications, different treatments—nothing really helped much. But we still kept looking for the best—hoping, praying.

Our son was late in speech. He was four when he started to talk. This then affected him in his social skills, communication, understanding, and his behaviors.

Then he started a new school and faced many challenges in a very competitive environment—and he acted out behaviorally. He found it hard to focus in class, and to normally interact with his classmates. Someone had to be always there to help him. And academically, our son was below average. So, we provided him with as much help as possible. And involved him in as many activities as possible. But he liked swimming and riding his horse most. So, we encouraged that.

Month by month he was improving, but it was very, very slow, and frustrating. That is, until we met Dr. Levinson. And only after our son started Dr. Levinson's treatment did we start to see positive changes—very quickly at first.

My son began to change for the better. He is calmer now. This helps him a lot with controlling his behaviors, which then improves his ability to socialize and focus in class. And now other kids can accept him. Most important, we can now see him as a happy and healthy boy, responsible for himself, newly confident, and living a normal life.

Dr. Levinson: We will forever thank and pray for you,

–Mrs. X.

Three Photos of Abe: Riding, Studying, Lecturing

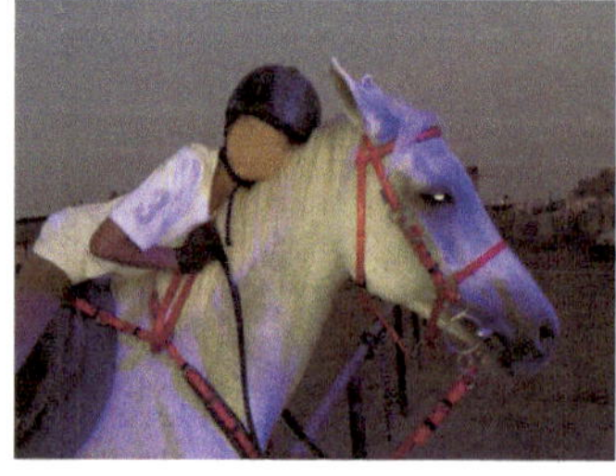

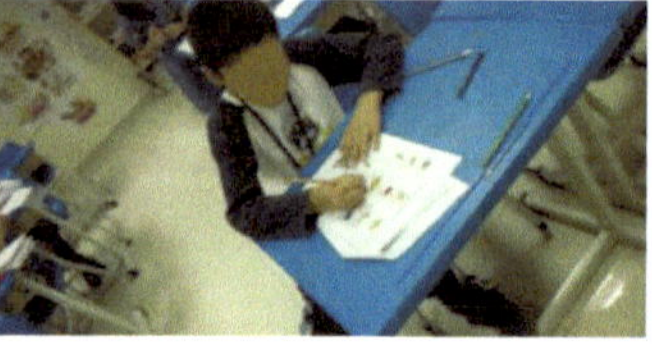

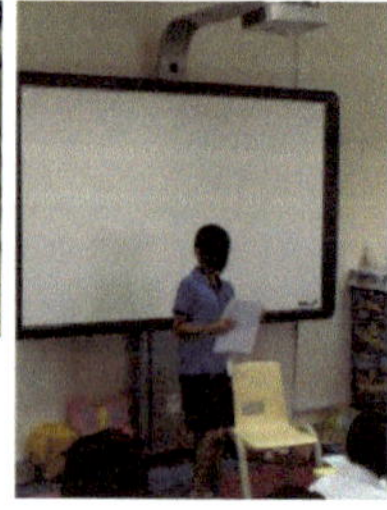

Bender-Gestalt Designs and Goodenough Figure Drawings: One Year Apart

Before concluding this case, I'd like to present Abe's *before-treatmen*t and *after-treatment f*igure drawings and copied illustrations. These were done when I initially examined Abe and then again on his follow-up on-meds revisit a year later. The differences are obviously remarkable—especially considering that these changes likely occurred much earlier than when the testing occurred.

Based on my clinical experience with these graphomotor test methods, the amazing changes that you'll see below do not occur by chance or after a relatively short time interval—even a year—in autistic children due only to possible maturation. Indeed, these changes most likely arose in conjunction with Abe's other favorable medication-triggered improvements.

Just to reemphasize: Although Abe's maturation didn't significantly change or regress over a year, his responses to specific meds and circumstances varied dramatically—both up and down. Accordingly, the below changes must be considered med-related—especially since his med-triggered, improved graphomotor (fine motor writing coordination) performance decreased when his meds failed.

Normal BG Designs

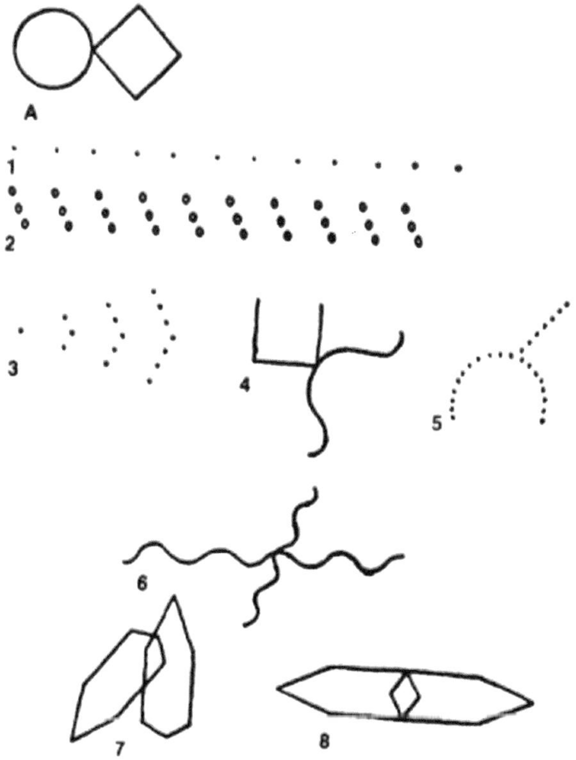

Abe's BG Designs Pre-treatment

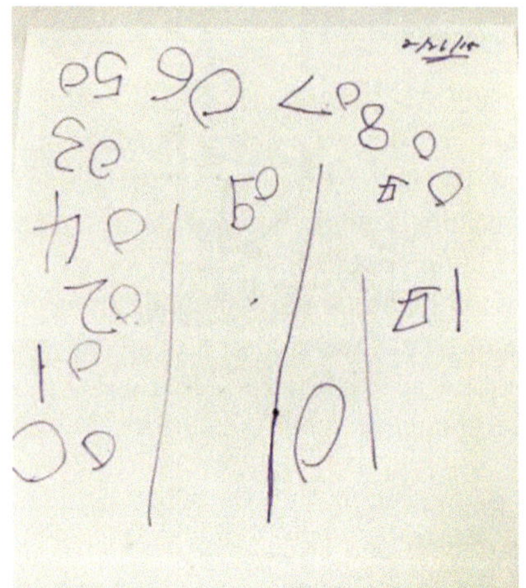

Abe's Goodenough Figure Drawing Pre-Rx

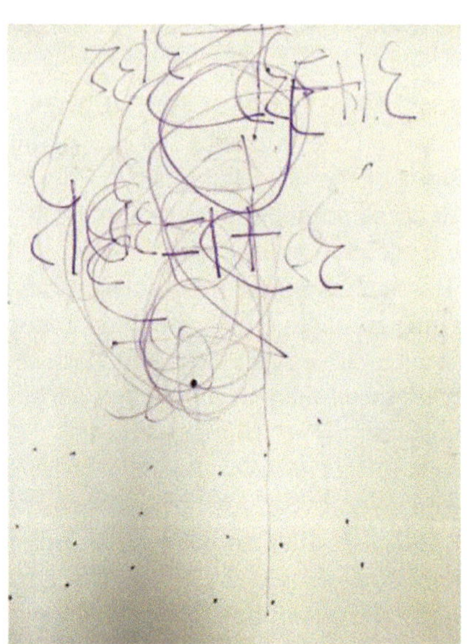

Abe's BG Designs Post-Rx

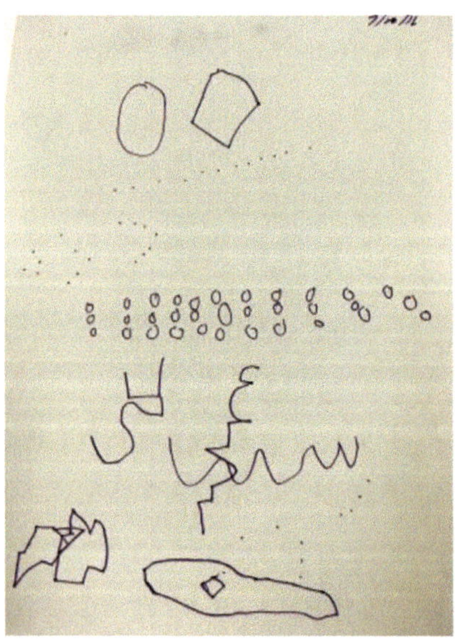

Abe's Goodenough Figure Drawing Post-Rx

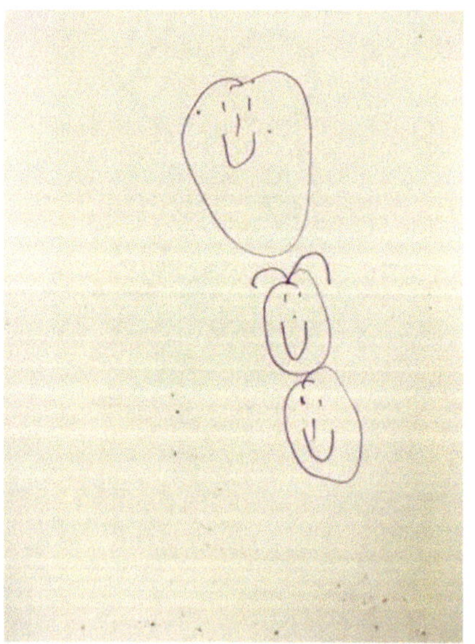

Jack

Jack is an 11-year-old, bright, artistically gifted autistic boy recently brought to me for testing and treatment. He resides in Beijing, China, with his Harvard-trained parents. Although he just began treatment, his response to the initial doses of his first med was encouraging. His parents report:

> *Although we are reluctant to use meds and rely on organic-health foods, we felt it worthwhile trying your treatment, which, after we researched it, seemed safe and well worth the risk and our anxieties. Well, we were especially surprised and pleased to note that Jack's use of words had somewhat improved after two weeks on the meds—absolutely no side effects. We both noticed that Jack became more verbal and/or curious, spontaneously asking such never-before questions as: "Why are you doing that?" and "Dad, are you going to work today?" And one of his unexpected comments was the most surprising of all—indicating a solid grasp and use of language. When discussing an important and deep artistic concept, he stunned us by commenting: "Like a big whale swimming under water?" These are comments he never before voiced—never. In fact, he seldom speaks—keeping mainly to himself and preoccupied with his computer games.*
>
> *He seems to have greater verbal and mental capacity. Thus, he appears to better comprehend and so respond to longer word chains than before. Since his improvements appear sporadic, they can best be judged by how often they pleasantly surprise us. Before treatment, we were seldom, if ever, pleasantly surprised.*

Since it's possible that Jack's initial speech/language improvements are not med-triggered or related, it might be helpful to consider that he did not similarly respond to two other meds he tolerated very well from the same therapeutic family. And that after he became ill and his med was stopped, his improved verbal responses lessened—perhaps due to his sore throat? After recovery, however, his prior improvement returned with resumption of his med.

An Explanatory Comment

CVS dysfunction is present but not the cause Many earlier investigators of severe autism reported inner-ear or vestibular dysfunction in their patients long before the moderate- and high-functioning part of the spectrum was considered, thereby explaining their characteristic balance and coordination problems. Some researchers even initially postulated that autism had an inner-ear/vestibular origin—which I disagreed with for clinical reasons that will soon become obvious. None had considered the cerebellum as an important determinant—until decades after I reported my CVS findings and improvements and after neuroimaging studies were belatedly initiated.

Having examined and successfully treated thousands of patients with the dyslexia or CVS syndrome—typical of the many cases thus far presented—it should be crystal clear to all readers that even the high-functioning Asperger-like cases, and/or those just seen, represent non-dyslexic disorders—even though ASD manifests CVS dysfunctioning.

As Maria, in the opening pages, simply explained: Those with the dyslexia syndrome have only one CVS-determined signal-scrambling "demon." By comparison, those with autism or ASD must have two separate but interacting "demons." One demon causes major primary brain sensing, transmission, and processing impairments resulting in autism or ASD—triggering characteristic and defining symptoms of a non-dyslexic nature. And a second coexisting and interacting minor CVS demon triggers signal-scrambling symptoms typical of those with the dyslexia syndrome.

Improving CVS vs. ASD symptoms Importantly, because of this CVS overlapping with ASD, I demonstrated that some autistics can now be helped with CVS-enhancing meds, as were Jordan, Abe, and Jack. And the same favorable responses are possible for those suffering with such other major processing brain disorders as *mental retardation, Down syndrome, cerebral palsy, traumatic brain injury, schizophrenia,* etc.—*where CVS dysfunctioning is a minor but often treatable co-conspirator.* No cures—but some definite improvements. *And for all of those favorably affected, this partial medical treatment, however minimal, is considered a godsend.*

The latest insights derived from fMRI and other neuroimaging studies may also help explain why the CVS meds work and fail in those with ASD—depending on a great many variables. These determinants likely include the severity and/or specific sites of the cerebellar and related brain pathology independently discovered to be impaired in ASD and/or how *disrupted their interconnected circuits* are when transmitting important information to, and from, vital autistic-related brain sensing and processing structures. In fact, one neuroimaging study reported different cerebellar sites involved with dyslexia, ADD/ADHD, and autism.

Eventually, I reasoned that when the autistic demon does not severely impair the language, cognitive, social, and IQ centers of the brain, as in Asperger's and other higher functioning individuals with ASD, favorable CVS improvements are more likely to occur and/or become evident. By contrast, in severe autistics where the above brain areas and transmitting circuits are significantly more impaired, as are the emotional sensing, transmitting, and processing centers, then favorable therapeutic outcomes are less probable and apparent, especially if there is also greater collateral brain involvement.

Other therapies Because of the above independently confirmed insights into the cerebellum and other lower-brain involvement in autism, in addition to likely higher brain processing disruption, it would seem important to supplement the effective cognitive therapies (especially ABA or applied behavior analysis) with both medical and non-medical cerebellar-vestibular-enhancing and related helpful lower-brain modalities so as to maximize improvements.

Before Concluding

I'd like to emphasize that all three of my presented cases here were male—and so is Barrow—the fourth to come. This supports the well-known clinical finding that males significantly outnumber females in ASD, more so than for any other neurodevelopmental impairment. Needless to say, the reasons determining this male dominance are under active study—as are other possible clues to the causes of ASD—by many highly gifted, altruistic, and determined researchers. And these researchers really know what they're looking for since they are using advanced neuroimaging techniques unavailable to the old time dyslexia researchers—myself included. Thus, I anticipate that all the rapidly accruing research data, including that presented here, will lead to more significant help—*sooner rather than later.*

A Fourth Vital Last Minute Addition: Barrow Maxwell Williams—A Gifted Autistic Trait-Disordered 16-Year-Old

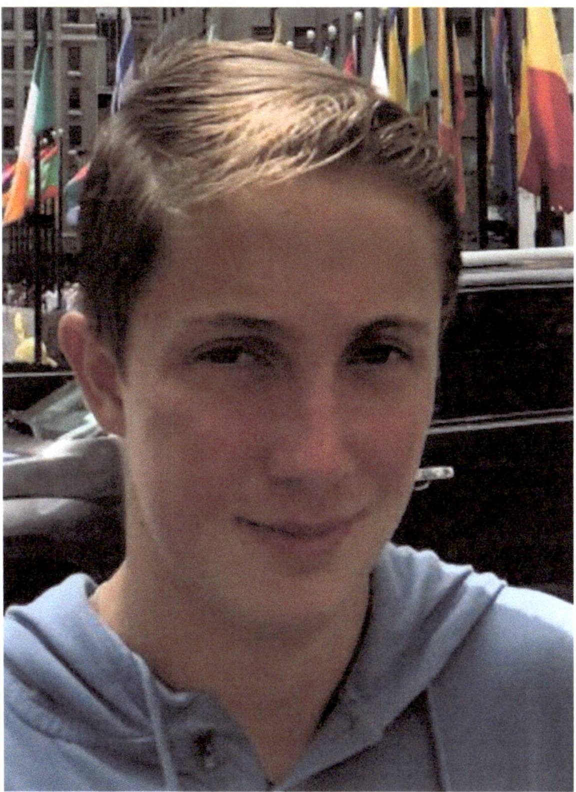

To better clarify autism, it's crucial to understand autistic lookalikes or those variations manifesting minor autistic traits and having the dyslexia/CVS syndrome. By analyzing the stimming and other quirky personality symptoms that characterized a 16-year-old gifted and affable *autistic trait-disordered* youngster named Barrow Williams, it appeared that his symptoms seemed best explained by a little known neuronal oversensitivity theory named Dabrowski's overexcitabilities (OE),[1] as well as by my own cerebellar insights.

It is important to emphasize that Barrow did not manifest most of the diagnostically typical verbal or nonverbal communication, empathic, or social difficulties typical of ASD. Just the opposite: He was highly empathic, made friends easily, and was readily accepted by all others. And like Jenny in Chap. 20, he avoided eye contact only to minimize overloading—since it's difficult for some CVS-impaired to look and accurately listen at the same time. Thus, an ASD diagnosis remained in limbo. And so, he was termed *autistic trait-disordered (ATD)* or *pseudo-autistic.*

Most importantly, Barrow was given Dramamine for motion sickness by his pediatrician, who happened to be his mom. And he responded so well that he, on his own, initially discontinued Ritalin, which had been previously needed for his concentration, distractibility, and activity/impulsivity symptoms.

Barrow's CVS Neurological Imbalance and Dyscoordination

Perhaps readers might be interested in learning just how the CVS might be impaired in ASD or ATD (autistic trait disorder)—since this was the primary basis for my attempting to treat this "demon" with the CVS enhancing meds many years ago.

Impaired balance and coordination on neurological examination Barrow's balance was significantly impaired, even with his eyes open and both feet grounded. Although very tall and lean, physically built for basketball, it became readily clear why he avoided playing.

When asked how he felt upon closing his eyes, standing with outstretched arms and feet together, he replied: "I feel as if the ceiling air conditioner's fan is blowing me over." He manifested difficulties with all the other CVS diagnostic neurological

---

[1] Dabrowski describes five clinically apparent overexcitable neuronal forms: psychomotor, sensual, emotional, imaginational, and intellectual. However, he skips over a possible neurophysiological cause of the neuronal sensitivities—cerebellar mechanisms involving inhibition, disinhibition, and facilitation of specific circuits and signals.

Psychomotor OE manifests as an enhanced neuromuscular excitation resulting in excessive energy and a need for—and satisfaction from—physical action.

Sensory/Sensual OE manifests as an intensified experience of pleasure or displeasure triggered by one or more of the five senses. Conversely, there may be extreme pain and disgust.

Intellectual OE manifests as an extreme desire to seek understanding and truth, to gain knowledge, and to analyze and categorize information. Children with this characteristic frequently love thinking purely for the sake of thinking.

Imaginational OE manifests as an intensified play of the imaginations. Often children high in Imaginational OE do not differentiate between truth and fiction or are absorbed in their own private world with imaginary companions and dramatizations.

Emotional OE is characterized by heightened, intense feelings and responses of various kinds. Children with this characteristic show strong emotional attachments to people, places, and things. They are empathetic, compassionate, and extremely sensitive.

Perhaps the following blog review will be helpful: https://positivepsychologyprogram.com/dabrowskis-positive-disintegration/, https://en.wikipedia.org/wiki/Overexcitability

parameters discussed in Chap. 19—Four Steps to a Certain Diagnosis. His findings included a clinically obvious, CVS-determined ocular-motor fixation and tracking impairment, which I initially and over-simplistically considered to be solely responsible for causing visual scrambling and dyslexia, way, way back in 1973.

Dr. Williams Describes Barrows' Improvements (My comments are italicized.)

As we started the protocol, Barrow was self-motivated to take the Dramamine because it helped him feel calmer in his head, and better able to interact with peers. *(He felt less overloaded and calmer, less anxious, as well as better focused, less distracted and mentally overactive. His confidence—self-esteem— then improved, especially since speech, memory and other functions that are needed to comfortably and properly socially interact improved as well; perhaps he even experienced enhanced auditory processing, although this needs verification. Indeed, these favorable CVS-enhancing med improvements also explain why meds are also helpful in those with true ASD, as noted previously.)*

Barrow wanted to find the right dose and medication combination that would help him to engage better in activities and complete work without getting distracted or overly restless. *(Clearly, it's also difficult to socially interact when unable to concentrate and perhaps experiencing brain fog and anxiety. And when your thoughts are fuzzy or not properly sequenced. To reemphasize: the CVS enhancers are also helpful in ASD by improving those coexisting CVS fine-tuning functions facilitating socialization and communication.)*

Upon Dr. Levinson's recommendations, Barrow was later placed on another CVS enhancer, cyclizine. His focus and concentration further improved, which then may have enabled him to significantly overcome his math difficulties. However, a new tutor was also very helpful. (*Yet Barrow did not respond favorably to meclizine, although this med is almost structurally/chemically identical to marezine. This shows just how amazingly specific the chemical triggers and responses are.*)[2]

[2] *Placebo* vs. *Non-Placebo*—Once again, it's important to emphasize just how unexpected and specific the favorable response to meds often are. And the same holds true for which symptomatic targets the meds hit. To date, none of the meds have significantly reduced Barrow's hyperactivity symptom. Yet most all have enhanced his concentration—the antihistamines more so than the stimulants.

Thus, until further clarified by necessary double-blind controlled studies, I will continue to suspect that these responses are non-placebo. And since the responses remain favorable over time, the ultimate verdict doesn't clinically matter to the patients or their families or their MDs. In fact, Dr. Jana Williams, also having exceptional pharmacological expertise, fully agrees with my views.

Once a med is approved by the FDA for efficacy and safety, clinicians never consider whether the improvements and/or side effects per patient are due to placebo positives or negatives. Importantly, all the CVS antihistamines used were approved for inner-ear symptoms and the stimulants for ADD/ADHD.

Chapter 23
Kathy's Favorable Response to Medical Treatment

Just when I once again thought this book was complete, and even "artistically" flavored with a touch of symmetry, I received a fascinating progress report from Kathy—the gifted woman whose amazing self-description filled Chap. 6.[1] Despite Kathy's incredible ability to describe her dyslexic symptoms, I initially considered leaving her therapeutic responses out—to symbolize the unknowns and the open-ended nature of this and all other clinical research efforts.

However, the illuminating vibrancy of Kathy's report created a slight artistic vs. clinical dilemma. And as you might well have guessed by now, there is very little artistic ability in my clinical makeup. So, I decided to zag once again and change my game plan. After all, how could I not include Kathy's favorable responses here? Wouldn't you and all other readers be interested in what became of this gifted dyslexic woman? And how her favorable responses to treatment validated this book's basic tenets? I certainly was!

Kathy's Self-Description of Her Response to Treatment

> *My life has changed in so many ways since our first encounter that I scarcely know where to begin. I'm sending this progress report and anticipating my yearly check-up at the end of June. The simple antihistamines and nutrients have greatly expanded my possibilities. However, I wonder what my story and that of my family's would have been like had I begun therapy at the beginning—when a child.*

---

[1] This book was initially begun many years ago and then put away for quite awhile. Thus, it includes just a few patients from the first version—Kathy being one of them. So her favorable response appeared at the end of my first draft. Needless to say, this new version is completely different and contains mostly new patients and my latest insights. Older patients were included for several reasons: They were especially interesting and informative and so provided a natural bridge to the present. And most importantly—I promised to include them when this book was completed. As you may remember from my Brooklyn beginning—I learned to forever remember and respect altruism and loyalty. This is my payback and respect for my patients' altruism.

H. N. Levinson, *Feeling Smarter and Smarter*,
https://doi.org/10.1007/978-3-030-16208-5_23

Overall Improvements – *The most dramatic change has been my ability to return to work as a physical therapist after a seventeen-year departure—and full time. I no longer feel as rushed or as far behind and overwhelmed by the simplest of things—things as easy to others as breathing. And when I challenge my patients' boundaries, I simultaneously challenge my own—for nothing was easy and reflexive or automatic for me! Previously I spent my days attempting to figure out the world and trying to fit into it. My dyslexic world entailed endless work and effort, where perceptions were a constant puzzle and the movement of my own body involved a conscious and deliberate effort. Walking, climbing stairs, reading, writing, tying shoes, blow-drying hair, driving, doing a day's work are no longer Herculean tasks. No longer do I get lost attempting to find my car or driving home—despite years and years of prior practice, maps, etc.*

Reading and Music – *Besides the amazing improvement I feel in the complex abilities involved in caring for stroke and brain-injured patients, there have been other positive changes in two areas I have always loved despite great challenges: reading and music.*

I can now read and play my piano for hours at a time without headaches. I still read slowly, but the letters no longer flicker, nor do I lose track of them as before. I still wear my tinted glasses and use my finger, but the words seem more likely to stick to the page rather than "move down a drain" past my focal point, as before.

Reading music is so much easier, too. I can now determine where the note is on the line or space—and thus, don't make the mistakes I used to. I remember the note I played and can reach for the correct interval to the next notes—without looking. And I can play pieces that frequently change key.

Occasionally I've played a piece completely—every last note, from beginning to end. And I can find the next line of music, without repetition. Sometimes I even play in the composer's chosen tempo (and not at the speed in which he wrote the composition). In other words, I play better. Everyone has noticed this difference.

Besides those things, there are countless little improved niceties now—like not falling up stairs or curbs so often, being able to spend hours in a store with tightly stacked, endless shelves of merchandise (no longer getting overloaded, light sensitive, claustrophobic, etc.), riding escalators without a thought to my personal safety, mechanically adjusting equipment (wheelchairs, platform walkers, etc.) with greater ease, even remembering where I parked my car and how to get home, etc.

Thank you,
Kathy

A Final Comment or Two

There is much to note about Kathy's favorable responses to inner-ear-enhancers, besides her improved reading, concentration, and anxiety/phobic symptoms. However, there is one outstanding characteristic worthy of significant emphasis. Before treatment, Kathy, similar to most dyslexics, had to compensate for her CVS inability to reflexly or autonomously function both mentally and physically—by using severe amounts of conscious, repetitive, and tiring thinking-brain effort. By contrast, after favorably responding to the inner-ear/cerebellar-enhancers, much of her autonomous or reflex CVS functioning improved—so, she no longer needed to exert all that conscious compensatory, cerebral energy.

Do not these simple observations help further substantiate the notion that Kathy's thinking brain is superb and in fact *compensated* for her CVS (or lower brain)-determined dyslexia syndrome and its reflex, autonomous functioning, rather than *caused* it?

Chapter 24
Summary

Having now completed the main content of this book, the next major question to resolve is: How can I effectively and interestingly summarize all the amazing qualities and diversities of the patient-derived insights you've read about, while avoiding boring repetition?

No doubt you've once again guessed my solution. As you will see, I've decided to finish this presentation as I began it—using information provided by patients (and/or their parents) who've agreed to use real photos and often real names, as well as to graciously reveal their diverse symptoms and favorable responses to a groundbreaking medical treatment.

By "listening" to the symptoms and favorable therapeutic improvements of these many altruistic volunteers who now can be seen and so deemed *alive and real*, I believe you will be rewarded with the best possible review and summary of the dyslexia syndrome as well as of this book's vital clarifications and discoveries.

So, I will now present these patients as a vivid flashback—brought to life by their photos, young and old, in random order—just the way I saw them when they initially came to me for help. Since they are all on my website (http://www.dyslexiaonline.com/treatment/patient_responses.html), I've decided to include only a handful here and summarize their content so as to facilitate your review.

H. N. Levinson, *Feeling Smarter and Smarter*,
https://doi.org/10.1007/978-3-030-16208-5_24

Zoe Friedman

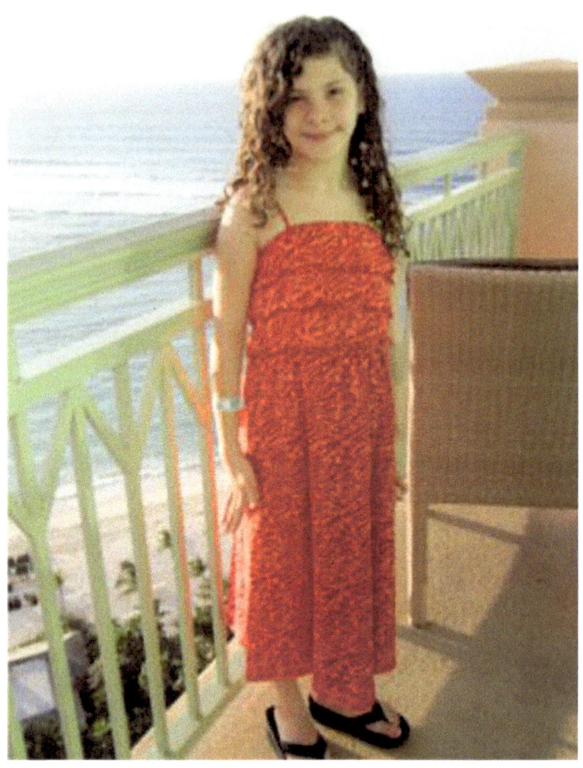

Dr. Levinson has been instrumental in helping my daughter achieve goals that we thought were far beyond her reach. Once he evaluated her and she began on her regimen, we immediately saw improvement in her tracking during reading and her handwriting legibility. Once we added in additional medication, her progress was even greater — she was able to sit through class, and it became much easier and clearer for her to comprehend what she was learning. Her focus greatly intensified and she feels better about herself in general. We feel so fortunate to have found Dr. Levinson and his unique approach to helping our daughter reach her maximum potential.

Mrs. Allison Friedman

Bethany S.

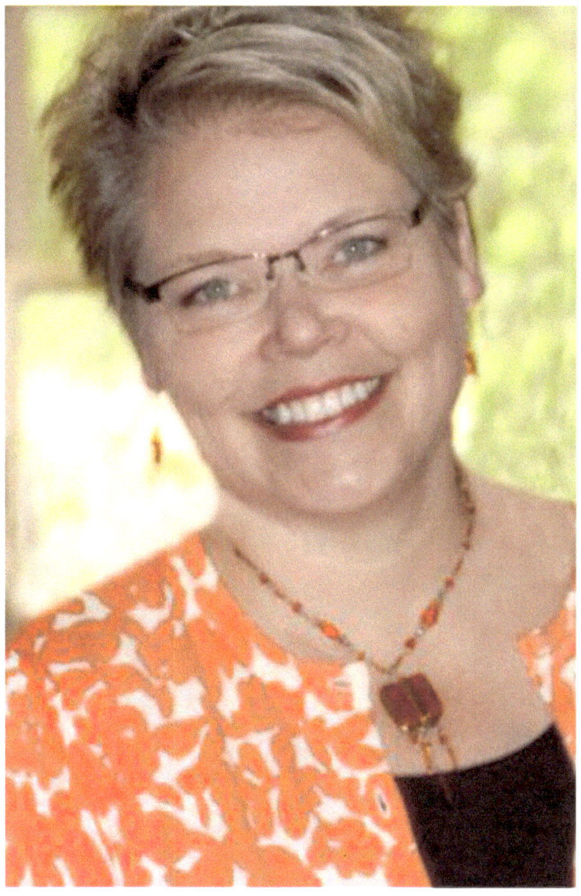

Stupendous!... It's like my spell check was broken before.

Bethany Shackelford is a highly gifted, 50-year-old artist and designer. Within several weeks of treatment, her improvement was "stupendous." Her organization, memory, and auditory processing dramatically improved—the latter resulting in handling phone messages more rapidly, without avoidance. Spelling suddenly became much easier. Now she's reading books instead of just magazines. Her headaches are gone as is motion sickness. She's no longer as fatigued and is more upbeat. Even better, improvements still continue to evolve months after therapy began. Best of all, her son Teaghan has also dramatically improved.

Teaghan S.

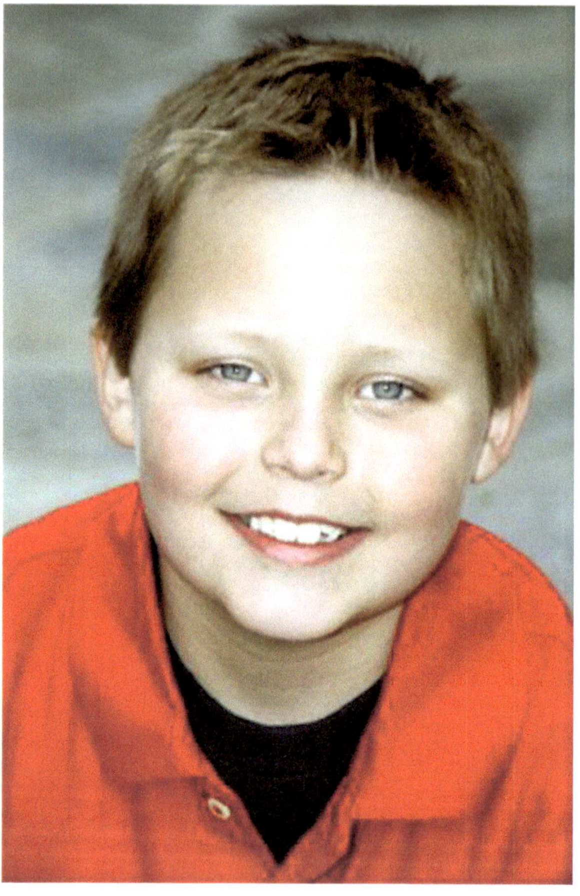

Teaghan, 9 years old, was recently examined and treated for dyslexia. Although brilliant, he was behind in several key areas. His needed improvement was both rapid and dramatic. Teaghan's handwriting samples before and after treatment reflect a wide range of other amazing changes.

Teghan's Handwriting Before Treatment.

Teaghan's Handwriting Shows a Dramatic Improvement Just One Month After Treatment Began

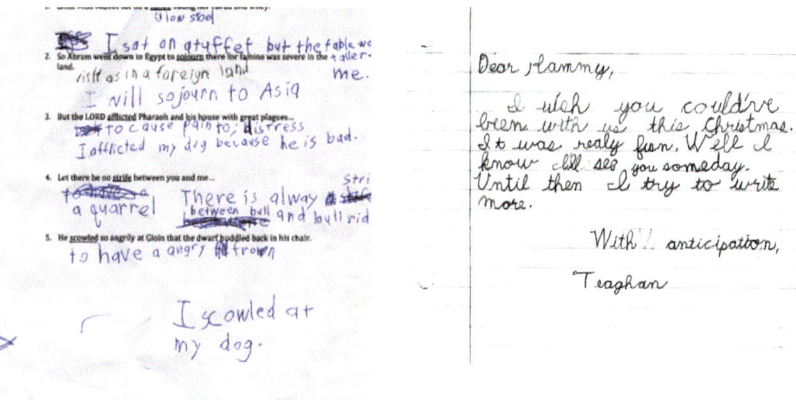

slow stod

I sat on a tuffet but the table was taller than me.

2. So Abram went down to Egypt to sojourn there for famine was severe in the land.

visit as in a foreign land

I will sojourn to Asia

3. But the LORD afflicted Pharaoh and his house with great plagues...

to cause pain to; distress

I afflicted my dog because he is bad.

4. Let there be no strife between you and me...

a quarrel

There is alway strife between bull and bull rid

5. He scowled so angrily at Gloin that the dwarf huddled back in his chair.

to have a angry frown

I scowled at my dog.

Dear Sammy,

I wish you could've been with us this Christmas. It was realy fun. Well I know I'll see you someday. Until then I try to write more.

With anticipation,

Teaghan

Robert White

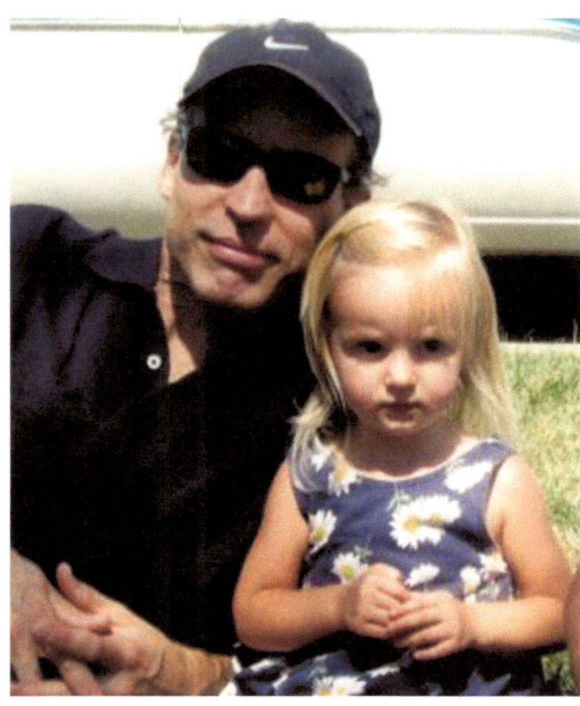

Dr. Levinson's diagnosis and treatment has completely transformed my life. This is no exaggeration on my part. After thirty-plus years of being aware that something was not quite right in my life and after twenty years of searching for the answer in books and in the offices of various medical professionals with no relief and often a worsening of my reality and the realities of my loved ones, I emerge, phoenix-like, from the ashes of some very real suffering.

After one month of treatment I experienced a complete cessation of my CV dysfunction symptoms. Bless you, Dr. Levinson. I can't thank you enough.

—Robert White

Nicole Barbee

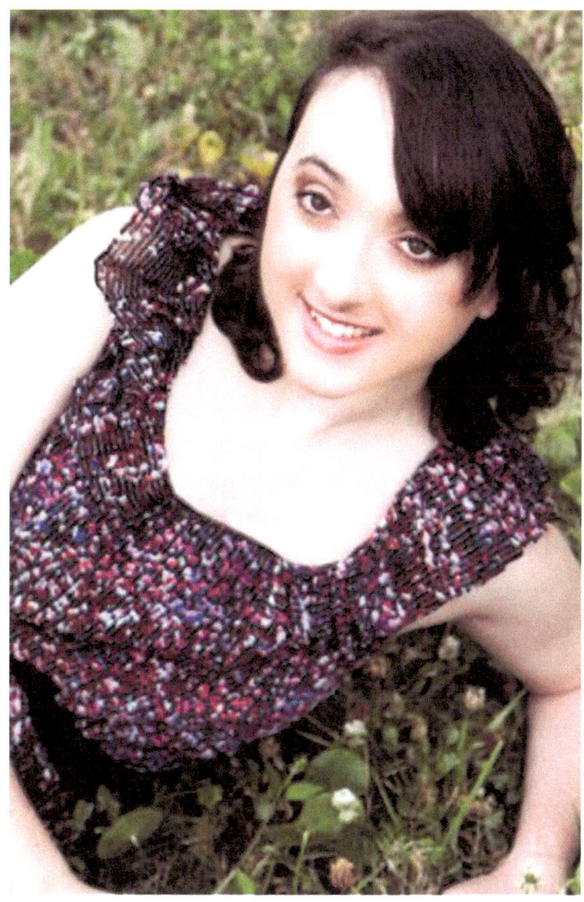

Shortly after treatment began, there resulted significant improvements in fifteen-year-old Nicole whose pre-existing symptoms had intensified after acquiring mononucleosis at thirteen. Her reading, writing, math, memory, speech and auditory processing, direction, concentration, balance, anxiety... all responded favorably to inner-ear enhancing medications.

—Anita Barbee

Luke Schubert-Brown

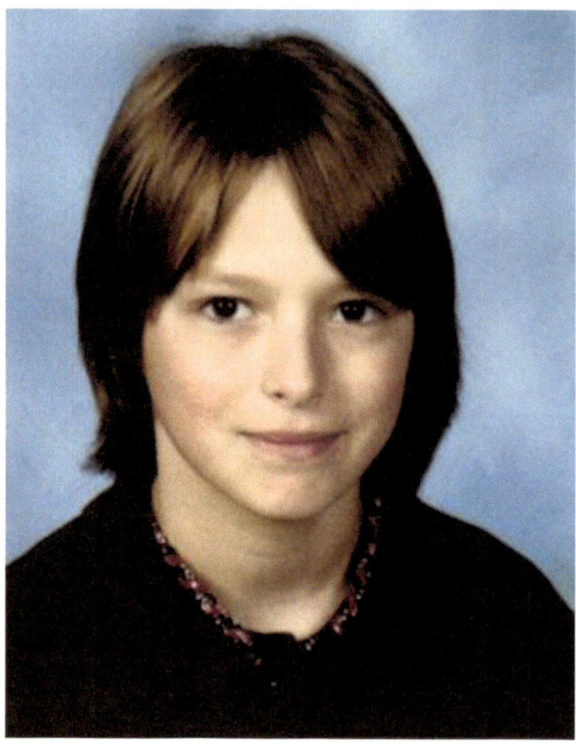

Luke is a very bright, determined-but-frustrated 10-year-old dyslexic. According to his mother:

> *Almost instantly...he stopped tripping...dozing out and began telling us what happened each day. It's like he suddenly showed up for his life.*

Rachel Snead

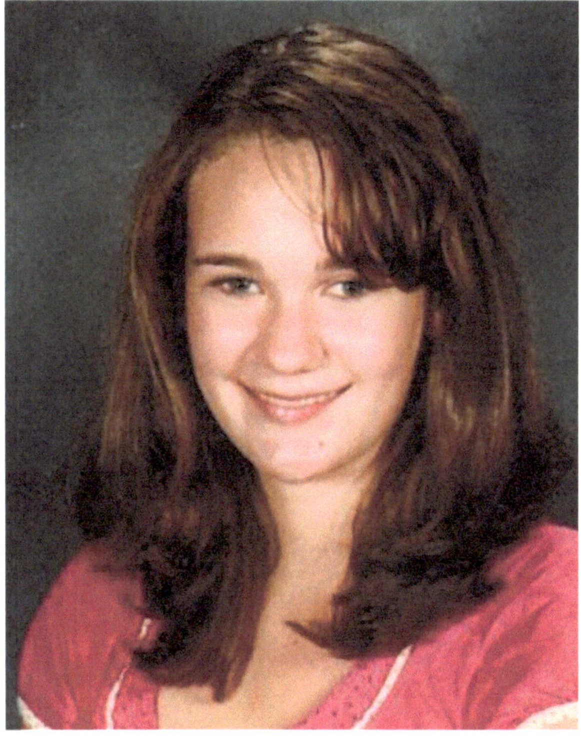

Rachel was 12 when she initially sought help. Her response to inner-ear-enhancing medications was rapid and dramatic—soon she was obtaining A's and A+'s in all her subjects. She has just received a scholarship to American University, studying International Relations.

Andrea C.

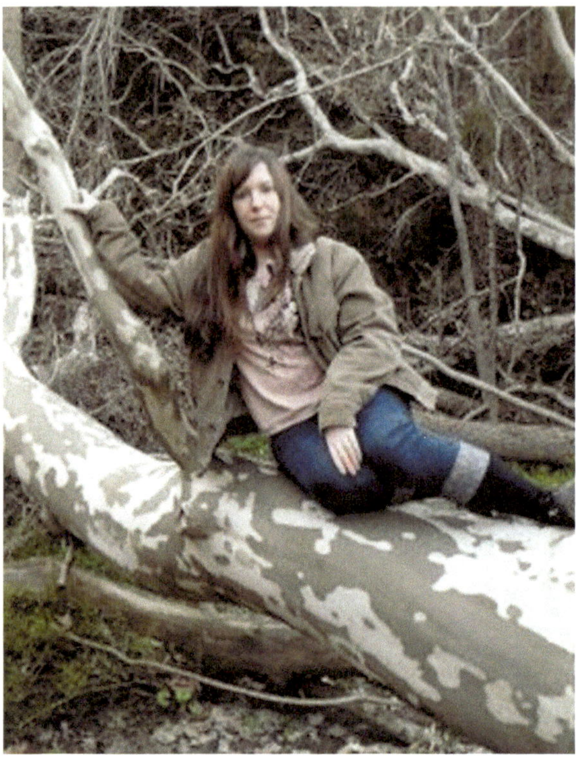

Since starting on inner-ear-enhancing medication, 37-year-old Andrea's panic attacks have disappeared during the day and while sleeping. Her overall anxiety and agoraphobia are now minimal. Her vertigo is gone. And Andrea completed reading her first book ever (500 pages), with greater speed and recall than in her past reading attempts.

Cal Martin

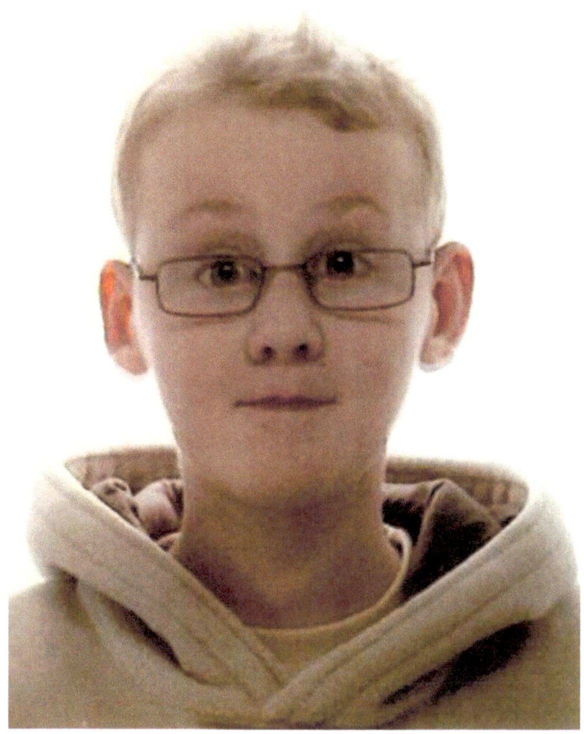

Cal was diagnosed with dyslexia/ADD when he was 11 years old. His eye tracking, clarity, and reading responded very well to medication, as did math, concentration, and mental focus. His muscle tone, balance/coordination, and sports improved, too, while accident proneness sharply decreased. His anxiety and emotional reactivity normalized.

Ethan S.

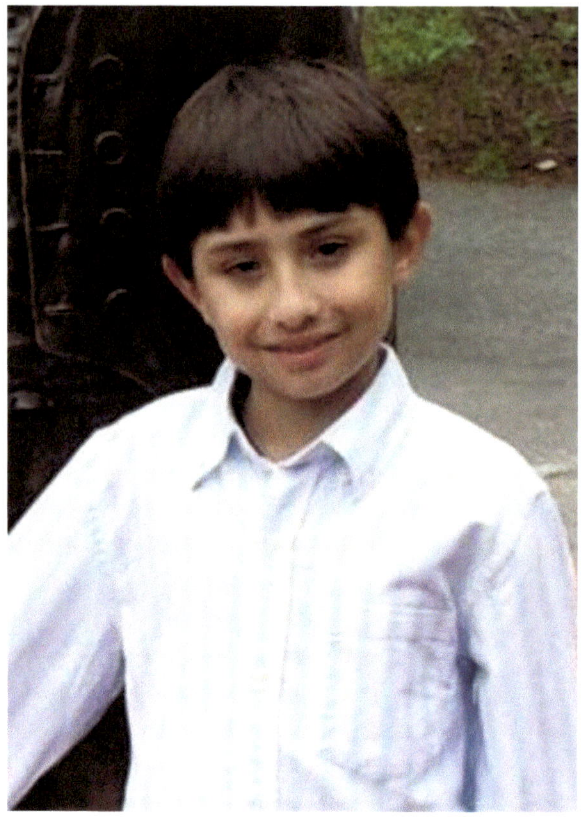

One week after starting the first antihistamine, Ethan picked up a Dr. Seuss book and read it by himself. We were absolutely astonished. Previously, he couldn't read a sentence and refused help. He also suddenly became more outgoing socially—wanting to be funny and make others laugh. His eye contact dramatically improved and his prior tics lessened and then completely disappeared. Also, his memory noticeably improved.

—Ethan's Mom

Carolyn Bernache

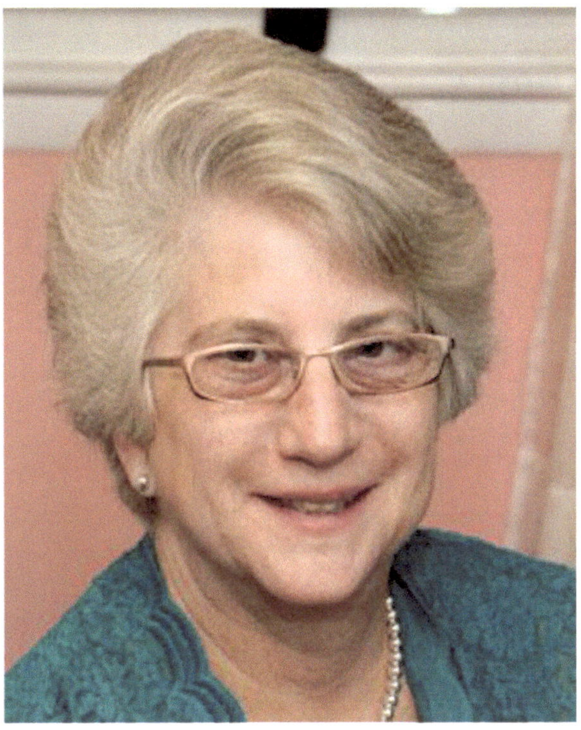

It's been a year and a half since I first saw you for severe panic attacks. Your treatment improved my inner ear, lessened my driving anxiety, and gave me the insight needed to drive. Knowing I wasn't crazy or wouldn't suddenly lose control was enormously helpful. But I still had to overcome my prior anticipation that my old panic would suddenly and terribly reoccur. It took me all this time of continually trying, testing, and succeeding to finally drive through my ever widening "safety bubble."

Thanks, Dr. Levinson, for Phobia Free *and freeing me of my driving phobia and panic.*

P.S. A quarter or third of an antihistamine leaves me more nervous than I want to be. Feels like my insides are on over-drive. It's back to half a pill for the time being. Thanks again, again, and again.

—Carolyn Bernache

Nicholas Aronne

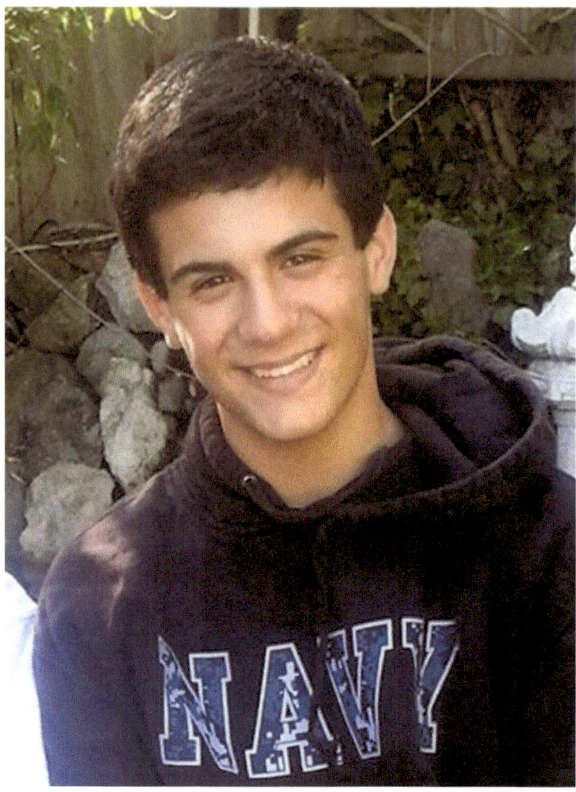

Nicholas was 10 years old when initially diagnosed and successfully treated for dyslexia and associated ADHD and phobias/anxiety. After a recent bout of obsessive overconcern was rapidly overcome with the nutrient GABA, his mother Lana offered the following to help others:

> *After Dr. Levinson's initial diagnosis of dyslexia/ADHD, a regimen of both medications and symptom-specific vitamins was started. There was a significant and rapid improvement in Nick's reading and writing skills as well as in balance/coordination. His fears and anxieties also lessened.*
>
> *He began seeing reading content in 3-D and was no longer afraid of the dark.*

Kevin Collins

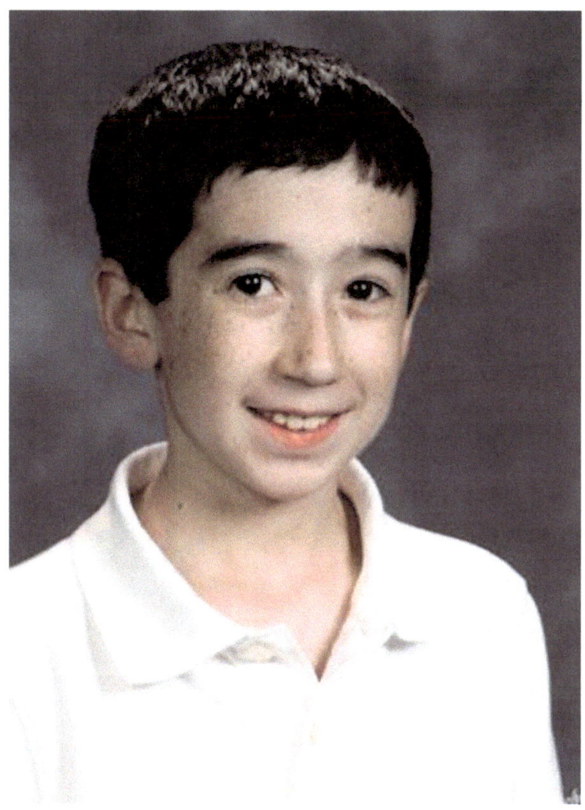

Kevin was in fifth grade when we first consulted Dr. Levinson. His response to Dr. Levinson's treatment plan was very quick. Within two weeks we saw an improvement in his reading and communication. He no longer suffers from severe eyestrain following homework nor the feeling that his eyes "locked" and he'd have to "shake them loose." Within two months, he was reading at grade level for the first time since first grade. His reading speed increased due to better tracking, faster processing and enhanced memory. For the first time ever, he wrote a fiction story and typed it into his computer. In fact, he now claims writing to be his favorite subject. Although his concentration was always good, it's now even better and lasts longer. He's less frustrated and no longer gets meltdowns by suppertime.

Eric R.

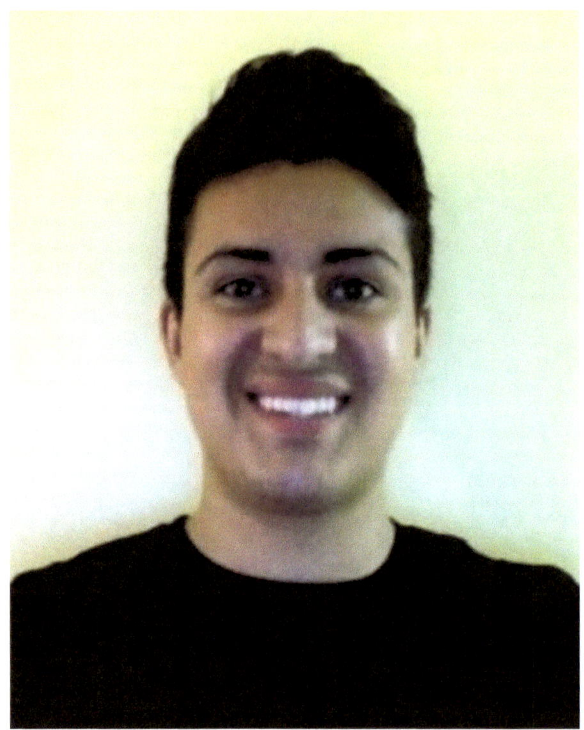

Written exactly one year after being treated by Dr. Levinson:

> *I first visited Dr. Levinson in August after struggling with symptoms of brain fog, panic attacks, lightheadedness. and dizziness. Within a few weeks of simple medications, I had noticed a dramatic shift in my symptoms. My panic attacks had lessened to almost none. My brain fog, lightheadedness and dizziness disappeared. I was very relieved to say the least.*
>
> *Today I can say I have put these terrible symptoms behind me and am living a productive, symptom-free life. And I've been off medications for the past three months.*
>
> —Eric R.

Gabriella Welzmuller

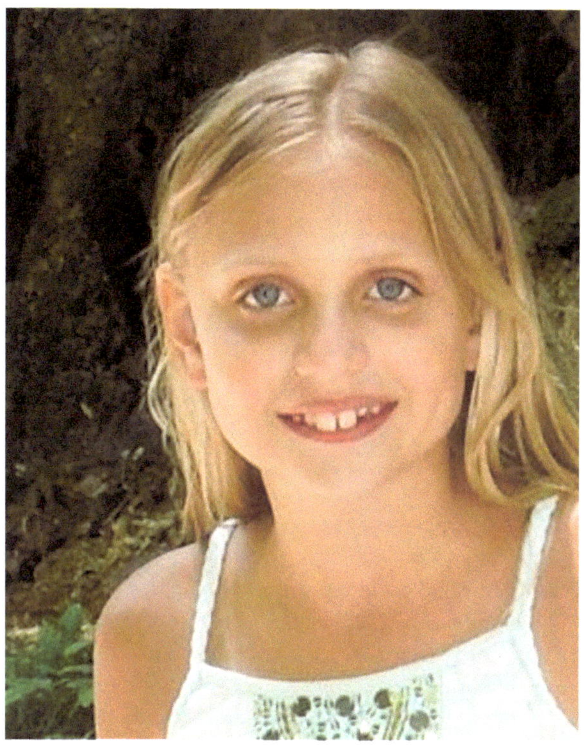

Gabriella was brought for treatment when she was 8 years old. She experienced academic difficulties, as well as symptoms of inattentiveness, overactivity, and anxiety, especially before bed. Within one month, she was described as "amazingly improved at home." She became mellow, compliant, and caring, as opposed to high strung, self-centered, and defiant. Her reading, writing, and ability to work independently advanced, and her motion sickness completely disappeared. Her energy level remained robust, albeit controlled. Most importantly, Gabriella felt and acted normal. During our last consultation, when I asked how things were, her mom said it all in one word: "GREAT!"

Gary Howell

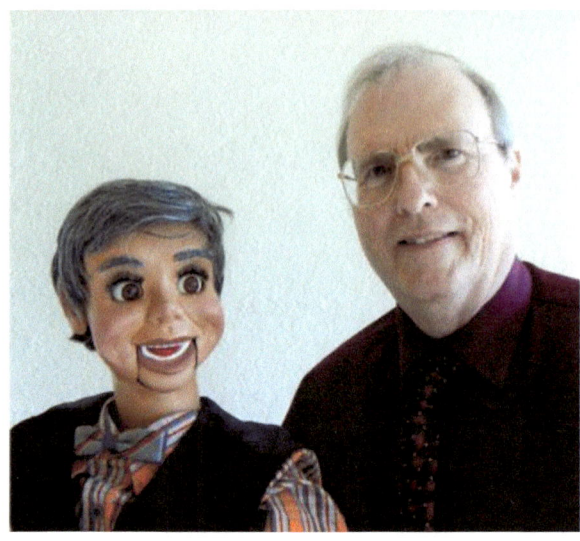

Gary's dyslexia manifested in many different symptoms, but *speech impairment* was the most bothersome of all. Fortunately, both his dyscoordinated motor mechanisms and his processing mechanisms of speech sounds rapidly improved on inner-ear-enhancing medications.

After a ventriloquist performance, a woman praising my show said, "It's amazing; your dummy talks better than you."The difference was that my dummy didn't have a dyslexic speech impairment when he learned to speak, and so, he doesn't have to unlearn poorly coordinated articulation mechanisms.

After only a few days on Dr. Levinson's treatment, I quickly saw the improved changes in my ability to use my tongue, jaw and lips when speaking. A few weeks later, I started to hear sounds used in the English language that I had never heard before.

Because of my improvements, I was encouraged to become a ventriloquist. Imagine that — probably belongs in "Believe It or Not." This would have been completely impossible before I visited Dr. Levinson.

By listening to prior tapes and comparing them to those I've recently recorded, I can really hear the progress I've made. And by concentrating on how I project my voice onto my dummy, the dummy is helping recondition me to speak better and better.

Occasionally I think back or reread my journal about all the obsessive, compulsive, phobic, anxious symptoms I had prior to visiting you. I am thankful for all the improvements your treatment provided me. Today, it's hard to imagine I was that way. It's a very different world for me now. I marvel at my new skills in speaking, hearing, memory, and many other areas.

Thanks again.

—Gary Ray Howell (https://youtu.be/E4L_AIKrXno)

Chapter 25
Closure: The End Is Just a New Beginning

All too often in science—as in life—you don't fully know what you're looking for or missing until after you've found it. As you've read in this book, all of my patients—collectively and surprisingly—provided me with every one of the vital insights needed to solve the many riddles of dyslexia and its syndrome of related disorders, including the discovery of a "lifesaving" treatment. Without their help, I'd still be orbiting the planet *Alexia*, mistakenly believing it was *Dyslexia*—lost in space along with most other researchers. And even worse, I wouldn't even have known I was lost, since I didn't clearly know beforehand what I was looking for, until finding and thoroughly exploring planet *Dyslexia—guided there by thousands of dyslexic patients.*

In a similar way, only after I belatedly received Marylyn O'Hora's correspondence (below)— remarkably expressing her amazing determination as well as her newfound confidence and optimism—did I realize that this book could not have properly ended without her: *that she symbolized the needed closure.*

The heartfelt and inspiring words within her thank-you note, sent to me after she sailed far above and beyond her dyslexic impairment, made all of my lifelong research—and the painstaking efforts required to achieve and present this book's insights—totally and satisfyingly worthwhile.

My closing hope is that Marylyn and my many other successfully treated patients will inspire *a new beginning* for all dyslexics and their dedicated loved ones and healers. She writes:

> *Dear Dr. Levinson,*
>
> *In high school I was told that my symptoms were in my head, and that I was just lazy—not dyslexic as my mother thought. So, I gave up. Why should I work hard to achieve nothing? And after failing out at SUNY Oswego, I went to our local community college. And in English 101, I researched dyslexia—to find out if I was dyslexic or just lazy. After skimming the case histories in your books, I couldn't believe it. Their personal accounts were mine. And I came to realize that I had been right all along, and the system was wrong! After failing out of two colleges in two years, I told my mom that I needed to see you that summer. AND WE DID!*

H. N. Levinson, *Feeling Smarter and Smarter*,
https://doi.org/10.1007/978-3-030-16208-5_25

Since treatment began, I have made tremendous progress. Despite a prior GPA of 1.15, my fall semester was the best ever. I was taking 13 credit hours and got four A's and one B+. I was ecstatic. It was a lot of hard work, but I did it!!! It can't get better than that, right? BUT IT DID!

The spring semester was a lot harder. Despite very difficult classes, I hung in and got a 4.0!!! ALL A's!!! THANK YOU! Now my GPA is at 3.375. I am cum *laude. Hopefully by next year I'll be summa* cum *laude.*

This year I started tutoring others and love it. I am really making a difference in someone else's life, like you made in mine. There is only one problem: Now I can do anything!

Thanks again,
Marylyn O'Hora

Real Closure and Expectations

Marylyn's astonishing improvements, as well as those of so many of my other patients, occurred despite using almost century-old meds. Just imagine the incredible benefits that would be possible were new-generation, high-potency medications designed and developed specifically for those suffering from the dyslexia or inner-ear/CVS syndrome.

I can readily anticipate "lifesaving" improvements such as Marylyn's—even cures—for all dyslexics, including those with related CVS-determined ADD/ADHD, phobias, etc. I can imagine vastly improved help for many with ASD and other major processing brain disorders where CVS-triggered signal-scrambling is an overlapping but treatable impairment. I can even envision a time in the very near future when the early screening and pre-treatment of the CVS impairment in potential "dyslexics" will totally prevent symptoms from ever surfacing. We are almost there now. Only then will there be a true closure for my research and a new beginning for all those with the dyslexia or CVS syndromes and all those altruistic healers and scientists dedicated to making this life-changing reality happen.

Perhaps the best way to now "end" this forever expanding research effort and book is by presenting you with a deeply humbling and God-inspired realization that is as valid today—and tomorrow—as when I clinically derived it almost four decades ago:

God is cosmic and organismic mind,
Mind is an electromagnetic computer field,
Matter is energy transformed,
Earth is a spec in the cosmos,
Man is a cell in the dust,
Science is an electron in search of its orbit,
Theory is one of many orbits,
Fact is fiction in perspective,
The end is just a new beginning…

So, the best is yet to come!

Appendices

Appendix 1: The Anatomical and Functional Relationship Between the Inner-Ear, Cerebellum, and Cerebral Cortex: A Brief Sketch

As you by now know, an understanding of the inner-ear and cerebellum, as well as of the thinking brain or cerebral cortex, is crucial to explaining dyslexia and its many and diverse symptoms. So, you may be wondering why I placed this summarized explanation within the Appendix, rather than right up front where it traditionally and “logically” belongs?

It’s because I believe that the patient-based clinical insights needed to properly understand the dyslexia syndrome and its treatments were so important and complex that they needed priority time alone, especially as they may go counter to all you may have previously learned. Thus, in the opening pages, I merely presented a general “treasure map” of the named gross brain structures I repeatedly mention throughout this book. This up-front visual is initially required to better guide you to the hidden golden solution to the dyslexia riddle—without adding distracting and overloading neuroanatomical details.

Don’t get me wrong. The detailed neuroanatomy is important. But it is best understood now—after you have learned the origins of dyslexia and its complex syndrome. In fact, were it not for my research, the opening map would have shown you only the cerebral cortex or thinking brain. And even after understanding all its detailed neuroanatomy, this map would only have led you to dead ends—as it did all others.

Perhaps being somewhat oppositional and mathematical by nature, I always choose to grasp concepts first, if possible, and then fill in and/or correct prior insights and details.

So, I simplified the neuroanatomical explanations and placed them at the end—within this Appendix for easy access whenever needed. No doubt, this read will now be easier and more comprehensible and thus provide added depth and foundation—and perhaps even excitement.

H. N. Levinson, *Feeling Smarter and Smarter*,
https://doi.org/10.1007/978-3-030-16208-5

Hopefully the following neurophysiological foundations and facts will make more sense now than had you studied them beforehand—as merely an isolated dry neuroanatomy lesson before knowing just how vital they were in solving the dyslexia riddles.

The Inner-Ear and Its Vestibular System

Having been trained psychiatrically and somewhat neurologically, most of my understanding of the inner-ear was of a simple clinical nature. This understanding increased substantially after I recognized that the inner-ear appeared to play a vital role in both explaining and causing the eye-tracking, spatial, and orientation mechanisms responsible for the reading, writing, concentration, balance, and related symptoms and signs that characterized my dyslexic patients.

The Inner-Ear

As the drawing illustrates, the inner-ear is a maze of tubes and passages resembling a labyrinth. Within it can be found the cochlea and vestibular systems.

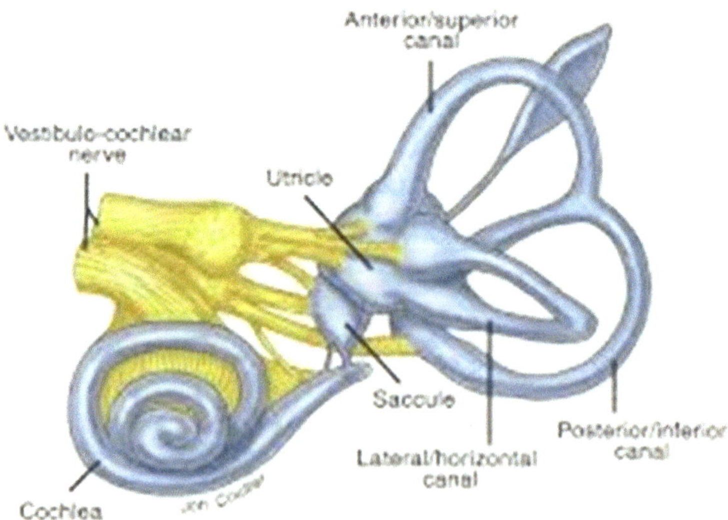

The Cochlea (the part that resembles a snail shell)

In the cochlea, sound waves from the outer and middle ears are transformed into electrical impulses. They are then sent on to the brain via the auditory nerve so they can be translated into recognizable sounds.

The Vestibular System

The vestibular part of the inner-ear registers the head's and body's movements in space so that we can maintain our balance. It consists of three ring-shaped passages—called the semicircular canals—filled with fluid. They are directed in three different spatial planes so as to triangulate all our movements of the head and body. Hair fibers within these canals react to the movement of the fluid and send impulses to the "brain" (the cerebellum and cerebral cortex, etc.) for decoding. (Sometimes little calcium crystals referred to as "otoliths" or "canaliths" form within the semicircular canals and create dizziness which may intensify dyslexic symptoms. These may be easily removed by a simple positional method called the Epley maneuver.)

The vestibular system also works with the eyes and visual system, as well as joint and muscle receptors, especially within the neck—thus, enabling normal orientation and balance.

Vestibular Symptoms

As might be expected, the greatest insights into all the intricate inner-ear functions are obtained by recognizing and analyzing their symptoms and mechanisms—when normal functions fail.

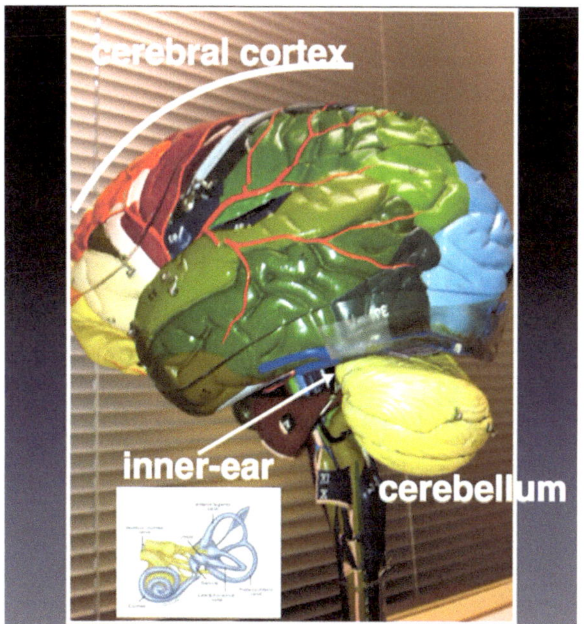

The Cerebellum

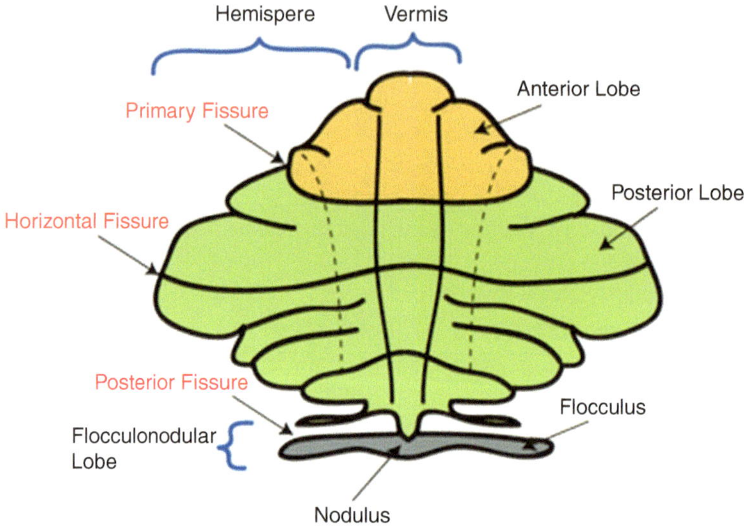

Traditionalist Cerebellar Views

Until recently, the cerebellum had been viewed as a brain structure primarily involved in planning and executing movement. Clinically, its pathology was recognized by detecting impaired motor functions involving balance, coordination, and rhythm. Nobel Laureate Sir John Eccles had also shown this highly complex organ to be capable of highly skilled motor learning as well as regulating brain signals—primarily by inhibiting them at receptor sites so as to properly modulate them and so also avoid overloading.

Also, the cerebellum was known to regulate motion and proprioception—the latter telling us where our muscles, tendons, and body parts are located in space and time. Lord Sherrington (1906), in fact, called the cerebellum the head ganglion of the proprioceptive system. In order for the brain to properly execute motor functions, it is crucial to know exactly where all body parts are. This function is termed *proprioception*.

My Clinically Derived Cerebellar Views

Having no direct anatomic or research experience with the cerebellum, most of my initial insights about this brain structure were obtained by reading the work of well-respected traditionalists in the field. That was how I first proposed that dyslexia was due to an inner-ear/cerebellar-vestibular motor dysfunction—based on the fact that only balance, coordination, and rhythmic diagnostic signs were found in my dyslexic patients and those of other clinicians.

Because my training was primarily clinically vs. neuroanatomically based, I merely followed the dyslexia facts wherever they led—rather than being biased by prior traditionalist neurophysiological *dyslexia* = *alexia* beliefs and neuroanatomical details. In Huxley's words, I followed the clinical facts wherever they led. And so, I solved all the prior dyslexia-related riddles, including a new and entirely unexpected one—*higher cerebellar (cerebral-like) functioning*.

Contrary to most dyslexia experts who apply known neuroanatomical and neurophysiological facts to better explain traditionalist theories—leading them nowhere new, I pursued the clinical dyslexic facts and so discovered/validated their hidden CVS-determining neurophysiology and corresponding anatomy.

Clinically based reasoning Although I discussed this content earlier in the book within Chapters 9 and 10, and especially Chap. 11, I would like to review and expand upon the topic a bit here because of its incredible importance. Simply put:

1. If only inner-ear and cerebellar neurological dysfunction are found in dyslexics, then it was reasonable to assume that all the dyslexic symptoms favorably responding to inner-ear- and cerebellar-enhancing medications might be of cerebellar/inner-ear origin, unless proven otherwise. Accordingly, by discounting some of the more obvious spatial and orientation symptoms clearly traceable to the inner-ear, as well as some of their related balance, steering, and motor signs, it seemed reasonable to suspect that the majority of the remaining *sensory* and *higher* functions described in the Self-Diagnostic Test in Chap. 7 were probably of a primary cerebellar origin. Some of these higher functions involved memory; concentration; speech and communication; clarity and sequenced thought; learning (reading, writing, spelling, math, grammar, etc.); emotions; sense and perception of time, direction, and space; and "socialization." Equally as important, it became obvious that the cerebellum must play a vital role in modulating all sensory *input* brain signals, just as it was previously known to play in modulating the total motor *output*.

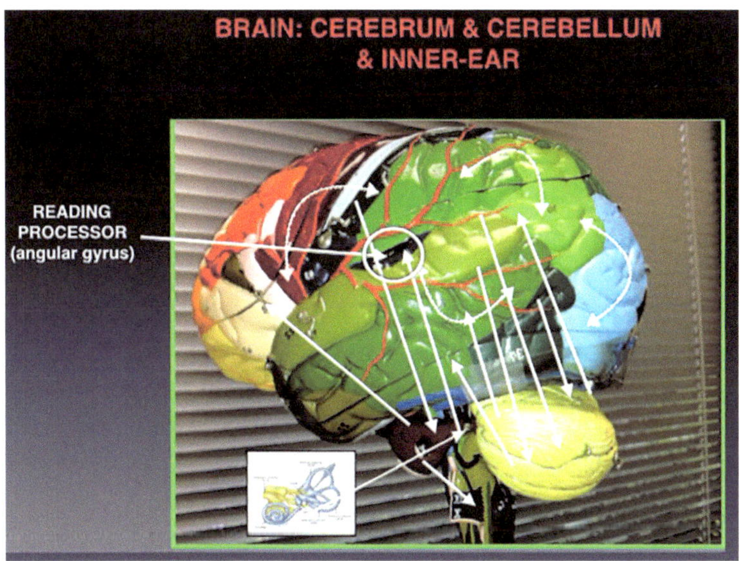

2. My clinically derived concepts of *higher* and *total sensory* cerebellar processing functions were consistent with observations that many animal species possessing only a primitive cerebellum are capable of various degrees of the above higher functions. And some have exceptional degrees of sensory processing.

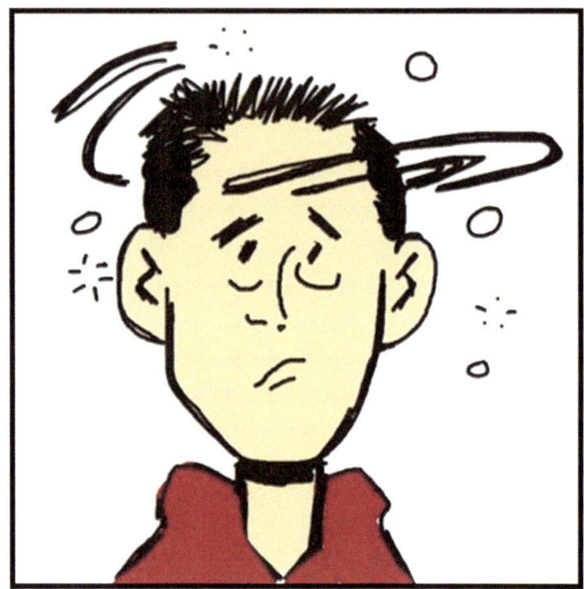

3. In addition, spinning non-dyslexic humans around till dizziness occurs often triggers all the dyslexic symptoms listed in the Self-Diagnostic Test. And pre-treatment with inner-ear-/cerebellar-enhancing meds prevents these dyslexic symptoms from arising or minimizes them—likely validating these new and challenging cerebellar concepts.

Finding a concept to fit the facts Although my above clinically derived observations and reasoning were as simple and logical as my dyslexic concepts, I had to further expand my cerebellar concepts to completely account for the hundreds of dyslexic symptoms that characterized this complex syndrome:

1. By recognizing that spinning and dizziness could transiently create the entire dyslexic syndrome, I reasoned that the brain's signals must become "dizzy" or scrambled in dyslexics.
2. I then expanded Nobel Laureate Eccles' concept of cerebellar signal inhibition and thus, modulation. I reasoned that the cerebellum modulates *all* input and output brain signals, not just the ones at receptor sites that prevent overloading. Thus, I hypothesized that one fine-tuning cerebellar impairment can radiate hundreds of scrambled signals to multiple normal processing structures in the brain

and so may *secondarily* trigger scores of corresponding symptoms and their determining mechanisms.

3. To explain, for example, why the CVS-enhancing stimulants worked better for those with ADHD whereas the CVS antihistamines were more effective for the more typical academic symptoms, I reasoned it was likely that distinct cerebellar substructures communicated with different brain areas for the varied impairments characterizing the dyslexia syndrome. Interestingly, this idea was confirmed by neuroimaging studies, such as the one by C. Stoodley in 2014, indicating how specific cerebellar areas contribute to dyslexia, ADHD, and autism.

Summary

My dramatically expanded views of cerebellar functioning were derived from the clinical study of many thousands of dyslexic patients and their amazing favorable responses to inner-ear-/cerebellar-enhancing meds, not from prior theory. Thus, it was no surprise that these new and unique concepts proved fully capable of encompassing and explaining all the many and varied symptoms comprising the dyslexic syndrome. However, these “highly original” (as one reviewer called them) cerebellar and dyslexia concepts challenged the traditionalists’ concepts, and so, resistance to these ideas reigned supreme for several decades. And it still does to a large extent, despite the vast number of neuroimaging publications supporting my contentions. As just presented, a growing number of fMRI and related studies now report cerebellar involvement in dyslexia, ADD/ADHD, anxiety, and some depressive disorders—and even autism.

Unfortunately, these new-age neuroimaging scientists appear stuck with a scientific conflict they seem unable to recognize and resolve: They believe that dyslexia is a reading disorder of primary cerebral origin—and yet they often obtain both cerebellar and cerebral findings. Perhaps this book’s insights will help resolve their conflict and better enable them to explore new and unique solutions.

Initially Validating My Hypothesis of Higher Cerebellar Functioning

My search of the neurophysiological literature revealed studies in the 1940s by Johns Hopkins cerebellar researchers Ray Snider and A. Stowell, and others, that supported my ideas. They demonstrated sensory as well as motor feedback circuits from the cerebellum of animals to the cerebral cortex. These findings were magnificently portrayed by Snider in a 1958 Scientific American article entitled, “The Cerebellum.” However, there was a problem. In a personal conversation with Sir John Eccles many years ago, he claimed the above authors’ results could not be replicated. But I knew from my clinical data that the findings of Snider and Stowell were correct—even if they couldn’t be replicated by others, Sir John Eccles included.

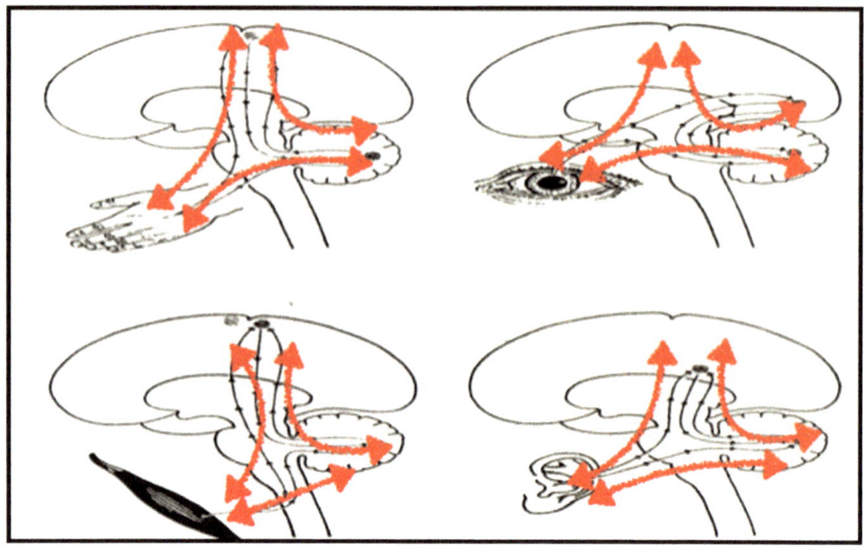

Ray Snider: Signal projections from the sensory organs to the cerebellum and cerebral cortex, and back (Scientific American 1958)

Later Validation

Fortunately, all of my clinically derived cerebellar deductions were later independently validated by such outstanding neuroscientists as Leiner, Leiner, and Dow. In their groundbreaking paper entitled, "Does the cerebellum contribute to mental skills?" (*Behavioral Neuroscience*. August, 1986), these authors claim:

> "The phylogenetically newest structures of the cerebellum may contribute to mental skills in much the same way that the... older structures contribute to motor skills. Signals from the older part of the dentate nucleus certainly help the frontal cortex to effect the skilled manipulation of muscles, and the newest part... may help the frontal association cortex to effect the skilled manipulation of information or ideas. The validity of this new concept can be tested on humans by means of tomographic brain scans."

And in a 1991 Behavioral Brain Research publication, they state:

> "The role of the cerebellum in these (cognitive and language) human functions has tended to be obscured by the traditional preoccupation with the motor functions of the cerebellum which have been widely observed in other vertebrates as well... Anatomical evidence and behavioral evidence combine to suggest that this enlarged cerebellum (in the human brain) contributes not only to motor function but also to some sensory, cognitive, linguistic, and emotional aspects of behavior."

Validating cerebellar cognitive functioning I also came across a piece in the scientific journal, *Neuron* (Volume 80, Issue 3), called, "The Cerebellum and Cognitive Function: 25 Years of Insight from Anatomy and Neuroimaging," in which Randy Buckner summarized the important fMRI and related neurophysiological research over the previous 25 years that proves the existence of higher cerebellar functions in man. This independent validation of my clinically derived higher cerebellar concepts, which I initially recognized and reported in the 1970s, also tends to indirectly confirm the validity of my dyslexia research. Were my dyslexia concepts incorrect, there is no way I would have accurately derived these groundbreaking neurophysiological concepts about higher cerebellar functioning more than two decades before others—including Eccles.

Dual cerebellar functions Only recently did I postulate, for simplicity sake, that the cerebellum has dual or split functioning. The older cerebellum appears more involved with the inner-ear and so, when impaired, may contribute to signal scrambling and related motor functioning. The higher cerebellum is significantly involved with cerebral functions via feedback loops and involved with cognition, memory, learning, communication, concentration, and compensatory descrambling. However, from a realistic point of anatomic view, there are many more cerebellar subdivisions and splits.

Abundant MRI Validation

A wide range of fMRI and other studies began verifying the role of the cerebellum in dyslexia. The 1989 study by Rae and colleagues in the journal, *The Lancet*, is typical of many others except for one important oversight: In recognizing the role of the cerebellum in dyslexia, Rae directly quoted evidence of balance and coordination dysfunction in dyslexia from one of my research papers to support her findings. And she noted the improvements in reading when using my concept of "cerebellar-vestibular stabilizers":

> "*Dyslexic people are often uncoordinated with poor balance and delayed motor milestones such as crawling, walking, and learning to ride a bike. Antimotion-sickness medications which may be considered 'cerebellar-vestibular stabilizers,' have been shown to improve reading performance in dyslexia. The present study has shown significant metabolic abnormalities in the cerebellum in dyslexia.*"

Four Bias Errors: Freudian vs. Random

*S*o, the study validated my findings. But due to the first dyslexic or Freudian error, Rae mistakenly credited her colleague, although quoting me. And because of a second Freudian error, she refused to correct it when asked to do so! Although the first error may have been purely neurophysiological in origin, the second one had a psychological component and so was definitely of Freudian origin.

There was a third error that was/is typically made by most all traditionalist researchers—the "triple-blind" one—mistakenly identifying dyslexia with only its reading impairment. And a fourth one too—*The Lancet*—refused to correct this error despite recognizing it from my documented submission.

Motivation Considering the importance of these errors, and the ease of correcting them, then why were they made? And why were they left in place? Hopefully, all readers can by now answer these questions—except for those still preferring denial.

Reinterpreting Cerebral Cortical fMRI Data

It is crucial to highlight that neuroimaging data has revealed abnormal patterns in the thinking brains of dyslexics as well as in the cerebellum. And some studies have even demonstrated these cerebral patterns in young pre-reading children—suggesting that their findings are primary rather than due to the secondary effects of reading vs. non-reading.

But in my opinion, these gifted researchers may have overlooked a crucial alternative hypothesis that only my signal-scrambling theory of dyslexia could explain. *Might cerebellar-determined signal-scrambling secondarily affect the thinking brain, thus, explaining the presence of fMRI cerebellar findings in young pre-readers?* Or stated another way, might there be a scrambled cerebellar-cerebral circuit or loop? And so, the findings were noted at the cerebral site tested, rather than the CVS site of origin.

The Thinking Brain or Cerebral Cortex

The cerebral cortex is the largest part of the human brain, associated with higher brain functions such as thought and action. It is divided into four sections or "lobes": the frontal lobe, parietal lobe, occipital lobe, and temporal lobe.

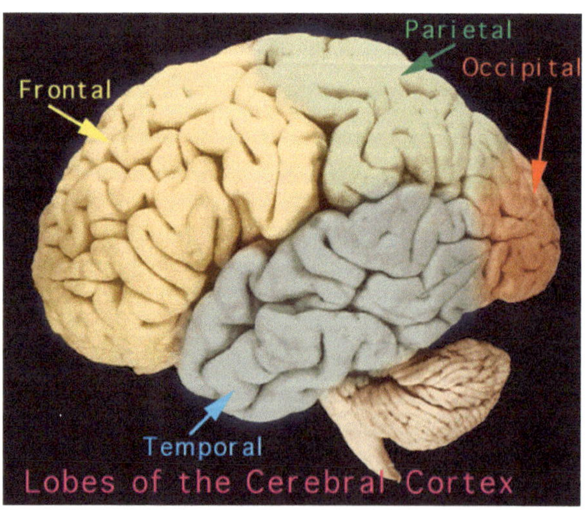

The functions of these lobes:

- *Frontal lobe*—associated with reasoning, planning, parts of speech, movement, emotions, and problem-solving
- *Parietal lobe*—associated with movement, orientation, recognition, and perception of stimuli
- *Occipital lobe*—associated with visual processing
- *Temporal lobe*—associated with perception and recognition of auditory stimuli, memory, and speech

The Importance of the Cerebral Cortex in Dyslexia and Its Syndrome

Although the thinking brain was mistakenly believed to be the primary cause of dyslexia for over a century, thousands of my dyslexic patients, and all the research summarized within this book, suggest otherwise. In fact, a normal thinking brain plays an important *compensatory* role in the dyslexia syndrome. *It creates the symptoms defining the dyslexia syndrome only when secondarily failing to descramble the "dizzy" or distorted signals received from an impaired CVS fine-tuner.*

My further research suggests that the higher cerebellum, together with the thinking and related brain structures, is also involved in this overall process—possibly via a primary decoding deficit. And as previously stated, it's possible a combined cerebellar-cerebral circuit may be involved in those with the dyslexia syndrome, including ADD/ADHD.

The thinking brain is important in the dyslexia syndrome As repeatedly noted, I've come to better appreciate the potent descrambling and compensatory role of the thinking-brain processors and those of the higher cerebellum in co-determining CVS-triggered dyslexic reading and non-reading symptom formation and outcomes. And I've repeatedly emphasized my evolving belief that a lapse or failure of cerebral/super-higher-cerebellar inhibition is likely responsible for varied dyslexic-related slips and thinking/reasoning errors—as well as subconscious thoughts and mechanisms—popping into, and even shaping, our conscious thinking and actions, as well as facilitating phobias, including the universal ones; and even OCD.

The thinking brain in general, not just its reading processor, together with the super-higher cerebellum, may likely play an *active* predisposing role in the dyslexia or CVS syndrome—especially for ADD/ADHD. And not the passive one I initially postulated way back in 1973 or even my later idea that the initially normal thinking brain may have been secondarily altered by the continually active primary CVS-signal-scrambling it receives. The latter concept evolved so as to better explain the accruing neuroimaging data indicating both cerebral and cerebellar findings.

In Summary

I believe these unfolding clarifications of the neural structures involved in the dyslexia syndrome, based on the data illuminated, will allow you to more deeply understand all dyslexics as well as their complex syndrome and underlying mechanisms. In addition, I hope you will recognize how a valid hypothesis often leads to new and exciting breakthroughs. Based on the above insights, I was able to devise new inner-ear/cerebellar-related methods of screening, diagnosis, treatment, and prevention.

And finally, via a clinical analysis of patients suffering from the dyslexic syndrome, I was able to hypothesize and correctly predict the presence of a vast array of sensory and higher cerebellar functions more than 20 years before anyone else. And I did so without the benefit of specialized neurophysiological expertise and complex neuroimaging and other techniques. In other words, the simple anecdotal technique of listening to dyslexics describe their symptoms while observing their performance errors as well as their favorable responses to CVS-enhancing medications proved as valuable, if not more so, than the most sophisticated neurophysiological investigative techniques currently known to man.

Moreover, my technique was better able to capture holistic portraits of both the cerebellum and the dyslexia syndrome. By comparison, the fMRI-related neuroimaging techniques captured only microscopic—albeit vital—bytes of the complex holograms under investigation. And these insights led to upgrades in my theory so that they may better encompass and explain dyslexia data. Years ago, I actually advised integrating both our techniques so that neuroimaging might more accurately pinpoint and explore involved areas/circuits within the inner-ear/cerebellum as well as in the interacting cerebral brain.

Appendix 2: Classification of Smart Chemicals in Dyslexia and Related ADD and Phobic Disorders (Many Meds and Nutrients Can Be Combined for Maximum Results)

I CVS-Enhancing Medications

A: **Antihistamines/Antimotion-Sickness Medications**
First Line

- Antivert—*meclizine hydrochloride*
- Dramamine—*dimenhydrinate*
- Marezine—*cyclizine hydrochloride* or *lactate*

Miscellaneous Anti-vertigo/Antimotion-Sickness/Antiemetic Medications
Second Line

- Piracetam—*nootrophil*

- Transderm-Scop—*scopolamine*
- Phenergan—*promethazine hydrochloride*

General Antihistamines
Third Line

- Older Generation—more tiredness and other side effects
- Atarax—*hydroxyzine hydrochloride*
- Benadryl—*diphenhydramine hydrochloride*
- Chlor-Trimeton—*chlorpheniramine maleate*
- Dimetapp—*brompheniramine maleate, phenylephrine hydrochloride, phenylpropanolamine hydrochloride*

Newer Generation—less tiredness and side effects
First Line

- Claritin—*loratadine*
- Allegra—*fexofenadine hydrochloride*
- Seldane—*terfenadine*
- Tavist—*clemastine fumarate*
- Zyrtec—*cetirizine hydrochloride*
- *Others*

ADHD Stimulants and Related Meds
First Line *(All short- and long-acting forms of stimulants)*

- Dexedrine/Dextrostat—*dextroamphetamine sulfate*
- Adderall—amphetamine salts
- Vyvanse—*lisdexamfetamine*
- Ritalin—*methylphenidate hydrochloride*
- Concerta—*methylphenidate hydrochloride* (extended-release)
- Metadate—*methylphenidate hydrochloride* (extended-release)

Second Line

- Desoxyn—*methamphetamine hydrochloride*
- Provigil—*modafinil—used primarily for wakefulness and narcolepsy*
- (Cylert—*pemoline—no longer manufactured. Was great long-acting stimulant*)

Third Line

- Sudafed—*pseudoephedrine hydrochloride*
- Caffeine
- Theophylline
- Ephedra

Fourth Line—*non-stimulant for ADHD. Not nearly as effective as stimulants*

- Strattera—*atomoxetine hydrochloride*
- Kapvay—*clonidine*
- Intuniv—*guanfacine*

Antidepressants/Antianxiety Medications
Second and Third Lines
A. Older Tricyclic Antianxiety and Antidepressants

- Elavil—*amitriptyline hydrochloride*
- Norpramin—*desipramine hydrochloride*
- Pamelor—*nortriptyline hydrochloride*
- Tofranil—*imipramine hydrochloride*
- Sinequan—*doxepin hydrochloride*

First Line: Mainly for Anxiety and Depression
B. Newer Selective Serotonin Reuptake Inhibitors (SSRIs)

- Prozac—*fluoxetine hydrochloride*
- Paxil—*paroxetine hydrochloride*
- Zoloft—*sertraline hydrochloride*
- (Many other SSRIs)

Serotonin Norepinephrine Reuptake Inhibitors (SNRIs)

- Effexor—*venlafaxine hydrochloride*
- Cymbalta—*duloxetine*
- (Many other SNRIs)

Other First Line—For Mild Depression and Concentration

- Wellbutrin—*bupropion hydrochloride*

C. Miscellaneous
Second Line

- Desyrel—*trazodone hydrochloride*
- Ludiomil—*maprotiline hydrochloride*
- Serzone—*nefazodone hydrochloride*
- *Others*

Antianxiety/Anti-panic Agents
First Line
Benzodiazepines

- Ativan—*lorazepam*
- Librium—*chlordiazepoxide hydrochloride*
- Serax—*oxazepam*
- Tranxene—*clorazepate dipotassium*
- Valium—*diazepam*
- Xanax—*alprazolam hydrochloride*
- *Others*

B. Beta Blockers: Useful for General Anxiety, Stage Fright, and Social Anxiety

- Inderal—*propranolol hydrochloride*
- Tenormin—*atenolol*

C. Miscellaneous Antianxiety Meds/Nutrients

- Buspar—*buspirone hydrochloride*
- GABA—a great and effective nutrient
- L-Tyrosine—a calming nutrient

II CNS Signal and Processing/Regulating Enhancers

A. Miscellaneous

- Deaner—*deanol acetaminobenzoate*
- DHA—*docosahexaenoic acid*
- DMAE—*dimethylaminoethanol bitartrate*
- Ephedra (Ma-Huang)
- Ginkgo
- Hydergine—*ergoloid mesylate*
- Lecithin
- Long-chain unsaturated fatty acids (i.e., Efalex-F)
- Mentalin—*gotu kola* and *bacopa decoction*
- Vitamins/minerals—niacin, calcium, magnesium, etc.

B. Anti-impulsive Behavior Medications/Regulators

1. Beta-blockers (i.e., Inderal and Tenormin)
2. Non-stimulant ADD/ADHD meds—helpful for impulsivity (also listed above)
   - Strattera—*Atomoxetine hydrochloride*
   - Kapvay—*Clonidine hydrochloride*
   - Intuniv—*Guanfacine*
3. *Antiseizure Rx*
   - Tegretol—*carbamazepine*
   - Depakote—*valproic acid*
   - *Many others*

Appendix 3: Helpful Vitamins and Nutrients

Since I began my research over 50 years ago, I've stumbled over a number of nutrients that have been investigated and reported by others to help some of the functions impaired in the dyslexia syndrome. Having never been trained in this area, I received my initial education from adult patients and/or parents who investigated some of these substances on their own and then reported improvements. Thus, I was educated about nutrients in the same way I was about dyslexia—from suffering patients and their loved ones desperately searching for help. And from an investigatory angle, the fatty acids have appeared most helpful.

In more recent years, the nutrient industry has exploded. And so, products were developed that often contained combinations of those ingredients most commonly reported to be helpful. So, for your convenience, I will report them here as well as those specific nutrients most likely to be helpful as indicated by reviewers. I do this not as an expert—since this is a field that requires a doctorate on its own. However, as a medical clinician rather than a trained and experienced nutritionist or unlicensed "jack-of-all-trades," it appears that these nutrients may help somewhat (from what some patients have reported prior to my treating them)—but seldom, if ever, dramatically so. Thus, I test-use them as helpful adjuncts to increase my odds of more frequent and better wins while causing no loss to patients (side effects are rare).

The nutritional substances advised by reviewers include Provasil, Neuroflexyn, Focus Power, Lipogen PS, Brain Essence, and other products. The various ingredients within these products are deemed by sources listed below (which I am unqualified to personally and objectively judge) to help such functions as memory, concentration and focus, energy, and overall neurotransmitter and brain health.

Provasil and Neuroflexyn are abstracted from two unknown and personally unverified sources noted below:

Provasil is designed to help improve memory while increasing focus and concentration. It contains the following:

- *Vitamin C* is an antioxidant that may improve memory and help combat stress, dementia, and depression.
- *Folic acid* is believed to enhance brain health and combat memory loss.
- *Vitamin B12* also promotes brain health and supports the central nervous system.
- *Phosphatidylserine* may promote memory and cognitive function.
- *L-Glutamine* is used to treat ADHD and may help with moodiness and anxiety.
- *Resveratrol* is an antioxidant that is thought to help prevent nerve damage and possible help counter Alzheimer's.
- *DHA* is a fatty acid that is believed to aid overall brain function.
- *Choline bitartrate* helps to improve concentration and alertness.
- *L-Tyrosine* improves* alertness and brain health.
- *N-Acetyl carnitine* increases acetylcholine levels in the brain and enhances* memory and recall.
- *Bacopa* benefits the brain by improving the learning ability.
- *Ginkgo* is an antioxidant and improves* the blood circulation.
- *Phosphatidylcholine* slows down the aging process of the brain.
- *Panax ginseng root* is an ancient medicine that provides* improved* brain function (abstracted from https://www.provasil.com/the-provasil-formulation.html).

Neuroflexyn is designed to help improve mental vision, memory, focus, and concentration by enhancing neurotransmitter stability in the brain. It includes phosphatidylcholine; bacopin; omega-3; GABA; Ginkgo biloba; vitamins E, B6, and B12; folate; alpha lipoic acid; and eleuthero ginseng:

- Vitamins such as B6 and 12, both of which help support the nervous system.
- Alpha lipoic acid elevates the metabolism, helping to supply the brain cells with energy needed to stay alert throughout the day.
- Vinpocetine, along with the traditional substance Ginkgo biloba, increases the blood flow to the brain, giving the cells a boost of invigorating oxygen and the body—energy.
- GABA is a caffeine-free way to provide the system with energy but without causing jitteriness, relieving stress, and making concentration easier.
- Eleuthero ginseng boosts energy and overall health (abstracted from https://www.consumerhealthdigest.com/brain-enhancement-supplements/neuroflexyn.html).

Before concluding here, I'd like to mention two additional ingredients which may boost memory, Rhodiola and huperzine, and green tea—which can increase focus and relaxation.

I have just attempted to provide readers with additional insights into the limited but helpful power of nutrients. However, I do so hesitantly since my research experience has rendered me cautious about accepting conclusions I have no in-depth experience with. Thus, I suggest that all those interested in these substances consult with an experienced nutritionist.

Appendix 4: More on the Diagnostic Process

The diagnostic process I explained in Chap. 19 as well as the response pattern to medications may often suggest the presence of coexisting but hidden non-CVS (or non-Type III) determinants of symptom formation. In other words, improvements in CVS-determined neurophysiological measures suggest there should be a corresponding improvement in symptoms. When this improvement does not occur, emotional/educational and related "blocking" factors may be inhibiting positive responses and should be investigated.

Conversely, favorable therapeutic responses can occur without corresponding improvements in the testing parameters. What does this imply? Probably, that new parameters are needed to reflect the observed changes. As I've repeatedly said, very few initial assumptions held up following more extensive investigations. And so, follow-up theoretical modifications, and even corrections, were essential for my research progress to continue. This zigzagging process is analogous to the military truism: All intricate battle plans are invariably scrapped after the first shot is fired. So, zigzagging and reinvestigation are often absolutely essential determinants for any successful scientific outcome—certainly mine.

Needless to say, the traditional CVS diagnostic tests were initially very helpful in discovering the CVS neurophysiological origins of dyslexia and related ADD/

ADHD and anxiety/mood disorders. However, what I may not have mentioned is that I utilized the data I obtained from CVS-dysfunctioning patients to better understand, re-standardize, and redesign/enhance the efficacy of these well-accepted diagnostic test methods.

In other words, most clinicians use CVS tests to prove the presence of CVS dysfunctioning—as I initially did and still do. However, once I knew that all dyslexics had CVS dysfunctioning, I was then able to utilize this insight to correctly modify and enhance the diagnostic accuracy of the CVS test parameters.

In retrospect, this "back-and-forth" analytical method eventually led to an enhanced understanding of (1) dyslexic, ADD/ADHD, and phobic patients, (2) their CVS function and dysfunction, (3) traditionally used and accepted neurophysiological and neuropsychological diagnostic tests, and (4) new testing methods helpful in highlighting the hidden underlying mechanisms crucial for understanding the highly complex dysfunctioning vs. compensatory processes at work.

Appendix 5: Diagnostic ENG Testing: Illustrations

The following illustrations attempt to specifically highlight normal and abnormal inner-ear/cerebellar responses during electronystagmography and posturography testing. Hopefully these responses will enable interested readers—especially professionals—to better understand the interpretation of these test parameters as briefly reviewed within Chap. 20, Four Steps to a Certain Medical Diagnosis.

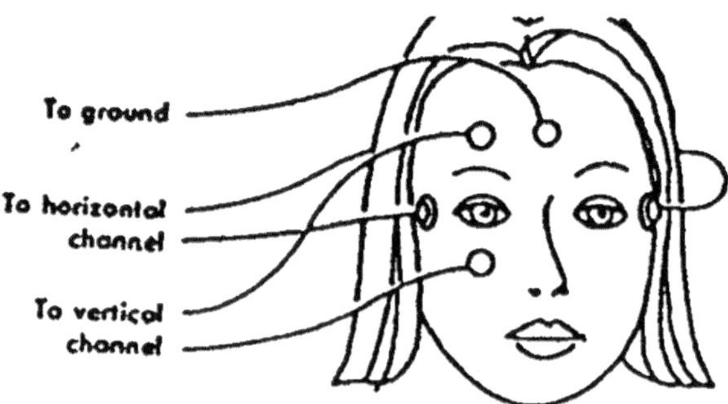

Fig. 1 Standard placement of ENG recording electrodes so as to record eye movements with eyes open and closed

Fixation and Tracking Tests

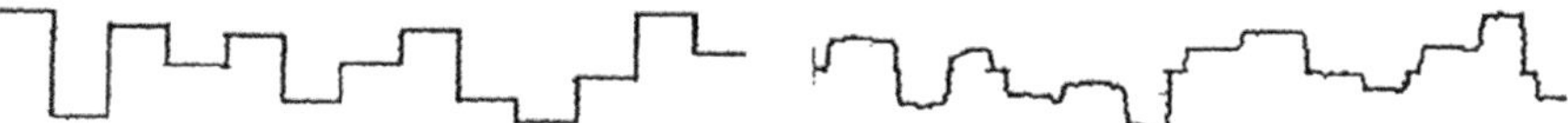

Fig. 2 The horizontal saccade test. A dot moves randomly on the screen, and the patient must "chase" it with his/her eyes. A saccade is a quick, jerky eye movement that positions a visual target on the retina. The cerebellum plays an important role in determining this tracking function (normal at left and abnormal at right)

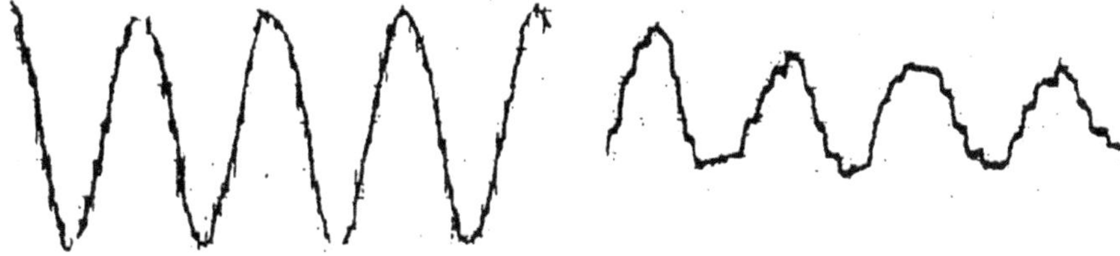

Fig. 3 The horizontal pursuit test. A dot cycles back and forth across a screen, and the eyes' ability to follow it smoothly is electronically recorded and measured (normal at left). An inner-ear or CVS dysfunction may result in the inability to produce smooth pursuit movements (abnormal at right)

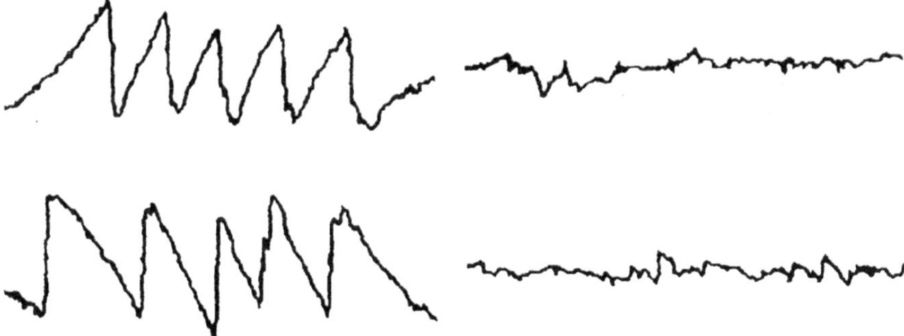

Fig. 4 Horizontal optokinetic test. A series of dots move across and then off a screen—left to right and then right to left. As the leading dot disappears, the eyes reflexly begin tracking the next in line—resulting in a to-and-fro eye movement pattern or nystagmus. This reflex is significantly modulated by the CVS (normal at left and abnormal at right; dots moving to the right on top and dots moving to the left on the bottom)

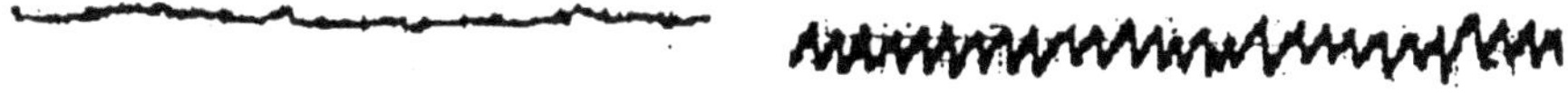

Fig. 5 The gaze test. The patient fixes his/her gaze on one point, first with eyes open and then with eyes closed. The appearance of spontaneous nystagmus or a rapid beating of the eyes back and forth—intensified or triggered with eyes closed—suggests a CVS dysfunction (normal at left and abnormal at right)

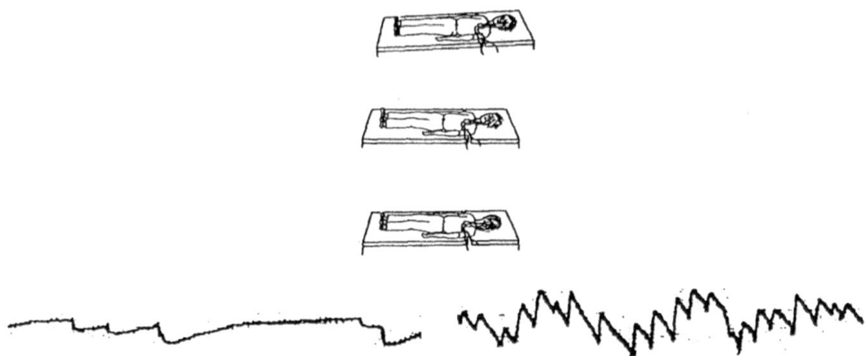

Fig. 6 Positional testing. The presence of horizontal or vertical nystagmus in varying positions of the head and neck suggests abnormal CVS functioning (normal at left and abnormal at right)

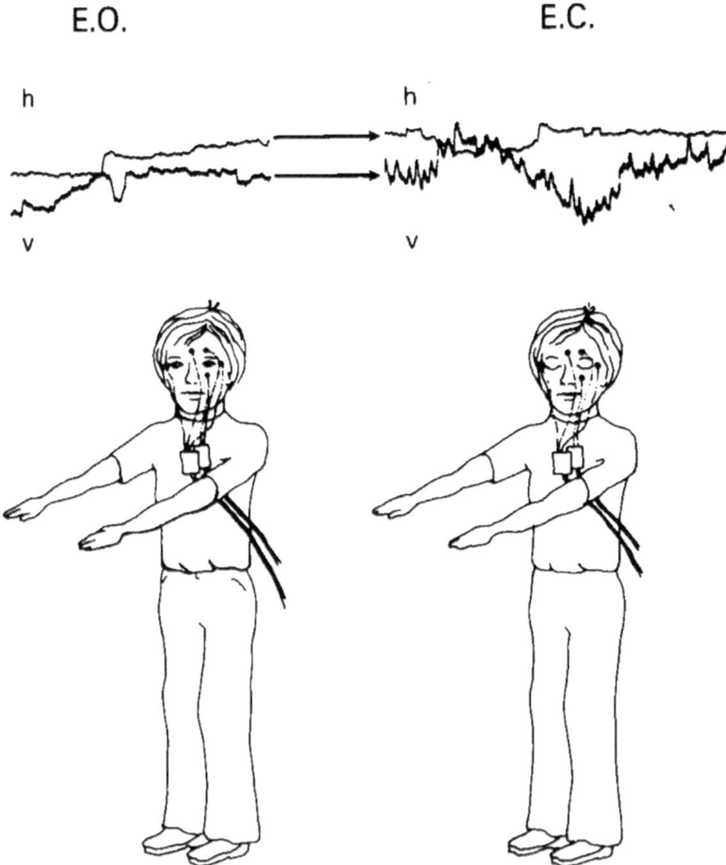

Fig. 7 Positional and Romberg testing. The presence of horizontal and/or vertical nystagmus suggests CVS dysfunctioning (EO—eyes open, EC—eyes closed, h—horizontal nystagmus, v—vertical nystagmus)

Rotation Testing

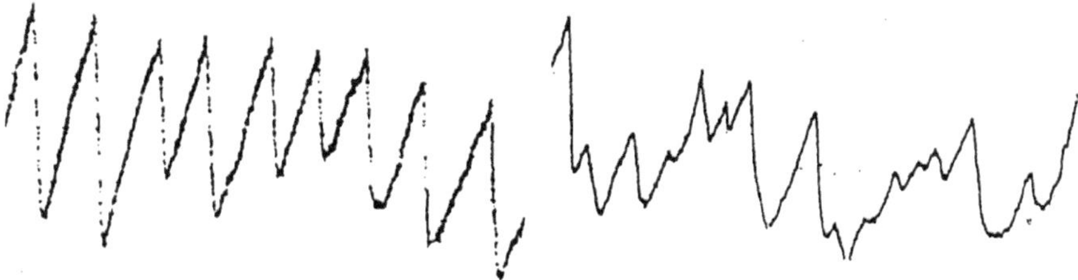

Fig. 8 Rotational testing. As illustrated, rotating individuals clockwise normally triggers a repetitive series of eye movements (nystagmus), and the opposite pattern occurs when rotated counter-clockwise (normal at left). Abnormal responses (at right) may be underactive, overactive, or dysrhythmic

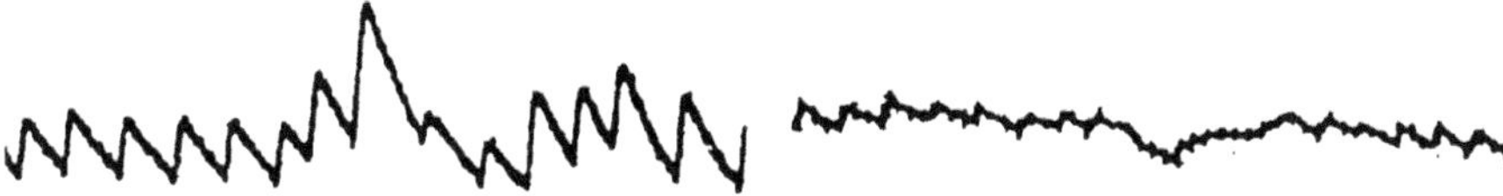

Fig. 9 Caloric stimulation of the right ear with warm water (44ºC). As illustrated in the graph on the left, stimulating the right ear with warm water normally triggers a rapid series of eye movement beats or nystagmus. The graph on the right shows a weak (abnormal) caloric response. These responses may also be abnormally overreactive or dysrhythmic. Cool water (30ºC) triggers an opposite nystagmus pattern

The Important ENG Test Parameters—Summarized

The following are several parameters that I use, depending on the presenting symptoms of the patient. Hopefully, these tests (detailed and previously illustrated) will provide you with an idea of the functions characterizing the CVS as well as how we attempt to indirectly measure its dysfunctioning:

Eye Movement Testing

- *The horizontal saccade test*—In this test, a dot moves randomly on the screen, and the patient must "chase" it with his/her eyes. A saccade is a quick, jerky eye movement that positions a visual target on the retina. The cerebellum plays an important role in determining this tracking function and, thus, its dysfunction.
- *The horizontal pursuit test*—In this test, a dot cycles back and forth across a screen, and the eyes' ability to follow it smoothly is electronically recorded and measured. A CVS dysfunction may result in the inability to produce smooth pursuit movements.
- *The horizontal optokinetic (OPK) test*—In this test, a patient is asked to watch a series of dots move across and then off a screen—left to right and then right to left. As the leading dot disappears, the eyes reflexively begin tracking the next in

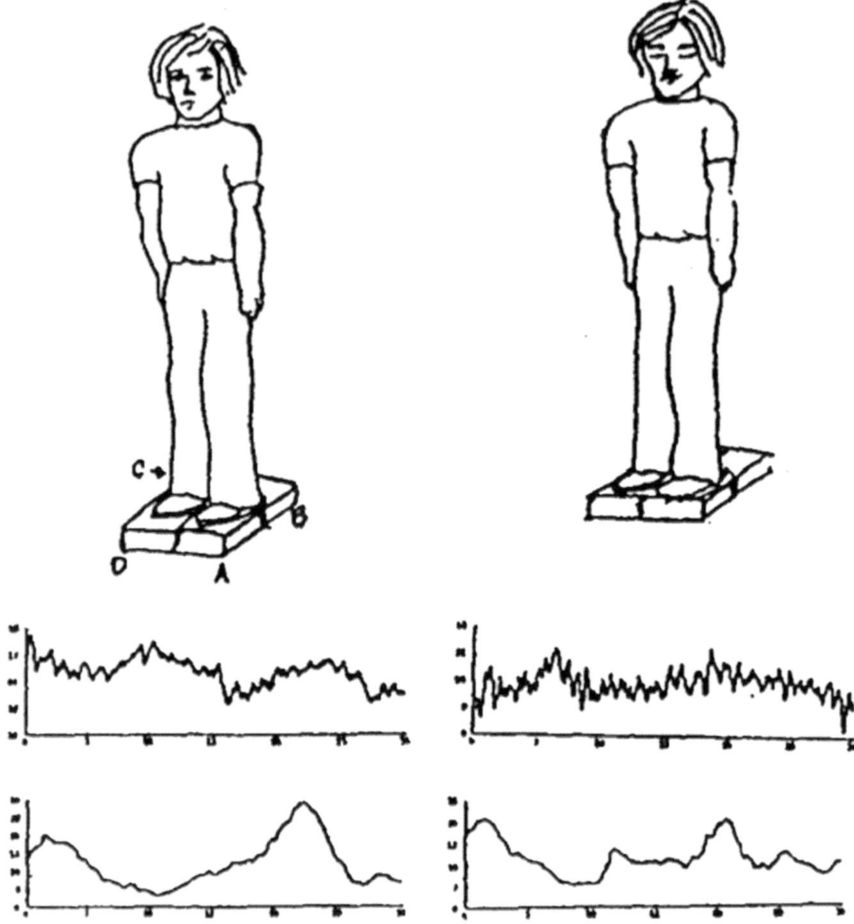

Fig. 10 Posturography (balance test). When patients are electronically tested for balance under varying conditions, the presence of instability is highlighted by abnormal herky-jerky-like movements (abnormal on top and normal on the bottom)

line—resulting in a to-and-fro eye movement pattern or nystagmus. The reflex is significantly modulated by the CVS.

- *The gaze test*—In this test, the patient fixes his gaze on one point, first with eyes open and then with eyes closed. The appearance of spontaneous nystagmus or a rapid oscillation of the eyes back and forth—intensified or triggered with eyes closed—suggests a CVS dysfunction.
- *Positional and Romberg testing*—These tests look for the appearance of nystagmus in varying positions of the body and head. The presence of nystagmus when none should exist is indicative of an inner-ear or CVS disorder.
- *Rotational testing*—This test measures vestibular or inner-ear responses to rotation. The patient is rotated in a chair, which normally induces a rapid, rhythmic

nystagmus. If the nystagmus is dysrhythmic, underactive, or overactive, then an abnormal vestibular system is suggested.
- *Caloric testing*—Nystagmus is normally triggered when the ears are rinsed with cool and warm water. Abnormal and asymmetric nystagmus responses suggest inner-ear or CVS dysfunctioning.

Appendix 6: Additional Insights into 3-D Scanners

3-D Optical Scanner Insights

I initially and simplistically assumed that the dyslexic reading disorder was due to a primary CVS-determined ocular fixation and scrambling dysfunction that secondarily confused cerebral processing. And the 3-D optical scanner statistically proved this assumption correct. However, there were severe dyslexics with high blurring speeds and the reverse. To explain these seemingly paradoxical results, as well as other atypical data, I personally tested hundreds—thousands—of dyslexics, getting nowhere.

Once again, a dyslexic solved this riddle—highlighting the clinical value of "living with patients" to best understand them. I vividly recall, during routine testing of an adult dyslexic about 40 years ago, I asking her to tell me the moment the elephants started blurring. "Which blurring event do you want?" she innocently replied. And suddenly I understood the answer I was looking for all along. And upon questioning, this bright woman replied: "First I blur out all five elephants at once. And then I continue seeing one elephant clearly until that finally blurs out." In this one simple answer, all the puzzling data suddenly became obvious.

This also explained why there was a significant discrepancy between the *blurring speed* and its more objective equivalent, the *recognition speed*. The latter occurred when a totally blurred sequence was slowed down until recognition occurred. Simple logic mandated that *blurring speed = recognition speed*. But as you recall, the simple logic that *dyslexia = alexia* was just as mistaken. Are we all not unwittingly misled into oversimplification and overgeneralization via kryptonite-like bias mechanisms?

In short, the first *sequential blurring speed* was the CVS diagnostic one—the one substantially reduced in dyslexics. However, the *single-targeting blurring speed* was a cerebral tracking compensatory one—and so was normal and even supernormal. Since these mechanisms were previously discussed, interested readers can pursue this content in my medical text, *A Solution to the Riddle Dyslexia*. And there is another insight that you may recall when I discussed the many dysfunctioning reading mechanisms in dyslexia (Chap. 16). Not all dyslexics have obvious, detectable, or even abnormal tracking mechanisms as I mistakenly and oversimplistically assumed initially. I hope you will now recognize the enormous benefits of clinical research as well as the value of attempting to understand both the statistical rule *and* especially its exceptions.

- As a result of these clarifications, the testing became more reliable and diagnostic—since I was able to separate out and independently study the compensatory masking component. Importantly, I also gained my first real insights into the complex, dysfunctioning vs. compensatory nature of the dyslexia reading (and non-reading) CVS disorder as well as the parameters needed for its definition and diagnosis.
- I had also simplistically assumed that diagnosing this impaired reading fixation and tracking mechanism with my 3-D optical scanner would identify potential reading-impaired dyslexics rather than simply those with CVS dysfunction. As it turned out, those with CVS dysfunction may or may not later develop reading impairments, due to a variety of reasons—especially since there are over 20 reading mechanisms in dyslexia, each having its own distinct dysfunctioning vs. compensatory potency. And also, some CVS-scrambled signals may not even hit the cerebral reading processor. And to my initial dismay, not all reading-impaired dyslexics have impaired and/or measurable eye-tracking disturbances, albeit a majority do.
- *In fact, I've yet to find one dyslexic or CVS diagnostic parameter or typical symptom in all patients with this syndrome. Variability rather than uniformity is the rule.* This finding no doubt explains why all dyslexia theories and definitions dependent on only one variable (e.g., severe reading score impairments, phonological dysfunctioning, eye-tracking difficulties, etc.) are, have been, and will be mistaken.

Although I discovered that repetition of the scanning exercise might improve the above visual mechanism, it might not significantly affect the reading disorder for the complex reasons just described.

3-D Auditory Scanner Insights

- Similar to the above, many dyslexics—but not all, as initially and oversimplistically assumed—were found to have delayed and/or distorted rapid auditory processing speeds for words listened.
- Because of compensatory and other complex auditory processing factors, my 3-D auditory scanning instrument did not detect all impaired auditory processing mechanisms—nor even all the rapid auditory dysfunctioning processing mechanisms tested for, as initially thought. So further research is needed.
- And by improving just one of many dysfunctioning auditory or phonological mechanisms, reading may or may not be significantly affected.

In retrospect, I can safely say that the vast majority of insights—many books' worth—that I've obtained to date were initially unexpected and thus would likely be considered atypical. Indeed, my research would never have gotten to first base had I not analyzed the *atypical* data with even greater diligence than the "expected" results—especially the so-called soft CVS neurological signs characterizing dyslexics. Sadly, the scientific tendency to "find and report only the statistically expected"—relying largely on denial to exclude the unexpected—helps explain why the research into dyslexia and related disorders led nowhere for over a century.

Appendix 7: Blurring Speed Visuals

To demonstrate and highlight these blurring phenomena, I measured the blurring speed reported by individuals observing a sequence of black elephants accelerating across a blank (Mode I) white background and then across a floral (Mode II) background. By and large, the reported sequential blurring speeds for Mode I and II gestalts were significantly lower in dyslexics vs. non-dyslexics (Figs. 1 and 2).

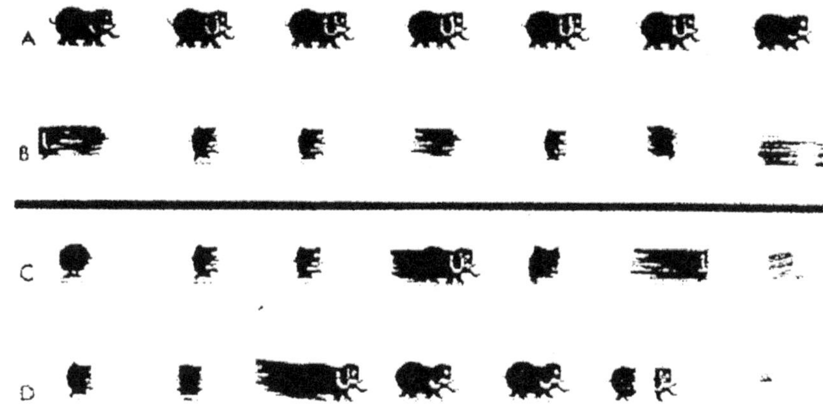

Fig. 1 (**A**) The elephant Mode I gestalt and (**B**) its blurring-speed endpoint. (**C**) and (**D**) are examples of single-targeting or tunnel vision. Mode I testing was used here to determine only the visual span during the perception of the stationary elephant sequence

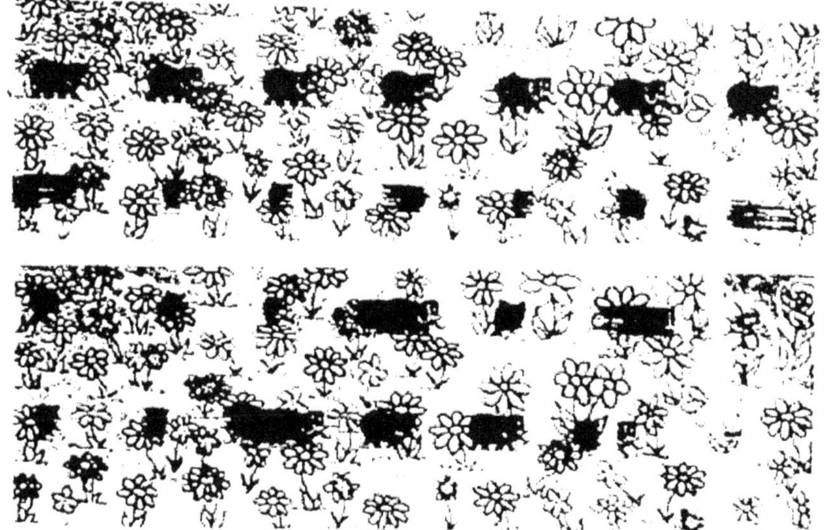

Fig. 2 (**A**) The elephant Mode II gestalt and (**B**) its blurring-speed endpoint. (**C**) and (**D**) are examples of single-targeting or tunnel vision. Mode II testing was used here to determine the blurring-speed endpoint as well as the visual span during optokinetic tracking of the moving elephants

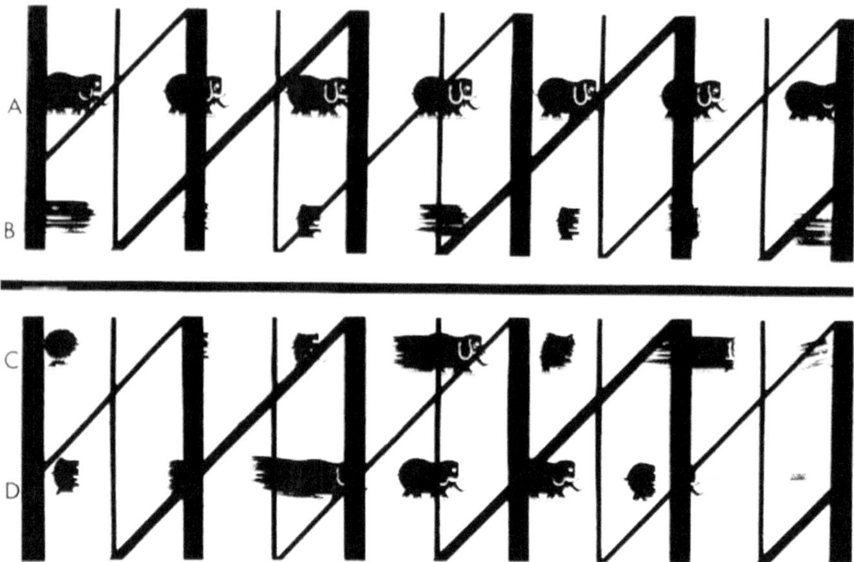

Fig. 3 (**A**) The elephant Mode III gestalt and (**B**) its Mode III blurring endpoint. (**C**) and (**D**) are examples of single-targeting or tunnel vision. Mode II testing here was used to determine the presence of background blurring, movement illusions, and the visual span during the movement of the optokinetic grid

Visual and motion illusions Since a majority of dyslexics reported word blurring and other visual illusions during reading, I decided to examine for these phenomena in a rather unique way. Thus, for example, while a moving picket-like fence is accelerated across a stationary sequence of black elephants (Mode III testing Fig. 3), many dyslexics report *visual elephant blurring and/or motion illusions*. In other words, they experience the clear stationary elephant sequence as blurred and/or these stationary elephants and/or themselves in motion. CVS normal non-dyslexics did not report these illusions (as frequently).

Tunnel vision During the reading process, many dyslexics reported seeing only one or two letters of a four-to-seven-letter word configuration at any given fixation or glance. Thus, for example, when attempting to read the word "letter," they would initially see only the "le" or "tt" or "er"—a phenomenon I called tunnel vision. And after responding favorably to mediations, these same individuals were often capable of seeing the whole word gestalt at a single glance. In order to test subjects for tunnel vision, I tested their visual spans, while they fixated the center elephant of a stationary seven-elephant Mode I sequence and were tracking the accelerating elephants (Mode I and Mode II) sequences. Variations aside, dyslexics were found to have smaller visual fixation and tracking spans than did CVS normal non-dyslexics, exceptions aside.

My research demonstrated that normal visual spans are composed of central cone vision and peripheral CVS-modulated rod vision. In the presence of CV dysfunction, the peripheral rod function is often diminished, and so, tunnel vision results. However, atypical exceptions once again materialized—to shatter my simple convictions. So, I was forced to realize that some dyslexics had super-peripheral vision, and why? They were either genetically or otherwise predisposed to this gifted tendency. Or, because of an impaired coordination of adaptive central and peripheral visual mechanism, the latter was turned on and left or stuck that way?

Correcting Misleading Diagnostic Parameters

As previously mentioned, just about every known characteristic thought to be absolutely diagnostic of dyslexia, including poor reading, turned out to be incorrect to explain all dyslexics. Were it not for my CVS fine-tuning theory of dyslexia, we would all still be attempting to reconcile seemingly irreconcilable facts about dyslexia. And denial of the seemingly atypical exceptions would still be the only comforting option available to cope with our scientific frustrations. So, riddles would have been created rather than solved. Needless to say, we would never have understood why there were so many conflicting objective studies refuting one another—including those stating that eye movements were and weren't important in diagnosing dyslexia. In many ways, conflicting study results were due to improper assumptions and convictions about dyslexia and thus, poor study designs and misinterpretation of what the results really meant. (Indeed, I've included some of these studies within the references.[1]) And these errors certainly explained why the APA was justifiably led to conclude that dyslexia didn't exist—meaning its oversimplified and mistaken concepts didn't exist.

Appendix 8: Reflex Therapy: Sally Goddard Blythe

Reflexes have long been used in medicine both to assess the functioning of the central nervous system (CNS) in the neonate and to identify signs of pathology.

Two types of reflexes—*primitive* and *postural*—are of particular interest to practitioners seeking to identify signs of immaturity in the functioning of the CNS and

[1] Thus, one diagnostic test reported by Professor Money of Johns Hopkins many years ago noted that dyslexics often have difficulty knowing right and left. And some have poor directional senses. So, he designed a maze test to tap this dysfunction. It didn't work! Why, you may ask? Because you could see how to escape the maze, whereas you can't see right and left. And, of course, many dyslexics do not have right and left or directional difficulties. Indeed, some have exceptional abilities. And he overlooked the compensatory factor, as well. As noted, I also designed 3-D optical and auditory scanners—and only belatedly recognized their initial limitations. So, it took years to correct some of my unwitting assumptions and convictions as well as my tunnel thinking. The phonological theorists, as discussed within this book, have yet to discover the one frustrating principle characterizing dyslexia research: that all known dyslexic characteristics differ among dyslexics—and so must be accounted for rather than denied.

its role in a variety of disorders including dyslexia, developmental coordination disorder (DCD), attention deficit disorder (ADD), educational underachievement, and the perpetuation of agoraphobia and panic disorder in the absence of exogenous causal factors.

Primitive reflexes emerge during life in the womb, are fully developed in healthy infants born at full term, and are gradually inhibited by higher centers in the brain in the first six months of life.

Postural reflexes (sometimes referred to as reactions) start to develop after birth up to three and a half years of age. Collectively, these later reflexes provide a repertoire of subconscious adaptive responses, which support posture, balance, and coordination, including a stable platform for centers involved in control of eye movements.

As there are developmental periods when these reflexes should be active, suppressed, and replaced, the assessment of primitive and postural reflexes in children of school age and above can provide "signposts" of maturity in the functioning of the CNS. Primitive and postural reflexes are not the primary cause of the presenting problems but provide tools with which to identify underlying mechanisms at fault. They are indicators of the developmental level from which physical remediation should start and thus are measures with which to assess improvements during and after an intervention program.

Psychologist Peter Blythe in the early 1970s developed a specific system of screening, assessment, and remediation that is now known as the INPP method.[2]

Blythe (1980) asserted that:

> *"The innate mechanistic processes involved in the inhibition, modification and transformation of the basic reflexes are observable, and more importantly* ***replicable*** *at any age, to assist in the rehabilitation of neurological impairment."*[3]

The theory of *replication* is the basis for all the reflex inhibition techniques used by INPP. It is possible to give the brain a second chance to register the inhibitory movement patterns which should have been made at the appropriate stage in development or to recapitulate a stage of development which may have been omitted during uterine life or infancy.[4]

Primitive and postural reflexes both reflect and affect the functioning of cooperative systems, particularly those relating to posture, balance, and associated eye movements. When using an effective reflex integration program, as there is a general maturation in the functioning of these systems, primitive reflexes remiss (inhibit) and postural reflexes develop, providing both markers of increased maturity and secure foundations for the functioning of all systems.

---

[2] Blythe P, NcGlown DJ, 1979. *An organic basis for neuroses and educational difficulties*. Chester. Insight Publications.

[3] Blythe P, 1980. An organic basis for neurosis and the existence, detection and treatment of secondary neurosis. (Monograph). Swedish Institute for Neuro-Physiological Psychology. Gothenburg.

[4] Goddard SA, 1990. A developmental basis for learning difficulties and language disorders. INPP Monograph Series.1/1990.

The INPP method is available as an individual (clinical) program, as part of teacher developmental screening and movement in schools,[5] and as a screening test for clinicians and health practitioners.[6]

Commentary

It is often uncanny how different parallel lines of clinical data, evaluation, treatment, and theories intersect. Thus, Peter Blythe and most other researchers and clinicians in the 1970s were completely unaware of the cerebellum in determining these reflexes and inhibiting/facilitating them. So, if these cerebellar changes were made and we look at the varied disorders helped by Blythe, then we might conclude that our separate or parallel concepts independently validate one another.

Similarly, the many symptoms and functions I determined were due to a CVS dysfunction and helped by the CVS enhancers (refer to the Self-Diagnostic Test in Chap. 7), and those obtained by VEDA were almost identical—yet arrived at differently and independently via separate parallel lines.

So, as a clinician and a former aspiring mathematician, I believe these highly improbable clinical occurrences could not have occurred by chance alone. Rather, similar theories were formulated to describe data obtained and validated via different methods.

Appendix 9: A Surprise Addendum: Fact Is Fiction in Perspective

> *"It's a learning disorder! It's a language disorder! It's brain damage! Is it alexia? Congenital word blindness? Minimal brain damage? Minimal cerebral dysfunction? No, it's strephosymbolia (twisted symbols), specific learning disorder, specific learning disability, ... No one has it! Everyone has it!*
>
> *It's a gift! It's a tragedy! It's normal! It's abnormal! It exists! It doesn't exist!"*

What if all these "ideas" and synonyms taken from Chap. 1 were somewhat correct, as were Critchley and all those theorists I have previously negatively critiqued? And they were—but their concepts required significant modifications. So, just in case you may have overlooked my prior explanations within the overloaded content thus far presented, let me once again put all of these fascinating insights into a proper, condensed scientific perspective before finally ending this book full of research surprises and zigzags.

---

[5] Goddard Blythe SA, 2012. *Assessing neuromotor readiness for learning. The INPP developmental screening test and school intervention programme.* Chichester. Wiley-Blackwell.

[6] Goddard Blythe SA, 2014. *Neuromotor in children and adults. The INPP screening test for clinicians and health practitioners.*

Further information

www.inpp.org.uk

Understanding anecdotal content Freud discovered many years ago that all anecdotal or reported content is meaningful, once properly understood, especially after first obtaining a holistic context. Accordingly, I believe my CVS theory is now capable of explaining everything about dyslexia—including the seeming nonsensical and contradictory content highlighted above, especially the importance of the thinking brain in dyslexia Thus, critics who mandate that only double-blind controlled content is valid, and nothing else, may be highly misled by kryptonite.

Reexplaining/reviewing the dyslexia synonyms and ideas As *dyslexia* = *alexia* = *"dyslexia"* does not exist, then no one has dyslexia (alexia). And since we all had the "embryonic" dyslexia or CVS syndrome and it remains inhibited/suppressed within our subconscious brain, then congenital dyslexia exists and so everyone had/has it.

Since CVS dysfunction may result in scores of differently named impairments included within the dyslexia syndrome, it is obvious that LD, SLD, as well as language/speech and even phonological disorders, are related to this syndrome, including their reversals or "twisted symbols" or strephosymbolia.

And compared to the diagnostic cerebral signs associated with major brain damage, resulting in adult alexia as well as other severe cerebral impairments, the CVS neurological deficit and its signs are considered minimal vs. major. Importantly, for those who overcompensate, dyslexia may be viewed as a gift—certainly it's abnormal for those who do not. And sadly, when misunderstood and untreated/mistreated, outcomes may be tragic.

Because the cerebral cortex and higher cerebellum are important in decoding CVS signal scrambling, the thinking brain likely plays a more important primary and/or secondary role in dyslexia than previously thought. So, the traditionalists were half right—rather than just wrong.

Nature's ambivalence It thus seems, in hindsight, as if nature provided us all with "ambivalent" clues as to dyslexia's origin and portrait—and so, we saw and heard them differently and very selectively. As a result, it took me over 50 years with the help of countless dyslexics to understand and explain most all. Each and every clue—however farfetched it seemed—likely had some validity, albeit initially leading us astray or to dead ends and certainly to bouts of frustration.

Although initially rejecting many of the above theories/ideas as nonsensical—especially since they first appeared as if merely disjointed forms and sounds lost/unsupported in endless space, I better comprehended and integrated them all only after eventually obtaining a vitally needed overall perspective of the dyslexia/CVS syndrome, such as the one eventually presented to you within Chap. 9.

In retrospect, nature's ambivalence—symbolized by Superman vs. kryptonite—resulted in some of these flawed ideas and so required continuous psychoanalysis and neuroanalysis: first to separate fact from fiction and then to determine the fact highlighted by the fiction as well as the distortions resulting from bias mechanisms.

Thus, I was forced to wonder: Are we not all mere puppets dancing alone against howling winds to nature's silent but infinitely complex tunes, many initially misleading?

Hopefully, you've enjoyed and understood the song—rather symphony—I eventually heard and have now played for you within this book. I truly gave it my very best effort, despite kryptonite continually throwing us all off course and key while also attempting to disconnect vs. unite us all. And this scientific confusion and conflict reigned for over a century—until now!

References

A: Independent Validating References—Typical of Thousands
B: Dr. Harold Levinson's Research Publications and Books
C: This Book's More Specific References

Because the independent validation of my CVS research is vital, I accumulated hundreds, perhaps a thousand, crucial references, in addition to this book's regular bibliography. Although the importance of the cerebellum was not scientifically recognized and validated until two decades after my initial publications and discoveries in the early 1970s, the previously denied importance of the cerebellum has since exploded exponentially. So, now there are thousands of studies—just way too many for a work of this type to cite. Yet they are all important.

So, I decided to simplify and compromise: I will provide just a "few" typical independent cerebellar references corroborating the insights that I've discussed in this book under their important functional and comorbid headings—providing additional vital ones on my website: *dyslexiaonline.com*.

And to make things even easier for interested readers, I will then separately add on my own publications as well. Finally, I will also include the references specific to this book's content, excluding most of the above. Although perhaps novel, I believe this method will enable readers to more readily benefit from these important studies and reviews.

A: Independent Validating References—Typical of Thousands

The Cerebellar Differences in Dyslexia, ADHD, and Autism

Stoodley CJ. Distinct regions of the cerebellum show gray matter decreases in autism, ADHD, and developmental dyslexia. Front Syst Neurosci. 2014;8:92.

The Higher Cerebellum and Dyslexia-Related Functions

De Smet HJ, Paquier P, Verhoeven J, Mariën P. The cerebellum: its role in language and related cognitive and affective functions. Brain Lang. 2013;127(3):334–42.

Leiner HC, Leiner AL, Dow RS. Does the cerebellum contribute to mental skills? Behav Neurosci. 1986;100(4):443.

Leiner HC, Leiner AL, Dow RS. The human cerebro-cerebellar system: its computing, cognitive, and language skills. Behav Brain Res. 1991;44(2):113–28.

Merhi D, Diana, DCH. Review of current concepts regarding the cerebellum. 2003;1–7.

Paradiso S, Andreasen NC, O'leary DS, Arndt S, Robinson RG. Cerebellar size and cognition: correlations with IQ, verbal memory and motor dexterity. Neuropsychiat Neuropsychol Behav Neurol. 1997;10(1):1–8.

Rapoport M, van Reekum R, Mayberg H. The role of the cerebellum in cognition and behavior: a selective review. J Neuropsychiatr Clin Neurosci. 2000;12(2):193–8.

Schmahmann JD, Sherman JC. The cerebellar cognitive affective syndrome. Brain J Neurol. 1998;121(4):561–79.

Schutter DJ, Van Honk J. The cerebellum on the rise in human emotion. Cerebellum. 2005;4(4):290–4.

Timmann D, Daum I. Cerebellar contributions to cognitive functions: a progress report after two decades of research. Cerebellum. 2007;6(3):159–62.

The Cerebellum and Dyslexia

Beaton AA. Dyslexia and the cerebellar deficit hypothesis. Cortex. 2002;38(4):479–90.

Eckert MA, Leonard CM, Richards TL, Aylward EH, Thomson J, Berninger VW. Anatomical correlates of dyslexia: frontal and cerebellar findings. Brain. 2003;126(2):482–94.

Kasselimis D, Margarity M, Vlachos F. Cerebellar function, dyslexia and articulation speed. Child Neuropsychol. 2008;14(4):303–13.

Rae C, Lee MA, Dixon RM, et al. Metabolic abnormalities in developmental dyslexia detected by 1H magnetic resonance spectroscopy. Lancet. 1998;351(9119):1849–52.

The Cerebellum and ADHD

Berquin P, Giedd J, Jacobsen L, et al. Cerebellum in attention-deficit hyperactivity disorder A morphometric MRI study. Neurology. 1998;50(4):1087–93.

Fliers EA, Franke B, Buitelaar JK. Motor problems in children with ADHD receive too little attention in clinical practice. Nederlands tijdschrift voor geneeskunde. 2011;155(50):A3559.

Mackie S, Shaw P, Lenroot R, et al. Cerebellar development and clinical outcome in attention deficit hyperactivity disorder. Am J Psychiatr. 2007;164(4):647–55.

Mackie S, Shaw P, Lenroot R, et al Brain development and ADHD. Clin Psychol Rev. 2006.

Shaw P, Ishii-Takahashi A, Park MT, et al. A multicohort, longitudinal study of cerebellar development in attention deficit hyperactivity disorder. J Child Psychol Psychiatry. 2018;59:1114–23.

The Cerebellum in Dyslexia and Coordination Disorder

Nicolson RI, Fawcett AJ, Berry EL, Jenkins IH, Dean P, Brooks DJ. Association of abnormal cerebellar activation with motor learning difficulties in dyslexic adults. Lancet. 1999;353(9165):1662–7.

O'Hare A, Khalid S. The association of abnormal cerebellar function in children with developmental coordination disorder and reading difficulties. Dyslexia. 2002;8(4):234–48.

The Cerebellum in Depression and Other Neuropsychiatric Disorders

Johnson CP, Christensen GE, Fiedorowicz JG, Mani M, Shaffer JJ, Magnotta VA, Wemmie JA. Alterations of the cerebellum and basal ganglia in bipolar disorder mood states detected by quantitative T1ρ mapping. Bipolar Disord. 2018;20:381–90.

Konarski JZ, McIntyre RS, Grupp LA, Kennedy SH. Is the cerebellum relevant in the circuitry of neuropsychiatric disorders? J Psychiatry Neurosci. 2005;30(3):178–86.

Linden DJ, Connor JA. Cellular mechanisms of long-term depression in the cerebellum. Curr Opin Neurobiol. 1993;3(3):401–6.

Wiser AK, Andreasen NC, O'leary DS, Watkins GL, Ponto LLB, Hichwa RD. Dysfunctional cortico cerebellar circuits cause 'cognitive dysmetria'in schizophrenia. Neuroreport. 1998;9(8):1895–9.

Comorbidity of ADHD and Dyslexia

Germanò E, Gagliano A, Curatolo P. Comorbidity of ADHD and dyslexia. Dev Neuropsychol. 2010;35(5):475–93.

ADHD with Comorbid Anxiety

Schatz DB, Rostain AL. ADHD with comorbid anxiety: a review of the current literature. J Atten Disord. 2006;10(2):141–9.

Comorbid ADHD/Dyslexia and Depression and Anxiety

Nelson JM, Gregg N. Depression and anxiety among transitioning adolescents and college students with ADHD, dyslexia, or comorbid ADHD/dyslexia. J Atten Disord. 2012;16(3):244–54.

The Cerebellum in Autism or ASD

Jaber M. The cerebellum as a major player in motor disturbances related to autistic syndrome disorders. L'Encephale. 2017;43(2):170–5.

McCarthy MM, Wright CL. Convergence of sex differences and the neuroimmune system in autism spectrum disorder. Biol Psychiatry. 2017;81(5):402–10.

Some Important Other Validating/Supporting References

The Role of Nutrition in Dyslexia, ADHD, and Autism

Carlton RM, Ente G, Blum L, Heyman N. Rational dosages of nutrients have a prolonged effect on learning disabilities. Altern Ther Health Med. 2000;6(3):85.

Richardson AJ, Ross M. Fatty acid metabolism in neurodevelopmental disorder: a new perspective on associations between attention-deficit/hyperactivity disorder, dyslexia, dyspraxia and the autistic spectrum. Prostaglandins, Leukotrienes and Essential Fatty Acids (PLEFA). 2000;63(1-2):1–9.

Richardson A, McDaid A, Calvin C, Higgins C, Purit B. Reduced behavioural and learning problems in children with specific learning difficulties after supplementation with highly unsaturated fatty acids: a randomised double-blind placebo-controlled trial. Paper presented at: Eur J Neurosci. 2000;12(Suppl 11):296.

The Role of Other Therapies

Goddard S, Blythe SG. The well balanced child: movement and early learning. Hawthorn; 2005.

Goddard Blythe S. Neurological dysfunction as a significant factor in children diagnosed with dyslexia. Paper presented at: Proceedings of The 5th International British Dyslexia Association Conference 2001.

Hill GT, Raymond JE. Deficits of motion transparency perception in adult developmental dyslexics with normal unidirectional motion sensitivity. Vis Res. 2002;42(9):1195–203.

McCredie S. Balance: in search of the lost sense. Brown: Little; 2009.

Solan HA, Shelley-Tremblay J, Larson S. Vestibular function, sensory integration, and balance anomalies: a brief literature review. Optometry Vision Develop. 2007;38(1):13.

Medical Treatment

Levinson JV, Stricker G, Levinson HN. The effect of treatment of dyslexic children on self-esteem and behavior — dissertation. The Gordon F: Derner Institute of Advanced Psychological Studies, Adelphi University; 2003.

NIH Clinical Research Studies, Protocol Number: 06-M-0234. The antidepressant efficacy of the anticholinergic scopolamine. https://clinicaltrials.gov/ct2/show/NCT00369915.

B: Dr. Harold Levinson's Publications

Books

Levinson HN. Dyslexia: a solution to the riddle. New York: Springer; 1980

Levinson HN. Smart but feeling dumb. New York: Warner Publications; 1984.

Levinson HN. Phobia free. New York: M. Evans and Company; 1986.

Levinson HN. Total concentration: how to understand attention deficit disorders with treatment guidelines for you and your doctor. New York: Evans; 1990.

Levinson HN, Sanders A. The upside-down kids: helping dyslexic children understand themselves and their disorder. New York: Harold Levinson; 1991.

Levinson HN, Sanders A. Turning around the upside-down kids: helping dyslexic kids overcome their disorder. New York: Harold Levinson; 1992.

Levinson HN. A scientific watergate, dyslexia: how and why countless millions are deprived of breakthrough medical treatment. New York: Harold Levinson; 1994.

Levinson HN. The Discovery of Cerebellar-Vestibular Syndromes & Therapies — A Solution to the Riddle Dyslexia, Stonebridge Publishing, Ltd., March 2000 (A re-titled and reprint of A Solution to the Riddle—Dyslexia) https://www.amazon.com/DiscoveryCerebellar-Vestibular Syndromes Therapies-Dyslexia/dp/0963930311

Levinson HN. Smart but feeling dumb: the challenging new research on dyslexia—and how it may help you. New York: Grand Central Publishing; 2003.

Published Papers

Frank J, Levinson HN. Auditory hallucinations in a case of hysteria. Br J Psychiatry, 1966 112(486), 523–523.

Frank J, Levinson HN. Anti-motion sickness medications in dysmetric dyslexia and dyspraxia. Acad Ther. 1977;12(4):411–24.

Frank J, Levinson HN. Seasickness mechanisms and medications in dysmetric dyslexia and dyspraxia. Acad Ther. 1976;12(2):133–53.

Frank J, Levinson HN. Compensatory mechanisms in CV dysfunction, dysmetric dyslexia, and dyspraxia. Acad Ther. 1976;12(1):5–27.

Frank J, Levinson HN. Dysmetric dyslexia and dyspraxia: synopsis of a continuing research project. Acad Ther. 1975;11(2):133–43.

Frank J, Levinson H. Dysmetric dyslexia and dyspraxia. J Am Acad Child Psychiatry. 1973;12:690–701.

The Above Six Papers Were Written with Dr. Jan Frank

Levinson HN. Abnormal optokinetic and perceptual span parameters in cerebellar vestibular dysfunction and learning disabilities or dyslexia. Percept Mot Skills 1989; 68(1):35-54E.

Levinson HN. The cerebellar-vestibular basis of learning disabilities in children, adolescents and adults: hypothesis and study. Percept Mot Skills. 1988;67(3):983–1006E.

Levinson HN. A cerebellar-vestibular explanation for fears/phobias: hypothesis and study. Percept Mot Skills. 1989;68(1):67–84.

Levinson HN. The cerebellar-vestibular predisposition to anxiety disorders. Percept Mot Skills. 1989;68(1):323–38.

Levinson HN. Abnormal optokinetic and perceptual span parameters in cerebellar-vestibular dysfunction and learning disabilities or dyslexia. Perceptual and Motor Skills. 1989; 68(1):3554E.
Levinson HN. The diagnostic value of cerebellar-vestibular tests in detecting learning disabilities, dyslexia, and attention deficit disorder. Percept Mot Skills. 1990;71(1):67–82.
Levinson HN. Dramatic favorable responses of children with learning disabilities or dyslexia and attention deficit disorder to antimotion sickness medications: four case reports. Percept Mot Skills. 1991;73(3):723–38.
Levinson H. Rapid mec1izine-induced reversal of cerebellar-vestibular dysfunction in adults with learning disabilities or dyslexia. Paper presented at: 144th annual meeting of the American Psychiatric Association, New Orleans 1991.
Levinson JV, Stricker G, Levinson HN. The effect of treatment of dyslexic children on self-esteem and behavior — dissertation. The Gordon F: Derner Institute of Advanced Psychological Studies, Adelphi University; 2003.

C: This Book's Bibliography

Because this book attempts to provide you with my latest CVS insights into the dyslexia syndrome—while also including the historical steps leading to its 50-year research solution—a detailed bibliography would be enormous and perhaps overloading; even impossible. So I decided to include here primarily those vital references referring to important content stated or clearly alluded to in this work—although there is some cross referencing or some better placed within the prior validating category. As a result, I urge readers to review the bibliographies attached to all my prior referenced research papers and books so that they may collectively and correctly provide you with the insightful light that awakened me from scientific darkness (refer to http://www.dyslexiaonline.com/media/papers.html).

Adler A. The work of Paul Schilder. Bull N Y Acad Med. 1965;41(8):841.
Adler-Grinberg D, Stark L. Eye movements, scanpaths, and dyslexia. Am J Optom Physiol Optic. 1978;55(8):557–70.
Adrian E. Afferent areas in the cerebellum connected with the limbs. Brain. 1943;66(4):289–315.
Agnew JA, Dorn C, Eden GF. Effect of intensive training on auditory processing and reading skills. Brain Lang. 2004;88(1):21–5.
Agras S, Sylvester D, Oliveau D. The epidemiology of common fears and phobia. Compr Psychiatry. 1969;10(2):151–6.
American Psychiatric Association. Diagnostic and statistical manual of mental disorders. Washington, D.C.; 2013.
Asmundson GJ, Larsen DK, Stein MB. Panic disorder and vestibular disturbance: an overview of empirical findings and clinical implications. J Psychosom Res. 1998;4(1):107–20.
Ayres AJ. Sensory integration and learning disorders. Los Angeles: Western Psychological Services; 1972.
Ayres AJ. Learning disabilities and the vestibular system. J Learn Disabil. 1978;11(1):30–41.
Baloh RW, Honrubia V, Sills A. Eye-tracking and optokinetic nystagmus: results of quantitative testing in patients with well-defined nervous system lesions. Ann Otol Rhinol Laryngol. 1977;86(1):108–14.
Bárány R. Some new methods for functional testing of the vestibular apparatus and the cerebellum. Nobel Lectures, Physiol Med. 1901;1921:500–11.
Baštecký J, Boleloucký Z, Skovroňský O. Psychotropic drugs in acoustic and vestibular disorders. Activitas Nervosa Superior (Prague). 1981;23:187–8.
Bauman ML. Neuroanatomic observations of the brain in autism. In: Baumann ML, Kemper TL, editors. The neurobiology of autism. Baltimore: Johns Hopkins University Press; 1994.
Bender L. A visual motor gestalt test and its clinical use. New York: Research Monographs, American Orthopsychiatric Association; 1938.

Benedikt M. Uber Platzchwindel. Allgemeine Wiener Medizinische Zeitung. 1870;15:488–90.
Berg R, Smedslund G. Effect of vitamins, minerals and other dietary supplements on mental health symptoms for people with ADHD, anxiety disorders, bipolar disorder or depression. 2011.
Bidwell LC, McClernon FJ, Kollins SH. Cognitive enhancers for the treatment of ADHD. Pharmacol Biochem Behav. 2011;99(2):262–74.
Black J, Collins D, De Roach J, Zubrick S. Smooth pursuit eye movements in normal and dyslexic children. Percept Mot Skills. 1984;59(1):91–100.
Blythe P, McGlown DJ. An organic basis for neuroses and educational difficulties: a new look at the old MBD syndrome: Insight Pub; 1979. p. 93–4.
Bodranghien F, Bastian A, Casali C, et al. Consensus paper: revisiting the symptoms and signs of cerebellar syndrome. Cerebellum. 2016;15(3):369–91.
Boniver R. Influence du Piracetam sur Ie fonctionnemenr du systeme vestibulaire. Acta Oto Rhino-LAryngologica Belgica. 1974;28:293–9.
Bouma H, Legein CP. Foveal and parafoveal recognition of letters and words by dyslexics and by average readers. Neuropsychologia. 1977;15(1):69–80.
Broad W, Wade N. Betrayers of the truth: fraud and deceit in the halls of science. New York: Simon & Schuster; 1982.
Brody J. Two doctors offer dyslexia theory: faulty link is suspected between brain and ear. New York Times. 1974;20
Brookler KH. Simultaneous bilateral bithermal caloric stimulation in electronystagmography. Laryngoscope. 1971;81(7):1014–9.
Brookler K, Pulec J. Computer analysis of electronystagmography records. Transact-Am Acad Ophthalmol Otolaryngol. 1970;74(3):563–75.
Buckner RL. The cerebellum and cognitive function: 25 years of insight from anatomy and neuroimaging. Neuron. 2013;80(3):807–15.
Bührle C, Sonnhof U. The ionic mechanism of postsynaptic inhibition in motoneurones of the frog spinal cord. Neuroscience. 1985;14(2):581–92.
Carlton RM, Ente G, Blum L, Heyman N. Rational dosages of nutrients have a prolonged effect on learning disabilities. Altern Ther Health Med. 2000;6(3):85.
Carr DB, Sheehan DV. Evidence that panic disorder has a metabolic cause. In: Bal-lenger JC, editor. Biology of agoraphobia. Washington, D.C.: American Psychiatric Press; 1984. p. 100–11.
Carter S, Gold A. The syndrome of minimal cerebral dysfunction. Pediatrics. 1972;15:879–82.
Cheek CW. Electronystagmography in children with specific learning disabilities. Unpublished doctoral dissertation, Wichita State University, Kansas, 1969.
Coffin JM. Cerebellar deficiency model of dyslexia upheld. Clinical Psychiatry News. 2000.
Cohen SC, Harvey DJ, Shields RH, et al. Effects of yoga on attention, impulsivity, and hyperactivity in preschool-aged children with attention-deficit hyperactivity disorder symptoms. J Dev Behav Pediatr. 2018;39(3):200–9.
Committee on Early Childhood, Adoption and Dependent Care, American Academy of Pediatrics. Middle-ear disease and language development. News Comment. 1984;35:5.
Conners CK, Werry JS. Pharmacotherapy. In: Quay HC, Werry JS, editors. Psychopathological disorders of childhood. New York: Wiley; 1979. p. 336–86.
Cope, S. Yoga and the quest for the true self: Bantam. 2018.
Cooper P, Pivik R. Abnormal visual-vestibular interaction and smooth pursuit tracking in psychosis:implications for cerebellar involvement. J Psychiatry Neurosci. 1991;16(1):30–40.
Corbett BA, Shickman K, Ferrer E. Brief report: the effects of Tomatis sound therapy on language in children with autism. J Autism Dev Disord. 2008;38(3):562–6.
Critchley M. The dyslexic child. Springfield: Charles C. Thomas; 1969.
Courchesne E, Townsend J, Saitoh O. The brain in infantile autism posterior fossa structures are abnormal. Neurology. 1994; 44(2), 214–214.
Dąbrowski K. Positive disintegration. Boston: Little Brown; 1964.
Dąbrowski K. Personality-shaping through positive disintegration. Brown: Little; 1967.
Dąbrowski K, Kawczak A, Piechowski MM. Mental growth through positive disintegration. London: Gryf Publications; 1970.

Dean W, Morgenthaler J. Smart drugs & nutrients: how to improve your memory and increase your intelligence using the latest discoveries in neuroscience, vol. 1: Smart Publications; 1990.
Dejerine J. Contribution a l'etude anatomo-pathologique et clinique des diffrerents varietes de cecite verbale. Comptes Rendus: Societe de Biologie. 1892;4:61–90.
Dejerine J. Sur un cas de cecite verbale avec agraphie suivi d'autopsie. Comptes Rendus: Societe de Biologie. 1891;3:197–201.
De Quiros JB. Vestibular-proprioceptive integration: its influence on learning and speech in children. In: Proceedings of the Tenth Interamerican Congress of Psychology, Lima, Peru, 1966. Mexico City: Editorial Trillas; 1967.
De Quiros JB. Diagnosis of vestibular disorders in the learning disabled. J Learn Disabil. 1976;9(1):39–47.
De Quirós JB, Schrager OL. Neuropsychological fundamentals in learning disabilities: Academic Therapy Publications; 1979.
Doehring P, Reichow B, Palka T, Phillips C, Hagopian L. Behavioral approaches to managing severe problem behaviors in children with autism spectrum and related developmental disorders: a descriptive analysis. Child Adolescent Psychiatric Clin. 2014;23(1):25–40.
Dow RS, Anderson R. Cerebellar action potentials in response to stimulation of proprioceptors and exteroceptors in the rat. J Neurophysiol. 1942;5(5):363–71.
Dow RS, Moruzzi G. The physiology and pathology of the cerebellum. Minnesota: U of Minnesota Press; 1958.
Duffy FH, Denckla MB, Bartels PH, Sandini G. Dyslexia: regional differences in brain electrical activity by topographic mapping. Ann Neurol. 1980;7(5):412–20.
Eccles JC. The cerebellum as a computer: patterns in space and time. J Physiol. 1973;229(1):1–32.
Eccles JC. Learning in the motor system. In: Progress in brain research, vol. 64: Elsevier; 1986. p. 3–18.
Eccles JC. Personal correspondence, 1976, 1987. And a letter to the Rodin Remediation Academy, 1989.
Eccles JC, Ito M, Szentagothai J. The cerebellum as a neuronal machine. New York: Springer-Verlag; 1967.
Einstein A. On the electrodynamics of moving bodies. 1905.
Elterman R, Abel L, Daroff R, Dell'Osso L, Bornstein J. Eye movement patterns in dyslexic children. J Learn Disabil. 1980;13(1):16–21.
Fagan JE, Kaplan BJ, Raymond JE, Edgington ES. The failure of antimotion sickness medication to improve reading in developmental dyslexia: results of a randomized trial. J Dev Behav Pediatr. 1988;96:359–66.
Fawcett AJ, Nicolson RI. Automatisation deficits in balance for dyslexic children. Percept Mot Skills. 1992;75(2):507–29.
Feingold BF. The Feingold cookbook for hyperactive children, and others with problems associated with food additives and salicylates. New York: Random House; 1979.
Fenichel O. The psychoanalytic theory of neurosis. London: Routledge; 2014.
Fenichel O. The psychoanalytic theory of neurosis. New York: W. W. Norton; 1945. p. 197, 202–203.
Ferenczi S. Further contributions to the theory and technique of psycho-analysis. London: Karnac Books; 1994.
Ferenczi S. Disease or Pathoneurosis. In: Richman J, editor. Further contributions to the theory and technique of psychoanalysis. New York: Basic Books; 1954.
Fernandes C, Samuel J. The use of piracetam in vertigo. South African Med J Suid Afrikaanse tydskrif vir geneeskunde. 1985;68(11):806–8.
Frank LM, Hartwig EL, editors. Perspectives on dyslexia— Special Issue, The Orton Dyslexia Society—Research Division, Maryland: The Orton Dyslexia Society, June 1983.
Fox S. Audiologists take on autism with auditory training. ADVANCE for Speech-Language Pathologists and Audiologists. 1992;6:10–1.
Frank J, Levinson H. Auditory hallucinations in a case of hysteria. Br J Psychiatry. 1966;112:19–26.
Freud, S. The psychopathology of everyday life. 1901.

Fuchs E, Flügge G. Adult neuroplasticity: more than 40 years of research. Neural Plast. 2014;2014:1–10.
Gabrieli JD. Dyslexia: a new synergy between education and cognitive neuroscience. Science. 2009;325(5938):280–3.
Galaburda AM. Neuropathological evidence for elective affliction of the magnocellular visial subsystem. Presented at The New York Academy of Sciences and The Rodin Remediation Academy, The XX Rodin Remediation Conference: Temporal In- formation Processing in the Nervous System: Special Reference to Dyslexia and Dysphasia, New York: September 12–15, 1992.
Galaburda AM, Kemper TL. Cytoarchitectonic abnormalities in developmental dyslexia: a case study. Ann Neurol. 1979;6(2):94–100.
Galaburda AM, Sherman GF, Rosen GD, Aboitiz F, Geschwind N. Developmental dyslexia: four consecutive patients with cortical anomalies. Ann Neurol. 1985;18(2):222–33.
Geiger G, Lettvin JY. Peripheral vision in persons with dyslexia. N Engl J Med. 1987;316(20):1238–43.
Geschwind N. Why Orton was right. Ann Dyslexia. 1982;32(1):13–30.
Geschwind N. Dyslexia, cerebral dominance, autoimmunity, and sex hormones. In: Dyslexia: its neuropsychology and treatment. New York: Wiley; 1986.
Gilbert LC. Functional motor efficiency of the eyes and its relation to reading. University of California Publications in Education. 1953;11:159–231.
Goddard S, Blythe P. Dyslexia-dyspraxia and other specific learning difficulties, UK.
Goethe J. Faust Hamburger Lesehefte Verlag. 29. Heft.
Goldrick SG, Sedgwick H. An objective comparison of oculomotor functioning in reading disabled and normal children. Am J Optom Physiol Optic. 1982;59:82.
Goodenough FL. Draw-a-man test: the measurement of intelligence by drawings. World Book: Yonkers-on-Hudson; 1926.
Goddard S, Blythe SG. The well balanced child: movement and early learning: Hawthorn; 2005.
Griffin DC, Walton HN, Ives V. Saccades as related to reading disorders. J Learn Disabil. 1974;7(5):310–6.
Guedry FE Jr, Lentz JM, Jell RM. Visual-vestibular interactions. I. Influence of peripheral vision on suppression of the vestibulo-ocular reflex and visual acuity. Aviat Space Environ Med. 1979;50:205–11.
Guye A. On agoraphobia in relation to ear-disease. Laryngoscope. 1899;6(4):219–25.
Hartwig EL, ed. Perspectives on dyslexia—medical research update, The Orton Dyslexia Society—Research Division, Maryland: The Orton Dyslexia Society, August 1984.
Hashimoto T, Tayama M, Murakawa K, et al. Development of the brainstem and cerebellum in autistic patients. J Autism Dev Disord. 1995;25(1):1–18.
Helfgott E, Rudel RG, Kairam R. The effect of piracetam on short-and long-term verbal retrieval in dyslexic boys. Int J Psychophysiol. 1986;4(1):53–61.
Hugues S. The Orton-Gillingham language approach. Res Rev 2007.
Huston AM. Common sense about dyslexia. Maryland: University Press of America; 1987.
Irannejad S, Savage R. Is a cerebellar deficit the underlying cause of reading disabilities? Ann Dyslexia. 2012;62(1):22–52.
Irlen H. Reading by the colors. Overcoming dyslexia and other reading disabilities through the Irlen method. 2005.
Ito M. The cerebellum and neural control. New York: Raven Press; 1984.
Jacob RG, Møller MB, Turner SM, Wall C. Otoneurological examination in panic disorder and agoraphobia with panic attacks: a pilot study. Am J Psychiatry. 1985;142:715–9.
Jongkees L, Maas J, Philipszoon A. Clinical nystagmography. ORL. 1962;24(2):65–93.
Jordan DR. Attention deficit disorder: ADHD and ADD syndromes. 2nd ed. Austin: Pro-Ed; 1992. p. 5.
Christensen L Jordan DR Attention deficit disorder: ADHD and ADD syndromes. Child Study J 1994; 24:169–169.
Kaga K, Suzuki JI, Marsh RR, Tanaka Y. Influence of labyrinthine hypoactivity on gross motor development of infants. Ann N Y Acad Sci. 1981;374(1):412–20.

Kane JM, et al. Panic and phobic disorder in patients with mitral valve prolapse. In: Klein DF, Rabkin JG, editors. Anxiety: new research and changing concepts. New York: Raven Press; 1981. p. 327–40.

Katzman MA, Bilkey TS, Chokka PR, Fallu A, Klassen LJ. Adult ADHD and comorbid disorders: clinical implications of a dimensional approach. BMC Psychiatry. 2017;17(1):302.

Kerr J. School hygiene, in its mental, moral, and physical aspects. J R Stat Soc. 1897;60(3):613–80.

Klein D. In: Klein DF, Rabkin JG, editors. Anxiety Reconceptualized in anxiety new research and changing concepts. New York: Raven Press; 1981.

Köhler T, Simon P. An experimental study on freudian slips. Psychother Psychosom Med Psychol. 2002;52(9–10):374–7.

Koestler A. The ghost in the machine. New York: Macmillan; 1968. p. 164.

Kohen-Raz R. Developmental patterns of static balance ability and their relation to cognitive school readiness. Pediatrics. 1970;46(2):276–85.

Kohen-Raz R. Learning disabilities and postural control. London: Freund Publishing House; 1986.

Kohl RL, Calkins DS, Mandell AJ. Arousal and stability: the effects of five new sympathomimetic drugs suggest a new principle for the prevention of space motion sickness. Aviat Space Environ Med. 1986;57:137–43.

Korner AF, Thoman EB. The relative efficacy of contact and vestibular-proprioceptive stimulation in soothing neonates. Child Dev. 1972;43:443–53.

Lambert NM, Sandoval J. The prevalence of learning disabilities in a sample of children considered hyperactive. J Abnorm Child Psychol. 1980;8(1):33–50.

Lannois M, Tournier C. Les lésions auriculaires sont une cause déterminante fréquente de l'agoraphobie. Annales des maladies de l'oreille, du larynx, du nez et du pharynx. 1899;14:286–301.

Lauter, JL., Lynch O, Wood SB, And L. Schoeffler. Physiological and behavioral effects of an Antivertigo Antihistimine in adults. Percept Mot Skills 1999; 88: 707–732.

Leiner H, Leiner A. Personal correspondence, June 3, 1991. Leiner, H. C., A. Leiner, and R. S. Dow. Does the cerebellum contribute to mental skills? Behav Neurosci. 1986;100:443–54.

Leiner HC, Leiner AL, Dow RS. The human cerebro-cerebellar system: its computing, cognitive, and language skills. Behav Brain Res. 1991;44(2):113–28.

Lentz JM, Collins WE. Motion sickness susceptibility and related behavioral characteristics in men and women. Aviat Space Environ Med. 1977;48:316–27.

Lenzi P, Milanesi I. Etude clinique d'un nouvel antivertigineux: la 2-pyrrolidone acetamide. Clinica Otorinolaringologa dell' Universita de Milano. 1969;24:513–21.

Lerer RJ, Lerer MP, Arner J. The effects of methylphenidate on the handwriting of children with minimal brain dysfunction. J Pediatr. 1977;91:127–32.

Lestienne FG, Gurfinkel VS. Postural control in weightlessness: a dual process underlying adaptation to an unusual environment. Trends Neurosci. 1988;11(8):359–63.

Lestienne FG, Gurfinkel VS. Posture as an organizational structure based on a dual process: a formal basis to interpret changes of posture in weightlessness. Prog Brain Res. 1988;76:307–13.

Levin AP, et al. Lactate induction of panic: hypothesized mechanisms and recent findings. In: Ballenger JC, editor. Biology of agoraphobia. Washington, D.C: American Psychiatric Association; 1987. p. 82–97.

Levinson HN. Comment on Richard Allington's review of a solution to the riddle dyslexia (the review of education). 7(2):153–8.

Levinson HN. Percept Mot Skills. 1991;73:723–38. pg 736 (an advised double blind study)

Levinson H. Dyslexia: does this unusual childhood syndrome begin as an ear infection. Infect Dis. 1974;15:15.

Linden M, Habib T, Radojevic V. A controlled study of the effects of EEG biofeedback on cognition and behavior of children with attention deficit disorder and learning disabilities. Biofeedback Self Regul. 1996;21(1):35–49.

Lindsay H. Cerebellar deficiency model of dyslexia upheld. Clin Psychiatr News. 2000.

Livingstone MS, Rosen GD, Drislane FW, Galaburda AM. Physiological and anatomical evidence for a magnocellular defect in developmental dyslexia. Proc Natl Acad Sci. 1991;88(18):7943–7.

Livingstone M. Segregation of form, color, movement, and depth processing in the visual system: anatomy, physiology, art, and illusion. Research publications-Assoc Res Nerv Mental Dis. 1990;67:119.

Llinás RR. The cortex of the cerebellum. Sci Am. 1975;232(1):56–71.

Lorusso ML, et al. Wider recognition in peripheral vision common to different subtypes of dyslexia. Vis Res. 2004;44:2413–24.

Lubar JF. Discourse on the development of EEG diagnostics and biofeedback for attention deficit/hyperactivity disorders. Biofeedback Self Regul. 1991;16(3):201–25.

Luria AR. Higher cortical functions in man. New York: Springer Science & Business Media; 2012.

Mann DMA, Iwatsubo T. Diffuse plaques in the cerebellum and corpus striatum in Down's syndrome contain amyloid 7 protein (A7) only in the form of A742. Neurodegeneration. 1996;5:115–20.

Marks I, Bebbington P. Space phobia: syndrome or agoraphobic variant? Br Med J. 1976;2:345–7.

Martin N, Oosterveld W. The vestibular effects of meclizine hydrochloride-niacin combination (Antivert). Acta Otolaryngol. 1970;70(1):6–9.

Masland RL. A review of smart but feeling dumb, reprinted from the New York Branch of the Orton Dyslexia Society Newsletter, Vol. VIII, No. 3, February 1985.

Masland RL, Upsrich C. A review of A Solution to the Riddle Dyslexia. Bull Orton Soc. 1981;31:256–61.

Menendez, M. Alexia [Internet]. Version 1. Clinical sciences. 2009 Oct 13. Medical Publishing Internet, Available from: https://clinicalsciences.wordpress.com/article/alexia-1bbsle13m97c0-111/.

McClure JA, Lycett P, Baskerville JC. Diazepam as an antimotion-sickness drug. J Otolaryngol. 1982;11:253–9.

Meadows T. 101 ways to do ABA! Practical and amusing positive behavioral tips for implementing applied behavior analysis strategies in your home, classroom, and in your community: CreateSpace Publishing; 2012.

Money J. Dyslexia: a post-conference view. In: Money J, editor. Reading disability: progress and research needs in dyslexia. Baltimore: Johns Hopkins University Press; 1962.

Morgan WP. A case of congenital word blindness. Br Med J. 1896;2(1871):1378.

Mosse HL, Daniels CR. Linear dyslexia: a new form of reading disorder. Am J Psychother. 1959;13(4):826–41.

Murphy JM. Review of a solution to the riddle dyslexia, understanding dyslexia: a story of scientific detection. Int Schools J. 1981;1:83–91.

Nicolson RI, Fawcett AJ, Berry EL, Jenkins IH, Dean P, Brooks DJ. Association of abnormal cerebellar activation with motor learning difficulties in dyslexic adults. Lancet. 1999;353(9165):1662–7.

Nicolson RI, Fawcett AJ, Dean P. Time estimation deficits in developmental dyslexia: evidence of cerebellar involvement. Proc R Soc Lond B Biol Sci. 1996;259:43–7.

Ocić G, Malobabić S, Marković-Jovanović Z. Alexia with agraphia. Neurologija. 1989;38(4):349–57.

Oosterveld W. The efficacy of piracetam in vertigo. A double-blind study in patients with vertigo of central origin. Arzneimittelforschung. 1980;30(11):1947–9.

Orton SP. Reading, writing and speech problems in children. New York: W. W. Norton; 1937.

Orton ST. Discussion of a paper by Dr. J. G. Lynn. Arch Neurol Psychiatr. 1942;47:1064.

Orton ST. Word-blindness in school children. Arch Neurol Psychiatr. 1925;14:581–615.

Othmer S, Othmer SF, Marks CS. Eeg biofeedback training for attention deficit disorder, specific learning disabilities, and associated conduct problems: EEG Spectrum; 1991.

Othmer S, Othmer SF, Marks CS. EEG biofeedback training for attention deficit disorder, specific learning disabilities, and associated conduct problems. EEG Spectrum. 1991.

Page N, Gresty MA. Motorist's vestibular disorientation syndrome. J Neurol Neurosurg Psychiatry. 1985;48(8):729–35.

Paradiso S, Andreasen NC, O'leary DS, Arndt S, Robinson RG. Cerebellar size and cognition: correlations with IQ, verbal memory and motor dexterity. Neuropsychiat Neuropsychol Behav Neurol. 1997;10(1):1–8.

Pavlidis GT. Do eye movements hold the key to dyslexia? Neuropsychologia. 1981;19(1):57–64.

Pavlidis GT. Erratic eye movements and dyslexia: factors determining their relationship. Percept Mot Skills. 1985;60(1):319–22.

Pellionisz A, Llinas R. Space-time representation in the brain: the cerebellum as a predictive space-time metric sensor. Neuroscience. 1982;7:2949–70.

Pincott J. Slips of the tongue, Psychol Today. 2012.

Polatajko HJ. A critical look at vestibular dysfunction in learning-disabled children. Dev Med Child Neurol. 1985;27(3):283–92.

Powers WH. Metabolic and allergic aspects of inner-ear dysfunction. In: Dickey LD, editor. Clinical ecology. Springfield: Charles C. Thomas; 1976. p. 637–44.

Rae C, Lee MA, Dixon RM, et al. Metabolic abnormalities in developmental dyslexia detected by 1H magnetic resonance spectroscopy. Lancet. 1998;351(9119):1849–52.

Rahko T. Alleviating dyslexia by treating benign positional vertigo and eye movement disturbances. Finnish Med J. 2003;39:3883–6.

Rapoport M, van Reekum R, Mayberg H. The role of the cerebellum in cognition and behavior: a selective review. J Neuropsychiatr Clin Neurosci. 2000;12(2):193–8.

Raymond JE, et al. Fixational instability and saccadic eye movements. Am J Optom Physiol Optic. 1988;65:174–81.

Redmond DE Jr. Alterations in the function of the nucleus locus coeruleus: a possible model for studies of anxiety. In: Hanin I, Usdin E, editors. Animal models in psychiatry and neurology. New York: Pergamon; 1977. p. 293–304.

Redmond DE, Huang YH. New evidence for a locus coeruleus—norepinephrine connection with anxiety. Life Sci. 1979;25:2149–62.

Robinson D. Adaptive gain control of vestibuloocular reflex by the cerebellum. J Neurophysiol 1979. 1976;39(5):954–69.

The Dyslexia Dilemma. Harper's Bazaar; 1988. p. 212, 243.

Sarley, Ilya and Garrett. Walking Yoga: Simon and Schuster, New York, 2002.

Schaaf RC, Dumont RL, Arbesman M, May-Benson TA. Efficacy of occupational therapy using Ayres sensory integration®: a systematic review. Am J Occup Ther. 2018;72(1):1–10.

Schilder P. The vestibular apparatus in neurosis and psychosis. J Nerv Ment Dis. 1933;78(1):1–23.

Shaywitz SE, Escobar MD, Shaywitz BA, Fletcher JM, Makuch R. Evidence that dyslexia may represent the lower tail of a normal distribution of reading ability. N Engl J Med. 1992;326(3):145–50.

Shaywitz SE, Shaywitz BA, Pugh KR, et al. Functional disruption in the organization of the brain for reading in dyslexia. Proc Natl Acad Sci. 1998;95(5):2636–41.

Silva PA, Kirkland C, Simpson A, Stewart IA, Williams SM. Some developmental and behavioral problems associated with bilateral otitis media with effusion. J Learn Disabil. 1982;15(7):417–21.

Silver LB. The 'magic cure: a review of the current contro- versial approaches for treating learning disabilities. J Learn Disabil 1987;20(8):498–505. Simpson E. Reversals. Boston: Houghton-Mifflin; 1979.

Snider R, Stowell A. Evidence of a projection of the optic system to the cerebellum. Anat Rec. 1942;82:448–9.

Snider, R., & Stowell, A. (1942). Evidence of a representation of tactile sensibility in the cerebellum of the cat. . Paper presented at the Fed. Proc. P. 82.

Snider RS, Eldred E. Cerebro-cerebellar relationships in the monkey. J Neurophysiol. 1952;15(1):27.

Snider RS, Stowell A. Receiving areas of the tactile, auditory, and visual systems in the cerebellum. J Neurophysiol. 1944;7(6):331–57.

Snider RS. Recent contributions to the anatomy and physiology of the cerebellum. Arch Neurol Psychiatr. 1950;64(2):196–219.

Snider R. (1943). A fifth cranial nerve projection to the cerebellum. Paper presented at the Fed. Proc. p. 46.

Solan HA, Shelley-Tremblay J, Larson S. Vestibular function, sensory integration, and balance anomalies: a brief literature review. Optometry Vision Develop. 2007;38(1):13.

Spinelli D, De Luca M, Judica A, Zoccolotti P. Crowding effects on word identification in developmental dyslexia. Cortex. 2002;38(2):179–200.

Stanley G, Smith GA, Howell EA. Eye-movements and sequential tracking in dyslexic and control children. Br J Psychol. 1983;74(2):181–7.

Stehli A. The sound of a miracle. New York: Avon Books; 1992.

Stein J. The current status of the magnocellular theory of developmental dyslexia. Neuropsychologia 2018.

Stein J, Glickstein M. Role of the cerebellum in visual guidance of movement. Physiol Rev. 1992;72(4):967–1017.

Stevens LJ, Zentall SS, Deck JL, et al. Essential fatty acid metabolism in boys with attention deficit hyperactivity disorder. Am J Clin Nutr. 1995;62(4):761–8.

Stevens LJ, Zentall SS, Abate ML, Kuczek T, Burges JR. Omega-3 fatty acids in boys with behavior, learning, and health problems. Physiol Behav. 1996;59(4–5):915–20.

Stockwell C, Sherard E, Schuler J. Electronystagmographic findings in dyslexic children. Trans Sect Otolaryngol Am Acad Ophthalmol Otolaryngol. 1976;82(2):239–43.

Stroud MH, Rauchbach E. Caloric and optokinetic nystagmus in cerebellar patients. Ann Otol Rhinol Laryngol. 1976;85(1):136–8.

Suttle CM, Barbur J, Conway ML. Coloured overlays and precision-tinted lenses: poor repeatability in a sample of adults diagnosed with visual stress. Ophthalmic Physiol Opt. 2017;37(4):542–8.

Tallal P. Improving language and literacy is a matter of time. Nat Rev Neurosci. 2004;5(9):721.

Temple E, Deutsch GK, Poldrack RA, et al. Neural deficits in children with dyslexia ameliorated by behavioral remediation: evidence from functional MRI. Proc Natl Acad Sci. 2003;100(5):2860–5.

Tichko P, Skoe E. Musical experience, sensorineural auditory processing, and rading subskills in adults. Brain Sci. 2018;8(5):pii. E77.

Tierney A, Kraus N. Music training for the development of reading skills. Prog Brain Res. 2013;207:209–41.

Townsend J, Courchesne E, Egaas B. Slowed orienting of covert visual-spatial attention in autism: specific deficits associated with cerebellar and parietal abnormality. Dev Psychopathol. 1996;8(3):563–84.

Turkington C, Harris J. The encyclopedia of learning disabilities. New York: Infobase Publishing; 2006. p. 174.

University GW. Was orton right? New study examines how the brain works in reading; offers key to better understanding dyslexia. ScienceDaily. 2003.

Valdois S, Bosse ML, Tainturier MJ. The cognitive deficits responsible for developmental dyslexia: review of evidence for a selective visual attentional disorder. Dyslexia. 2004;10(4):339–63.

Wender PH. Minimal brain dysfunction in children. New York: Wiley; 1971.

Wender PH. The hyperactive child, adolescent, and adult: attention deficit disorder through the lifespan. New York: Oxford University Press; 1987.

Wender PH. Minimal brain dysfunction: an overview. In: Lipton MA, DiMascio A, Kilan DF, editors. Psychopharmacology: a generation of progress. New York: Raven; 1978.

Vidyasagar TR, Pammer K. Dyslexia: a deficit in visuo-spatial attention, not in phonological processing. Trends Cogn Sci. 2010;14(2):57–63.

Wilsher CR, Bennett D, Chase C, Connors K, et al. Piracetam and dyslexia: effects on reading tests. J Clin Psychopharmachol. 1987;7:230–5.

Wilson V, Maeda M, Franck J. Inhibitory interaction between labyrinthine, visual and neck inputs to the cat flocculus. Brain Res. 1975;96(2):357–60.

Wiser AK, Andreasen NC, O'leary DS, Watkins GL, Ponto LLB, Hichwa RD. Dysfunctional cortico-cerebellar circuits cause 'cognitive dysmetria'in schizophrenia. Neuroreport. 1998;9(8):1895–9.

Wiss T. Vestibular dysfunction in learning disabilities: differences in definitions lead to different conclusions. Lear Disabil. 1989;22:100.

Wood CD, Cramer DB, Graybiel A. Antimotion sickness drug efficacy. Otolaryngol Head Neck Surg. 1981;89(6):1041–4.

Wood CD, Graybiel A. A theory of motion sickness based on pharmacological reactions. Clin Pharmacol Therap. 1970;11(5):621–9.
Yu D, Cheung S-H, Legge GE, Chung ST. Effect of letter spacing on visual span and reading speed. J Vis. 2007;7(2):2–2.
Zangwill O, Blakemore C. Dyslexia: reversal of eye-movements during reading. Neuropsychologia. 1972;10(3):371–3.
Zorzi M, Barbiero C, Facoetti A, et al. Extra-large letter spacing improves reading in dyslexia. Proc Natl Acad Sci. 2012;109(28):11455–9.
Zinkus PW, Gottlieb MI, Schapiro M. Developmental and psychoeducational sequelae of chronic otitis media. Am J Dis Children. 1978;132(11):1100–4.

Index

H. N. Levinson, *Feeling Smarter and Smarter*,
https://doi.org/10.1007/978-3-030-16208-5

E